The International Review of Child Neurology

SPINAL TUMORS IN
CHILDREN AND ADOLESCENTS

The International Review of Child Neurology

The International Review of Child Neurology

Spinal Tumors in Children and Adolescents

Ignacio Pascual-Castroviejo
Head, Child Neurology Service
Hospital Infantil, "La Paz"
Madrid, Spain

with contributions from:

David G. Ashley
Walter J. Curran, Jr.
Giulio J. D'Angio
Fred J. Epstein
Julio Escalona-Zapata
Marvin D. Nelson, Jr.
Hervey D. Segall

Raven Press   New York

Raven Press, Ltd., 1185 Avenue of the Americas, New York, New York 10036

Made in the United States of America

Library of Congress Cataloging-in-Publication Data

Spinal tumors in children and adolescents, I. Pascual-Castroviejo.
    p.   cm. — (The International review of child neurology)
    Includes bibliographical references.
    ISBN 0-88167-576-8
    1. Spinal cord—Tumors.   2. Tumors in children.   I. Pascual-Castroviejo,
I. (Ignacio). II. Series.
    [DNLM: 1. Spinal Cord Neoplasms—in adolescence.   2. Spinal Cord
Neoplasms—in infancy & childhood.   3. Spinal Neoplasms—in
adolescence.   4. Spinal Neoplasms—in infancy & childhood. WL 400 S78545]
RC280.S7S65   1988
618.92'99482—dc20
DNLM/DLC
for Library of Congress   89-10646
                                                  CIP

9 8 7 6 5 4 3 2 1

To the memory of my parents,
To the Alicias, my wife and my daughter,
They are my constant support and joy.
To the memory of my friend, John Stobo Prichard

Ignacio Pascual-Castroviejo

"To love is to serve"

Theresa of Avila

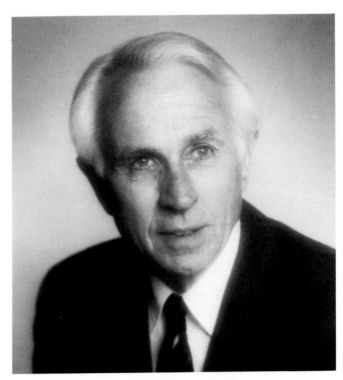

John Stobo Prichard
1914–1986

Foreword

This is the sixth volume of the International Review of Child Neurology, sponsored by the International Child Neurology Association. It is dedicated to the memory of Professor John Stobo Prichard of Toronto, first President of the Association and first Editor-in-Chief of the Review.

It is appropriate that the author of this volume should be a Spaniard since the Association was founded in Barcelona in 1973. The aim of the Association is to improve the quality of care that child neurologists and professionals in allied disciplines provide children with neurological disorders, to foster research in the prevention and treatment of these disorders, and to promote scientific exchange around the world by the dissemination of information through the written word and through personal contact at international meetings. Each volume of the International Review of Child Neurology is devoted to the in-depth examination of a particular topic relevant to child neurology. Previous volumes, written or edited by child neurologists from many countries, have encompassed disorders of higher cerebral function, progressive spinal muscular atrophy, brain tumors, epilepsy, and prenatal neurology.

This volume addresses the topic of neoplasms of the spinal cord. Dr. Ignacio Pascual-Castroviejo's extensive clinical experience enables him to review the subject broadly. This book is timely because it describes two revolutionary advances in the care of children with spinal neoplasms. The first is earlier, safer, more precise diagnosis provided by magnetic resonance imaging. Dr. Fred Epstein of New York describes the second, how the operating microscope enables the resection of previously inoperable lesions with a formerly hopeless prognosis. No doubt Dr. Prichard would have felt a secret pride knowing that the tree he had planted and nurtured, the International Review of Child Neurology, has produced yet another fruit.

Isabelle Rapin
Peter Procopis

Preface

The spinal cord is a critically important part of the central nervous system. Three of the most significant body functions—normal motricity, sphincteric control, and sexual potency—depend on the integrity of the spinal cord and nerve roots. Diseases of the cord and roots, notably extrinsic and intrinsic spinal tumors, may jeopardize any one or all of these functions. Clinical disease caused by spinal tumors is often very severe and occasionally requires urgent medical intervention. All too often, patients with spinal tumors consult specialists who do not recognize the nature of the problem and delay appropriate investigation and treatment. By then, loss of function may be irreversible and complete removal of the tumor no longer possible. Early diagnosis of spinal tumors is thus essential to the prevention of avoidable sequelae.

Neurologists with an adequate knowledge of the anatomy, physiology, and pathology of the spinal cord and of the neurologic syndromes resulting from spinal cord disease should have little difficulty suspecting a spinal mass. The spectacular advances of neuroradiology over the past two decades have revolutionized the diagnosis of spinal tumors. Metrizamide myelography, computerized tomography, and magnetic resonance imaging with the addition of paramagnetic contrast material now make possible reliable and detailed visualization of masses within the spinal canal, as well as those involving the spine, intervertebral foramina, and paraspinal tissues. These novel neuroimaging modalities have greatly decreased the need for painful and invasive diagnostic procedures. They provide the basis for a rational treatment plan that may include surgery, radiotherapy, and chemotherapy. Early clinical suspicion, prompt investigation, and aggressive management enhance the probability of cure in many spinal cord neoplasms.

This book is addressed first and foremost to child neurologists and neurosurgeons. I hope that it will also prove helpful to pediatricians and orthopedic surgeons and to all physicians who care for children with back pain, gait disorders, abnormalities of posture and movement, and unexplained deficits of sphincteric control.

Ignacio Pascual-Castroviejo

Acknowledgments

After I finished writing my book *Neurologia Infantil* (two volumes in Spanish), the Editorial Board of the International Child Neurology Association (ICNA) asked me to write a volume for the *International Review of Child Neurology* series. I accepted and chose the subject "Spinal Tumors in Children and Adolescents," a topic unfamiliar to many neuropediatricians. Using my personal experience and the help of eminent colleagues, I have tried to provide complete and clear information about the diagnosis and treatment of spinal tumors in young people. I thank the Publication Committee of ICNA and especially Dr. Isabelle Rapin for their support and trust in me to write a book in English.

Drs. Julio Escalona-Zapata, David G. Ashley, Marvin D. Nelson, Jr., Hervey D. Segall, Fred J. Epstein, Walter J. Curran, Jr., and Giulio J. D'Angio wrote very important chapters in this book. I greatly appreciate their confidence and help in the preparation of this volume.

I also want to thank my English teacher, Ms. Natalia Fracsek de Hernandez, and my colleague, Leonidas Perkikidis, who helped me edit the manuscript. My secretary, Julia Leon, who typed and retyped a manuscript written in a language unknown to her. Finally, on behalf of the readers, I wish to thank Dr. Isabelle Rapin whose linguistic efforts greatly improved the manuscript.

Ignacio Pascual-Castroviejo

Contents

Contributors

David G. Ashley *Department of Neuroradiology, Children's Hospital, Los Angeles, California, and University of Southern California Medical Center, 1200 North State Street, Los Angeles, California 90033*

Walter J. Curran, Jr. *Department of Radiation Therapy, University of Pennsylvania, Philadelphia, Pennsylvania 19104*

Giulio J. D'Angio *Department of Radiation Therapy, University of Pennsylvania, Philadelphia, Pennsylvania 19104*

Fred J. Epstein *Department of Neurosurgery, New York University Medical Center, 550 First Avenue, New York, New York 10016*

Julio Escalona-Zapata *Department of Pathology, Universidad Complutense, Madrid Hospital Provincial, Madrid, Spain*

Marvin D. Nelson, Jr. *Department of Neuroradiology, Children's Hospital, Los Angeles, California, and University of Southern California Medical Center, 1200 North State Street, Los Angeles, California 90033*

Ignacio Pascual-Castroviejo *Head, Child Neurology Service, Hospital Infantil, "La Paz," Paseo de la Castellana, 261, 28046 Madrid, Spain*

Hervey D. Segall *Department of Neuroradiology, Children's Hospital, Los Angeles, California, and University of Southern California Medical Center, 1200 North State Street, Los Angeles, California 90033*

The International Review of Child Neurology

SPINAL TUMORS IN
CHILDREN AND ADOLESCENTS

1

Epidemiology of Spinal Cord Tumors in Children

Ignacio Pascual-Castroviejo

EPIDEMIOLOGY

Prevalence

The prevalence of spinal tumors in children and young people depends on many factors. Any evaluation of these factors has to be regarded as tentative owing to the varying criteria used in the published accounts. An analysis of the incidence of spinal tumors must consider age, sex, site of lesions, and their histology, and to compare their frequency with that of brain tumors in children and of spinal tumors in adults.

In spite of the availability of a great deal of data in published accounts of spinal neoplasms in children (1–28), it is very difficult to arrive at a reliable estimate of their actual prevalence. Several factors contribute to this uncertainty. The ages of the patients differ in the various studies. Maximum cut-off age has ranged from 12 to 19 years. Most authors, however, have chosen 14 or 15 years as the cut-off in their analyses. The oldest age in the studies of Anderson and Carson (1), Dodge et al. (2), Klein (3), Richardson (4), Friedmann et al. (5), and Kordas et al. (6) is 14 years, whereas 15 years is used in the series of Hamby (7,8), Svien et al. (9), Grant and Austin (10), Haft et al. (11), Coxe (12), Dereymaeker et al. (13), Rougerie (14), Hutteroth and Gutjahr (15), and Di Lorenzo et al. (16). Also, a number of neoplasms are included in some series, but excluded in others. For example, Rand and Rand (17) included herniated discs and arachnoidal cysts; Rougerie (14) excluded only traumatic spinal cord compression.

The largest and most recent review is that of Di Lorenzo et al. (16) who analyzed 1,234 primary spinal neoplasms previously published in the literature, adding to this number 56 of their own cases. However, they excluded such interesting entities as intraspinal and bony metastases, tumors of the vertebrae, arachnoidal, bronchogenic, and neurenteric cysts, hematologic tumors (such as histiocytosis X and lymphomas), inflammatory granulomas, abscesses, and nontraumatic hematomas. These represent a significant number of space-occupying spinal masses; they require the same diagnostic studies and raise analogous therapeutic options. Several of these entities have been included in our series.

Spinal tumors account for 5 of every 2,000 new patients referred to a child neurology center. In our Child Neurology Service, a referral center for a major part of Spain, about 2,000 new patients are seen every year, and we encounter an average of five or six spinal tumors. After 20 years of operation (from August 1, 1965, to July 31, 1986), we have gathered a series of 116 cases between the ages of 0 and 12 years (Table 1).

Almost all of our patients were younger than 7 years (Fig. 1), which was the maximum age for admission to the children's hospitals of the Social Security until April 1, 1984. Since that date, the admission age was raised to 14 years. Fifty children (43%) were in their first year; 23 were neonates.

A higher incidence in the first year of life (almost 12%) was also reported by Di Lorenzo et al. (16), followed by the second and third year with an incidence of 7% and 8%, respectively. There was a tendency for the prevalence to decrease over the following 9 years, when it averaged between 3 and 7%. Although similar averages were reported in most series consulted for this review, some other series disagreed, notably Koos et al. (18) who added 107 of their own cases. In that series, a considerably higher incidence was observed in patients between 13 and 14 years of age. The series of Koos et al. was included in the review by Di Lorenzo et al. (16) who excluded spinal symptoms caused by hematologic diseases, herniated discs, vascular abnormalities, developmental lipomas, arachnoidal cysts, metastases of medulloblastomas, parasitic cysts, and localized chronic inflammations. All space occupying intrinsic and extrinsic spinal masses which may compress the spinal cord and/or roots, of whatever origin, are included in our series.

TABLE 1. *Spinal tumors; personal series*

Tumor	No. cases
Lipoma	54
Dermoid cyst	22
Neuroblastoma	8
Teratoma	7
Metastasis	5
Histiocytosis X	4
Astrocytoma	3
Ganglioglioma	2
Neurinoma	2
Hodgkin's	1
Rhabdomyosarcoma	1
Neurofibrosarcoma	1
Sarcoma of soft tissues	1
Inflammatory granuloma	1
Arachnoid cyst	1
Neurenteric cyst	1
Aneurysmal cyst	1
Muscular hemangioma	1
Total	116

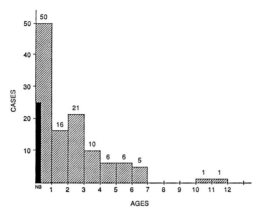

FIG. 1. Distribution of cases of tumor from ages 0 to 12 years.

Sex

Most series report an equal distribution across sexes. A 55% male to 45% female ratio was reported in the review of Di Lorenzo et al. (16). Distribution was equal in our own series and the series by Arseni et al. (19), and close to 50% in other series.

Segmental Level

No significant preference for any spinal segment is reported in most studies. The thoracic region is affected somewhat more often than the remaining segments, perhaps because it is longer. However, there are series that show a higher incidence in the thoracic region, such as 56% or 43%, with 25% located in the cervical and 25% in the lumbar regions. The disproportion is even higher in other studies that report 58% of tumors in the thoracic segments and 33% in the thoracolumbar zone. Other series, although distributed quite evenly, report a moderate lumbar predominance and a lesser prevalance in the thoracic region (20). In our series, there is a notable predominance in the lumbosacral region (74%) because of the numerous lipomas and dermoid and epidermoid cysts that occur preferentially in this location.

Location in the Horizontal Plane

It is very difficult to quantify data on the location of tumors of the spine and spinal cord because they are not published in journals of the same discipline. Bony tumors are usually described in orthopedic journals, whereas masses located in the spinal cord, meninges, or spinal nerves are commonly published in journals of

TABLE 2. *Prevalence of spinal and/or spinal cord masses by major series*

Series (ref)	Extradural tumors %	Intradural tumors %	Intradural and cauda equina tumors %
Hamby (7)	43.0	29.0	23.0
Hamby (8)	38.2	27.2	33.6
Rand and Rand (17)	37.5	16.7	41.7
Arseni et al. (19)	28.6	38.0	33.3
Koos et al. (18)	43.0	25.0	25.0
Grote et al. (25)	59.0	25.3	15.8
Kordas et al. (6)	40.0	35.0	25.0
De Sousa et al. (20)	36.0	29.6	34.6
Di Lorenzo (16)			
(personal series)	62.5	20.0	17.5
Our personal series	33.1	14.6	52.3
			(intra-extradural)

neurology or neurosurgery. According to the review of Di Lorenzo et al. (16), it seems that there is a clear predominance of extradural tumors (43%), while intra-medullary masses account for 31.4% and intradural extramedullary and cauda equina lesions for 24.4%.

Prevalences reported in the largest series are presented in Table 2. Astro-cytomas and ependymomas are the most frequent intramedullary tumors. To-gether, they constitute between 80 and 90% of all intramedullary masses in children as well as in adults. Lipomas, followed by dermoids and epidermoids are the most frequent extramedullary tumors.

Relationship Between Location and Histology

Although all spinal masses may be located at any level of the spinal canal, each type has a certain predilection for a specific zone. For example, astrocytomas commonly occur in the upper part of the spinal cord in the cervical, cervico-thoracic, and thoracic regions. Lipomas, especially cases with an important extra-dural component, are located in the lower part of the spinal canal, that is, in the dorsolumbar, lumbar, and lumbosacral regions. The same locations are observed for dermoids and epidermoids. Teratomas are found in the lumbar and sacrococ-cygeal regions. Sarcomas occur all along the spine, although more frequently in the thoracic region. Neuroblastomas are tumors commonly found in the tho-racolumbar and lumbar regions. Metastases are preferentially located in the tho-racic segments.

Prevalence of the Various Types of Masses

In order to obtain a reliable estimate of the various types of tumors, it is neces-sary to review studies from various parts of the globe encompassing patients ranging in age from newborns to 14 or 15 years. Each tumor has a predilection for a particular age. Teratomas, lipomas, and dermoids–epidermoids present clinically throughout the first three years of life, most of them during the first two years. Neuroblastomas also present mostly within the first three years. Neurinomas and meningiomas, which are common tumors of adults, are rare in children below age 10 years. Tumors of glial origin (astrocytomas and ependymomas), as well as sarcomas, have no preference for any particular age group and can be observed at any age.

In the series of 1,234 cases reviewed by Di Lorenzo et al. (16), gliomas (including ependymomas) were the most frequent tumors, with a prevalence of 30.1%; these were followed by sarcomas (18.6%), embryonal tumors (lipomas, teratomas, dermoids, and epidermoids) (18.5%), neurinomas and meningiomas (14.3%), and tumors of sympathetic origin (12.8%). The less frequent tumors were those originating in vertebrae (3.4%) and blood vessels (1.4%), chordomas (0.4%), and fibromas (0.2%); the reliability of these estimates is questionable, however.

The prevalences of spinal tumors differ markedly in children and in adults, in whom 18% of spinal masses are glial tumors, 9.3% sarcomas, 2 to 3% embryonal tumors, and 51 to 52% meningiomas and neurinomas. Adults also do not have tumors of sympathetic origin and they have a greater prevalence of bony and cartilaginous tumors which are very rare in children.

CLINICAL FINDINGS

Intramedullary tumors destroy or compress nerve tissue from their onset and cause neurologic symptomatology early on. Extramedullary masses, both intra- and extradural, also compress the spinal cord and cause more or less rapidly progressive neurologic symptomatology. Nerve roots are often affected before the spinal cord. Spinal tumors can cause neurologic symptomatology not only by destruction or compression of the spinal cord, but by the obstruction of spinal arteries or veins, with inadequate compensatory collateral circulation. These vascular mechanisms account for the occurrence of edematous or necrotic foci which often precede invasion of the cord by the neoplasm.

Intramedullary tumors are often quite circumscribed, while extramedullary masses, especially epidural ones, extend over several vertebral segments.

The clinical symptomatology depends on the spinal level of the mass and on whether it is intra- or extramedullary. Intramedullary tumors usually do not cause pain, but they may produce sphincteric alterations (incontinence or retention), sexual impotence or priapism, sensory disturbances, and motor symptoms with paraparesis or paraplegia (when the tumor occurs in the dorsal and lumbar segments), or tetraplegia (when the tumor is located in the cervical region). Pain is present only when the roots and, to a lesser degree the meninges are involved. External anomalies, such as lesions on the skin or deformities of the lower limbs (sometimes of an arthrogrypotic type), usually signal tumors of dysembryoplastic nature

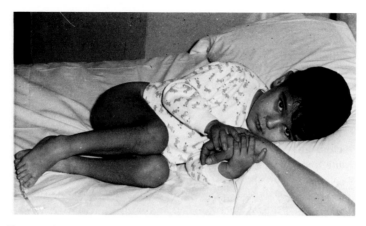

FIG. 2. Six-year-old boy with a malignant spinal tumor (yolk tumor). He presents an antalgic posture, holding his mother's hand.

(lipoma, dermoid or epidermoid cyst, etc.). Extradural tumors have a variable symptomatology depending on their malignancy. Malignant tumors produce persistent radicular or bony pain early on (Fig. 2), pain that is resistant to drugs, followed in a few days by sensory, pyramidal, and sphincteric symptomatology. Local swelling and a mass tender to palpation may also be found; patients adopt an antalgic posture and often lie in a preferred position. Although paraplegia or tetraplegia may be spastic at the beginning (Fig. 3), it becomes flaccid in advanced stages of the disease. These children appear severely ill, with dry skin and hair, shadows below their eyes, weight loss, irritability, and sadness, and complain almost continuously. Their sedimentation rate is elevated.

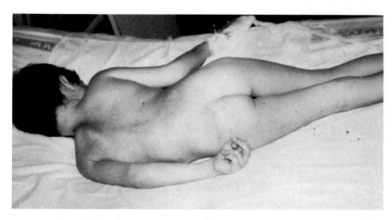

FIG. 3. Seven-year-old boy with a ganglioglioma affecting the entire dorsal spinal cord. He has a scoliosis and spasticity in the lower limbs. Both alterations are common findings in spinal cord tumors.

There are tumors that present with a radicular symptomatology because they compress a root (neurinomas and meningiomas). Embryonal tumors (lipomas, angiomas, pilonidal cysts, epidermoids, dermoids) are commonly associated with external malformations such as a dermal sinus, tuft of hair, or cutaneous angioma. Spinal tumors in children usually start with sphincteric disturbances and gait abnormalities, with pain appearing later. Neurinomas and meningiomas are seldom found in children (although they are very frequent in adults), hence the rarity of radicular pain in children. Radicular pain caused by these tumors increases after a lumbar puncture and the Queckenstedt test (elevation of the cerebrospinal fluid (CSF) pressure upon compression of the jugular veins) as well as during straining and coughing. Metastases may cause pain and produce motor disturbance within an interval of a few days.

Tumors located in the region of the occipital foramen can cause neck stiffness and uni- or bilateral diaphragmatic paralysis with respiratory disturbances. The symptomatology in "U" of cervical spinal cord compression is well known—an upper limb is affected first, followed by the lower limb of the same side, and later the lower and upper limbs on the opposite side. These tumors often cause muscular atrophies (Fig. 4) and arthrogrypotic upper limb deformities.

Compression below the cervical segments causes neurologic deficits only in the lower limbs, one side often being more severely affected than the other. Tumors of the conus and cauda equina (neuroblastoma, ependymoma, ganglioglioma, lipoma) affect several roots and cause more or less extensive muscular atrophy, whose neurogenic origin can be determined by electromyography (EMG). Sphincteric disturbances appear early when the mass is located in the lumbosacral region, but they occur late when the compression is higher. Both incontinence and

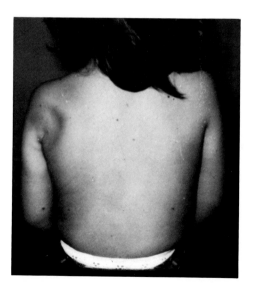

FIG. 4. Seven-year-old girl with histiocytosis X at the C6–C7 level on the left side. Severe muscular atrophy is seen in the left shoulder and upper part of the arm.

retention are observed. Tendon stretch reflexes are increased below the cord level affected by the mass, this increase being more pronounced on the side of the tumor when it is laterally placed. Unilateral or bilateral clonus and Babinski responses may be elicited. Flaccid tetraplegia or paraplegia mimicking spinal muscular atrophy (Werdnig-Hoffmann syndrome) may be present in cases with advanced tumor with spinal cord transsection. Paraplegia in flexion is occasionally seen.

When the tumor is located on nerve roots, the reflexes depending on these roots are diminished or abolished. Tumors located in the cervical region affecting sympathetic ganglia (stellate ganglion and thoracic chain) cause Horner's syndrome on the side of the tumor. Other signs of autonomic dysfunction (sweating, vasomotor reactions) occur in some cases. Subarachnoid hemorrhage and papilledema are occasionally found in some types of tumor (neurinoma, meningioma, ependymoma, highly vascularized tumors), especially those in the conus or cauda equina.

Mild pleocytosis and increased protein may be seen in the CSF. A complete block of the subarachnoid space commonly greatly elevates the CSF protein (Froin syndrome). The Queckenstedt maneuver may be useful in patients suspected of having an arachnoid block, but it should only be performed by experienced specialists. This maneuver is contraindicated when neuroimaging procedures are available.

Although the Brown-Séquard syndrome, hemisection of the spinal cord, is most frequently observed after a spinal cord trauma, it can also occasionally be found in spinal cord tumors. This syndrome is defined by: (a) impaired motor function on the homolateral side below the level of the lesion, (b) diminished or loss of vibration, pressure and position sense on the homolateral side of the body below the level of the lesion, and (c) loss of pain and temperature sense on the opposite side of the body below the level of the lesion, in some cases with segmental dysesthesia at the level of the lesion.

Pathophysiology

An expanding mass located in any portion of the spinal cord or the spinal epidural space impairs the function of the cord or spinal roots. Central or peripheral nervous tissues may be affected through direct effects of the tumor and by edema. This edema is probably of the vasogenic type, secondary to leaky blood vessels within the cord. The neoplasm diminishes the blood supply above, below, and at the level of the mass because of stasis in the venous system in the spinal cord and occlusion of the epidural venous plexus. The edema starts by involving the white matter, but the gray matter may also be involved in the later stages of compression. The spinal cord tolerates rapid compression very badly, but it can adjust to gradual compression over a period of weeks, months, and even years in cases of slow-growing benign tumors. Patients with widespread malignant tumors present very early signs of spinal cord compromise and undergo a rapid deterioration.

Differential Diagnosis

There are few diseases to consider in the differential diagnosis. Among them, the most frequent and an occasionally difficult one is acute or subacute transverse myelitis, which can cause neurologic disturbances similar to those observed in spinal tumors. The correct diagnosis often requires computerized tomography or nuclear magnetic resonance studies. Multiple sclerosis, especially at the time of first presentation, Guillain-Barré syndrome, hematomyelia, localized spinal cord edema after occult trauma, idiopathic scoliosis, spinocerebellar diseases, severe and chronic constipation, sciatica not preceded by a previous injection into the buttock, and impaired sexual potency of unknown origin are the main disorders to be ruled out.

REFERENCES

1. Anderson FM, Carson MJ. Spinal cord tumours in children. A review of the subject and presentation of twenty-one cases. *J Pediatr* 1953;43:190–207.
2. Dodge HW, Keith HM, Campagna MJ. Intraspinal tumours in infants and children. *J Intern Coll Surg* 1956;26:199–215.
3. Klein MR. Les tumeurs de la möelle chez l'enfant. *Acta Neurochir (Wien)* 1960;9:69–84.
4. Richardson FC. A report of 16 tumours of the spinal cord in children; the importance of spinal rigidity as an early sign of disease. *J Pediatr* 1960;57:42–54.
5. Friedman G, Thun F, Butzier HO. Röntgendiagnostik raumfordernder intraspinaler Prozesse im Kindersalter. *Fortschr Röntgenstr* 1972;117:408–412.
6. Kordas M, Paraicz E, Szensay J. Spinale Tumoren im Säuglings, und Kindersalter. *Zentrabl Neurochir* 1977;38:331–338.
7. Hamby WB. Tumours in the spinal canal in children: analysis of literature with report of a case. *J Nerv Ment Dis* 1935;81:24–42.
8. Hamby WB. Tumours in the spinal canal in childhood. II. Analysis of the literature of a subsequent decade (1933–1942); report of a case of meningitis due to an intramedullary epidermoid communicating with a dermal sinus. *J Neuropathol Exp Neurol* 1944;3:397–412.
9. Svien HP, Thelen EP, Keith HM. Intraspinal tumours in children. *JAMA* 1954;155:959–961.
10. Grant FC, Austin GM. The diagnosis, treatment, and prognosis of tumours affecting the spinal cord in children. *J Neurosurg* 1956;13:335–345.
11. Haft H, Ransohoff J, Carter S. Spinal cord tumours in children. *Pediatrics* 1959;23:1152–1159.
12. Coxe WS. Tumours of the spinal canal in children. *Am J. Surg* 1961;27:62–73.
13. Dereymaeker A, Van den Bergh R, Stroobandt G. Les tumeurs intrarachidiennes chez l'enfant. Statistique personelle. *Acta Neurochir* 1962;5:501–511.
14. Rougerie AD. *Les compressions médullaires non traumatiques de l'enfant.* Paris: Masson et Cie, 1973.
15. Hutteroth H, Gutjahr P. Kompression des Rückenmarks durch Tumoren. Ein pädiatrischer Notfall. *Med Kinderheilk* 1976;124:446–468.
16. Di Lorenzo N, Giuffre R, Fortuna A. Primary spinal neoplasms in childhood: analysis of 1234 published cases (including 56 personal cases) by pathology, sex, age and site. Differences from the situation in adults. *Neurochirurgia (Stutt)* 1982;25:153–164.
17. Rand RW, Rand CW. *Intraspinal tumors of childhood.* Charles C Thomas, Springfield, Ill., 1960.
18. Koos W, Laubichler W, Sorgo G. Statistische Untersuchungen bei spinalen Tumoren im Kindes- und Jugendalter. *Neuropädiatrie* 1973;4:273–303.
19. Arseni C, Horvath L, Iliescu D. Intraspinal tumours in children. *Psychiatr Neurol Neurochir* 1967; 70:123–133.
20. De Sousa AL, Kalsbeck JE, Mealey J Jr, et al. Intraspinal tumors in children. A review of 81 cases. *J Neurosurg* 1979;51:437–445.
21. Till K. Observations on spinal tumours in childhood. *Proc R Soc Med* 1959;52:333–336.

22. Ross AT, Bailey OT. Tumours arising within the spinal canal in children. *Neurology* 1953;3:922–930.
23. Matson DD. *Neurosurgery of infancy and childhood.* Charles C Thomas, Springfield, Ill., 1969.
24. Banna M, Gryspeerdt GL. Intraspinal tumours in children (excluding dysraphism). *Clin Radiol* 1971;22:17–32.
25. Grote W, Romer P, Block WJ, et al. Lang-zeitergebnisse in der Behandlung spinaler Tumoren des Kindes- und Jugenalters. *Med Kinderheilk* 1975;123:112–119.
26. Farwell JR, Dohrmann CJ. Intraspinal neoplasm in children. *Paraplegia* 1977–1978;15:262–273.
27. Iraci G. Intraspinal tumours of infancy and childhood: a review of 19 surgically verified cases. *J Pediatr Surg* 1966;1:534–545.
28. Intrau H, Usbeck W. Komprimierende Prozesse im Wirbelkanal bei Kindern. *Zentrabl Chir* 1971;36:1225–1230.

2

Pathology of Spinal Cord Tumors in Children

Julio Escalona-Zapata

The anatomic configuration of the spinal canal and its complex relationships with adjacent structures call for an inclusive definition of the concept of tumor when applied to these structures. The spinal cord lies inside a protective osseous compartment. The cord is separated from the vertebral column by several connective tissue structures (the meninges) that delimit the extradural and intradural spaces, encased in a semirigid membrane called the dura mater. The extradural or epidural areas contain sparse loose connective tissue, while the spinal intradural space has the same morphology as the intracranial one. The subarachnoid space around the spinal cord is a direct extension of its homologue around the brain and contains cerebrospinal fluid (CSF). The inner membrane of this space, which is applied to the surface of the spinal cord, is the pia mater. The anatomic complexity of the spinal cord is responsible for the development of certain classical neurologic syndromes not seen in tumors of glial origin. Extramedullary tumors produce a syndrome of segmental medullary compression at their level of origin.

Other structures to be considered are those that enter or leave the spinal canal through the intervertebral foramina. The two spinal nerve roots emerge from the spinal cord and fuse in the intradural space to form a common nerve trunk. The dorsal root ganglia are located on the posterior roots at each segmental level. The meninges provide the spinal nerves with their sheaths, after which the nerves leave the spinal canal to lie against the ribs in the thoracic region, and to form a plexus in the cervical and lumbosacral regions. The segmental vessels that enter and leave the spinal canal to irrigate the spinal cord through the anterior spinal artery (solitary) and the two posterior spinal arteries also traverse the intervertebral foramina.

Each one of these structures can be the seat of tumors, which may be purely intrinsic such as cord gliomas, or, like meningeal tumors, may cause an extrinsic spinal cord compression syndrome. Furthermore, the cord can also be affected by tumors originating in the fibrous and bony structures of the spine, not only through direct infiltration but occasionally through the mechanism of vascular ischemia. Finally, one needs to consider the "dumbbell" tumors, formed by neoplasms, some of which originate in the spinal canal and protrude through the intervertebral foramina, while others start outside the vertebral canal and penetrate it through the same route.

Consequently, spinal cord tumors must not be considered merely as a group of neoplasms originating in the spinal cord, but in a more extended sense, as all the space occupying processes affecting the cord, its coverings, and the spine, which may produce a spinal cord syndrome.

From a statistical point of view, cord tumors represent 20 to 25% of childhood nervous system tumors (1,2). In other series, they represent only 9.6% (3), 11% (4), and 13% (5). The overall prevalence varies with age during infancy and childhood, with a peak at age 3 years.

The prevalence is lower on both sides of the peak, being a little higher during the first and second years of life and slightly lower from 4 years of age onward. One should consult the monograph of Jänisch et al. (6) regarding statistics on fetuses and newborn children.

The relative prevalence of various tumors is remarkably different from that of adults. This is owing to two reasons: (a) the scarcity of carcinomatous metastases observed in children and (b) the predominance of malformative processes and dysembryoplasias in children.

In children, there is a higher prevalence of astrocytomas than of ependymomas, which, on the contrary, are more frequent in adults. Neurinomas and meningiomas are rare. The prevalence of metastasis differs from that of adults in whom carcinomas predominate; in children metastases of lymphomas and seeding from tumors of the brain and cerebellum, notably medulloblastomas, are more common. Finally, congenital processes and tumors of dysembryoplastic origin occur selectively in children and dominate the pathology of the first years. Comparative statistics between tumors in adults and children are cited in reference 7.

Owing to the above-mentioned anatomic considerations, the classification of cord tumors in children offers certain peculiarities. They can be classified in at least two ways: (a) topographically, according to their location in the spinal canal and their level along the spinal axis, and (b) histologically. Rigorous anatomopathologic and clinicopathologic correlations are required to devise an optimal therapeutic plan.

One can classify spinal cord tumors topographically as follows (8–10):

I.   Intramedullary tumors
II. Intradural extramedullary tumors
III. Extradural extramedullary tumors (including osseous and extraspinal neoplasias)

Depending on the series, intramedullary tumors constitute 22% (10), 25% (11), and 30% (2) of spinal tumors. Extramedullary intradural tumors represent 8% (9), 30% (2), and 44% (10). Reports on extradural tumors have the greatest variability, even though they are the most numerous, with reports of percentages of 34% (10), 40% (2), 50% (11), and 59% (9). The most stable figure is that for intramedullary tumors and the most variable for extradural neoplasias. This shows how difficult it is to arrive at statistically reliable figures in different areas of medicine. While intramedullary tumors are treated exclusively by neurosurgeons, extradural tumors may be treated by neurosurgeons, general surgeons, or even orthopedic surgeons. Consequently, the reported prevalence of the different pathologies varies with the medical team's specialization.

Another factor that must be taken into account is that each of these three types of tumors is not distributed homogeneously along the spine; this unequal distribution must be considered when attempting to collect reliable prevalence data. One needs to consider cervical tumors, thoracic tumors, lumbar tumors, sacral tumors, and tumors of the cauda equina. Of these, the prevalence of cervical tumors is reported to be 12% (8), 26% (12), 27% (9), or 28% (1); thoracic tumors: 32% (12), 41% (1), 43% (9), and 50% (8); and lumbar tumors: 20% (8), 24% (1), 27% (9), and 31% (12).

Figures on the prevalence of sacral or cauda equina tumors are particularly variable, because in some series the lumbosacral region is considered jointly and because tumors of the cauda equina are rare in children. It seems clear, however, that the highest prevalence of cord tumors is observed in the thoracic region, which comprises between one-third and one-half of all spinal tumors.

This macroscopic classification has its greatest application from a clinical, neuroradiologic, and neurosurgical point of view and, as will be seen later, it correlates highly with histologic diagnosis in each area.

The anatomic particularities previously mentioned, together with its histologic type, determine the course of each tumor. In this way, the following composite classification can be established:

I. Intramedullary tumors
    (a) Astrocytoma
    (b) Ependymoma
    (c) Medulloblastoma
    (d) Others
II. Intradural extramedullary tumors
    (a) Disembryoplastic tumors
        (1) Spinal teratoma
        (2) Dermoid and epidermoid cyst
        (3) Spinal neurenteric cyst
        (4) Intraspinal cyst
        (5) Spinal lipoma
    (b) Meningeal tumors
        (1) Meningioma
    (c) Tumors of the spinal nerves
        (1) Schwannoma (neurinoma)
        (2) Neurofibroma
    (d) Tumors and vascular processes

      (1)   Arteriovenous vascular malformation
      (2)   Spinal hemangioma
   (e) Metastatic tumors
      (1)   Extraneural (lymphoma)
      (2)   Of central nervous system origin
III.   Extradural tumors
   (a) Peripheral nerve tumors
   (b) Neurofibroma
   (c) Lymphoma
   (d) Osseous tumors

It is logical that some tumors occur exclusively in one region, while others, as in the case of lymphomas, metastases, nervous sheath tumors, etc., can occur in more than one area. Nevertheless, a classification that unites anatomic, topographic, and histologic features allows one (with a reasonable margin for error) to predict the probable histology of a particular tumor based on its clinical and radiologic features.

INTRAMEDULLARY TUMORS

Intramedullary tumors represent between 25 and 33% of infantile spinal cord tumors, compared with a 15% incidence in adults. They may appear at any level. This tumor group is formed by neuroectodermal neoplasias that are distributed as follows: astrocytomas, 47%; ependymomas, 24%; and malignant gliomas, 14%.

The sex distribution is 1:1 and the median age oscillates around 10 years. In general, there is a 2:1 proportion of astrocytomas to ependymomas (9). Oligodendrogliomas and medulloblastomas (13) are described occasionally, the latter being metastatic, or occurring by continuity in an infiltrative manner, from higher levels in the medulla and cerebellum.

Astrocytoma

Spinal cord astrocytomas are usually of the fibrous subtype (spongioblastoma, or piloid astrocytoma) (13–16), and they are preferentially localized in the cervical or the upper thoracic regions (1). They are most common between 3 and 5 years (2). They may be associated with von Recklinghausen disease. Macroscopically, they appear as a white or translucent mass, generally not well demarcated, that enlarges the cord diffusely. In one-third of cases, they are cystic, while, in the other two-thirds, they are solid, more compact, and firmer. They can spread along several segments, resulting in the so-called pencil-glioma that occupies the spinal cord longitudinally. Histologically, they are formed by fusiform or stellate cells with a uniform nucleus and sparse cytoplasm with long and short processes that usually end on a vessel. A number of cells may be bipolar with only two opposed processes. These cells lie randomly in an abundant interstitium in the cystic forms. The interstitium is more sparse in the solid forms.

Rosenthal fibers are uncommon. These tumors usually cause symptoms before reaching a sufficient size to compress the spinal cord. The vessels are commonly spared.

The rare malignant forms have a mixture of this basic pattern with greater cellular density, sparse atypias, and an admixture of smaller elements with hyperchromatic nuclei and poorly defined cytoplasm. This cellular mixture and the appearance of mitoses predominate in the aggressive forms, in which hyperplastic vascular alterations occur progressively. Necrosis is very infrequent. We believe that the majority, if not all, of the infantile glioblastomas of the cord described in the literature are really dedifferentiated astrocytomas. Malignant forms of astrocytoma are much less common in children than in adults (Fig. 1A).

Ependymoma

The proportion of ependymomas among all cord gliomas is 60% in adults, and only 20 to 25% in children (9,17). These tumors predominate in the lumbosacral region and in the conus medullaris, although the latter localization, frequent in

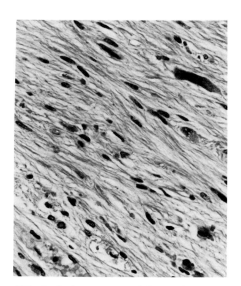 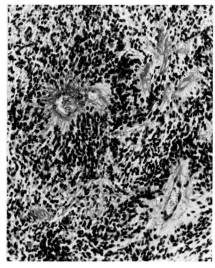

A,B

FIG. 1. A: Astrocytoma of the cord consisting of long, fusiform cells and isomorphous oval nuclei, arranged in parallel bundles. The vessels are well-formed capillaries. On the *right upper quadrant* there is a Rosenthal fiber (hematoxylin-eosin stain, 400 ×). **B:** Ependymoma of the cord. This is a cellular variant with gliovascular pseudorosettes centered around a vessel and cut in different directions. Around each, there is an acellular halo and crown of radial cells (hematoxylin-eosin stain, 200 ×).

adults, is rare in children. Macroscopically, ependymomas have the appearance of a lobulated, red, relatively well-delineated mass, and in the case of those of the conus medullaris, they are nodular and pediculated, lying between the roots of the cauda equina. In the rest of the spinal cord they are not so well demarcated, but there is almost always a cleavage plane; occasionally, they can be cystic. Histologically, the epithelial and cellular forms predominate in the cord, with a mixture of gliovascular systems (pseudorosettes) in which the cells are disposed radially around a vessel, leaving a clear acellular perivascular halo, and tubules lined by cylindrical ependymal cells lacking a basement membrane in which the cytoplasm seems continuous with the surrounding neuropil. In the conus medullaris, there is a characteristic myxopapillary variant, with development of papillae lined by ependymal epithelium, this time with a clear basement membrane. The cells are centered around a connective vascular axis of myxoid aspect and are replete with PAS-positive amorphous material. Even though malignant forms have been described (6), ependymomas are usually slow growing and of low malignancy. However, they may create problems because of their location and of local recurrences. Occasionally, they are capable of disseminating through the subarachnoid space, forming distant implants and blocking the flow of CSF (Fig. 1B).

The remaining spinal cord gliomas constitute a minute proportion of all gliomas. Exceptionally, medulloblastomas have been described, but, since they are usually metastatic subarachnoid seedings, they are dealt with later in this chapter (see the section on Extradural Tumors, below).

INTRADURAL EXTRAMEDULLARY TUMORS

Owing to the anatomic complexity of the intradural space, these tumors first require a careful classification. The following groups can be delineated:

(a) Tumors of a dysembryoplastic origin, commonly cystic and of variable complexity
    (1) Complex spinal teratomas
    (2) Dermoid and epidermoid cysts
    (3) Spinal neurenteric cysts
    (4) Intraspinal cysts of various types: arachnoid, dural, cysts of the spinal nerve roots, ependymal cysts
    (5) Lipomas
(b) Tumors of the meninges (meningiomas)
(c) Tumors of the spinal nerves
    (1) Schwannomas (neurinomas)
    (2) Neurofibromas
        (Both of these may appear in this area or in extradural locations.)
(d) Tumors and expansive processes originating from spinal vessels
    (1) Arteriovenous vascular malformations
    (2) Hemangioblastomas
(e) Metastases of tumors

(1) From the central nervous system (e.g., medulloblastomas)
(2) From extraneural tumors, which, in children, are dominated by lymphomas and leukemias (1,2,9)

Spinal Dysembryoplastic Tumors

Spinal Teratoma

Spinal teratomas represent the more severe maldevelopment, in comparison with dermoid and epidermoid cysts with which they are intimately related by a common pathogenic mechanism. Because of this, all these tumors are dealt with together in some studies. Therefore, obtaining reliable statistical figures is difficult. Furthermore, the existence of sacral teratomas without spinal cord symptomatology complicates the statistics. These tumors have a 2:1 predilection for the female sex. 68% of the cases appear under the age of 10 years, and they can even be congenital (18). In relation to the rest of the spinal masses of childhood, teratomas have a prevalence of 9% (1) to 10% (8), although, in some studies, these figures fall to 2.5% (9). A small percentage of these tumors are associated with other defects in the closure of the spinal canal, such as intracranial lipomas, dermal sinuses, Klippel-Feil syndrome, and, especially, spina bifida, supporting the hypothesis of their common dysembryoplastic nature. Spinal teratomas always occur in the lumbosacral region (8). They are located dorsally, although they can also be located intra- or extradurally and, occasionally, partially within the spinal cord. Macroscopically, they form well-encapsulated masses of variable size, sometimes considerable, with an indented surface and mixed colors; they cause a widening of the vertebral canal. Occasionally, they cause a secondary kyphosis (18). On the cut surface, solid and cystic areas alternate, the cystic ones with a clear or yellowish content. If the cysts contain hairs, the liquid is sebaceous and thick. The solid zones can be either rose colored and soft or white and firmer, depending on their content of fibrous tissue. Histologically, their aspect is very variable, resulting from the disordered mixture, in variable proportions, of tissues belonging to the three blastodermic layers. The endoderm is represented by bronchial or intestinal rudiments, the ectoderm by skin or its annexes and nervous tissue, and the mesoderm by fibrous, adipose, or even cartilaginous tissue, this last in relation to bronchial structures. Occasionally, muscular and osseous tissues can be observed (Fig. 2A).

Since it derives from abnormal closure of the spinal canal and not from derangements in the germinal cells, this type of teratoma behaves in benign fashion. Prognosis is determined by the degree of impingement on the cord and spinal compression or by the existence of an associated dysraphic pathology.

Dermoid and Epidermoid Cysts

These two types of cysts must be considered together because they represent different degrees of the same malformative process. They depend mainly on the persistence of tissular remains during development. The development of dermoid and epidermoid cysts results from disturbances similar to those that determine the formation of teratomas, although they appear later in embryologic development and, therefore, are of lesser complexity. Their morphology depends on the moment during embryonal life in which the defect arises. Earlier defects give rise to the more complex dermoid cysts and later defects give rise to epidermoid cysts. These processes may coincide with other malformative processes like spina bifida, a dermoid sinus, etc.

Their predominance during childhood is demonstrated by the fact that 45% of the cases are under 10 years of age (18). There is no predilection for either sex, and, globally, they constitute 10% of infantile spinal tumors. As a consequence of their pathogenesis, the dermoid and epidermoid cysts are localized dorsally and may occupy any of the compartments of the spinal canal. They are almost always extramedullary and intradural, but occasionally they can affect the spinal cord or present outside the dura. Their preferred location is the lower thoracic and lumbar regions.

Dermoid cysts appear macroscopically as soft masses, white, brilliant, and sometimes pearly, that separate the nerve roots and compress the spinal cord without infiltrating it. Their content is variable, from whitish to amorphous tan masses, depending on secondary alterations and the amount of hair follicles. Epidermoid cysts are similar, but of a more delicate aspect, with a finer capsule, and an unctuous, squamous, and white pearly content.

Histologically, both are lined by squamous epithelium, which, in the case of dermoid cysts, has various layers, usually with a thick granulosa and a thin squamous superficial layer that desquamates squamous epithelial plaques. In contrast, the epithelium that lines epidermoid cysts is thinner, not exceeding five cell layers. The granulosa is composed of only one cell layer, while the squamous epithelial layer is very thick, desquamating numerous keratinous plaques that, as they fill the cavity, give these tumors their typical pearly appearance (Fig. 2B, C).

Besides these differences in the epithelium, the clearest differential criterion is that, whereas epidermoid cysts are composed exclusively of squamous epithelium that lies directly over the connective tissue of the arachnoid, dermoid cysts, like the skin dermis, have their own stratum of connective tissue, in which sweat glands and hair follicles with sebaceous glands are found. Shedding of these products of secretion into the interior of the cyst and their mixture with hairy detritus are reasons for the morphologic differences in the cysts: in the epidermoid they are exclusively keratinous and in the dermoid they consist of a mixture of this material with the other previously mentioned elements.

The so-called inclusion epidermoid is an independent entity that develops in the subarachnoid space of the lumbar region in patients who have undergone repeated lumbar punctures without the use of a stylet, with the subsequent seeding of cutaneous epithelium into the subarachnoid space. This process was frequent during the period in which tuberculous meningitis was treated with intrathecal streptomycin. Because this type of treatment is now in disuse and because use of the stylet has become obligatory, the inclusion epidermoid is presently a rarity.

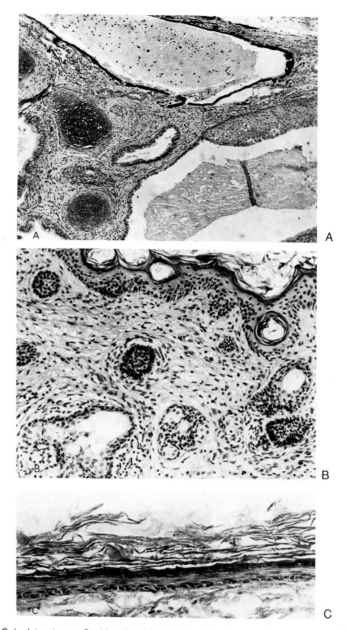

FIG. 2. A: Spinal teratoma. Cavities lined by partly cylindrical, partly squamous epithelium, areas of hyaline cartilage to the *left*, and a pigmented retinal "anlage" *above* may be seen. **B:** Spinal dermoid. A cavity, lined by sqamous cutaneous epithelium below which there are a dermal layer, hair follicles, and sebaceous glands (hematoxylin-eosin stain, 200×). **C:** Spinal epidermoid. The cavity of the cyst is lined by thin squamous epithelium of the epidermic type, with a thick granulosa and abundant keratinous plaques that lie superficially (hematoxylin-eosin stain, 400×).

Both dermoid and epidermoid cysts are benign, but they can cause problems owing to possible associated pathology, and because of adhesion to neighboring tissues that may complicate surgery. Another possibility is rupture of the cysts, with liberation of cholesterol, arising from the destruction of keratinous cells. This free cholesterol in the subarachnoid space is capable of producing an aseptic chemical meningitis, with the development of fibrous scars (arachnoiditis) and subsequent blockage of CSF flow.

Spinal Neurenteric Cyst

So-called neurenteric cysts of childhood are uncommon. They may occur occasionally up to the second decade of life. They are localized in the thoracic region and are always ventral. The cysts are the result of a broad spectrum of malformative processes that can include double vertebrae, intestinal duplications, and anomalous visceral and mediastinal cysts. Factors invoked in their pathogenesis are the incomplete separation of the notochord and the endoderm, giving rise to a diverticulum of the proximal intestine that usually impedes the fusion of the vertebral bodies (19). A second theory suggests herniation of the yolk sac or of the endoderm of the primitive gut with adhesion to the dorsal ectoderm (20). The severity of the defect determines the occurrence of either several or only one malformative processes. The height of the included portion of endoderm in the malformation determines the type of epithelium that lines the cyst. The epithelium can be of the respiratory type as well as of enteric type, more cubic, with a basal nucleus and cytoplasm filled with apical mucus (21).

The process is intrinsically benign and only produces symptoms when complicated by an associated malformation.

Intraspinal Cyst

A series of intraspinal cystic formations of variable morphology and different etiologies are grouped together under this title, including some types of unknown origin. They develop in the form of a cavity with a clear, aqueous content usually delimited by a fine wall. They grow slowly and slowly compress the cord. These cysts originate from the different coverings of the cord. This explains their position, sometimes intradural and other times extradural, sometimes anterior and, on other occasions, dorsal (22,23).

They have been well systematized in the following way (24):

(a)   Meningeal cysts
(b)   Arachnoidal cysts
(c)   Ependymal cysts
(d)   Dermoid and epidermoid cysts, and neurenteric spinal cysts.

As may be seen, the criterion applied is purely topographic and has a clinical orientation, since it unites dysembryoplastic processes previously mentioned such as dermoid and epidermoid cysts and postinflammatory lesions as the probable cause of arachnoidal cysts. All types may be found in infants and children, with the exception of the meningeal cyst, which we have not found in the literature. Whether spinal teratomas are included or excluded from the series, intraspinal cysts as a group represent an appreciable percentage, which, if dermoid and epidermoid cysts are included, can account for as much as 30% of the spinal cord tumors of childhood (1,10,12). On the contrary, if dermoid and epidermoid cysts are dealt with separately, cysts are restricted to the arachnoidal and ependymal cysts, which are rarer.

The Arachnoidal Cyst

Arachnoidal cysts are rare tumors that affect young adolescents. They are located preferentially at the thoracic level. Their frequency is difficult to determine, but they are quite rare. Their etiology is unknown, diverse factors being invoked, such as trauma, hemorrhage, and inflammatory processes, to which these cysts are attributed.

Macroscopically, they appear like sacks with semitransparent walls that contain clear liquid and communicate with the subarachnoid space. Histologically, they are constituted of a thin connective tissue membrane through which capillaries circulate, lined by a stratum of flat cells of arachnoid origin. This stratum may be absent in part or all of the cyst as a consequence of pressure in its interior.

Arachnoidal cysts are intrinsically benign, and their major clinical importance is their differential diagnosis with true intraspinal tumors.

The Ependymal Cyst

Ependymal cysts are also rare, representing a malformation of the ependyma that affects small children. They are localized in the ventral part of the intradural space. They produce symptoms of extrinsic cord compression. They are delimited by a wall of connective tissue lined by columnar or cubic epithelium, variably ciliated, of the ependymal type. They are benign processes whose extirpation is curative.

Intraspinal Lipoma

Intraspinal lipomas are rare tumors that may present in children or adults. Their growth is very slow. They are localized in the cervical and caudal regions, a thoracic localization being exceptional. These tumors are situated inside the spinal canal, in a dorsal position, occupying the subarachnoid space. They usally compress the posterior columns of the cord and grow between the nerve roots to which they adhere very tenaciously. Their anatomic limits are not well defined, and extirpation is difficult (25). Owing to their dysembryoplastic origin, they may coexist with associated anomalies such as dermal sinuses, meningoceles, and other dysraphic states.

Macroscopically, intraspinal lipomas appear as soft, yellowish masses that widen the posterior region of the cord and are admixed with the arachnoid and the spinal roots. Histologically, the findings are typical of a lipoma, with large adult adipose cells with an eccentric nucleus compressed against the cytoplasmic membrane. These cells lie packed, close to one another, with capillary vessels circulating between them. Externally, there is a capsule of variable thickness, but, in general, it is not very thick; frequently, nervous rootlets can be found in the periphery of the tumor, coming from the posterior roots of the spinal cord.

Prognosis is benign, unless there is poor demarcation of the tumor from the spinal cord or there is an associated malformation.

Tumors of the Meningeal Coverings

The only tumors originating from the meninges are meningiomas. Even though an intraspinal location is frequent in adults [prevalence about 28% of spinal tumors (26)], they are rare in children, appearing sporadically, primarily in young

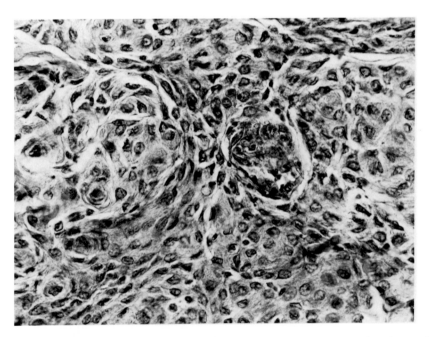

FIG. 3. Spinal meningioma. The tumor is formed of polygonal cells with a round nucleus and well-defined cytoplasm. The disposition in lobules is well defined, with a certain tendency to whorl formation on the left side (hematoxylin-eosin stain, 400×).

adolescents with a prevalence that oscillates around 2% of all intraspinal tumors (1,2). A thoracic location predominates in children (9), with a ratio of 2:1 in favor of females. Their macroscopic appearance is characteristic; they grow as sessile or flat nodular excrescences adherent to the internal face of the dura mater, compressing the spinal cord from without. This appearance helps differentiate them from schwannomas (neurinomas) of the region, which do not adhere to the dura and hang from the spinal nerve from which they originate. Histologically, the appearance of spinal meningiomas is similar to that of intracranial meningiomas. Meningocytic meningiomas are made up of solid nests of polygonal cells with uniform nuclei, frequent cytoplasmic inclusions, an opaque eosinophilic cytoplasm, and a well-defined membrane. These cells are arranged in whorls, forming concentric "onion sheath" structures. There is a scant stroma with well-vascularized fibrous bundles between the sheets of tumor cells. This meningocytic variant contrasts with other tumors with elongated cells, associated in more irregular whorls. This is the predominant fibrous, or en plaque, form (Fig. 3).

Meningiomas are consistently benign.

Tumors of the Spinal Nerves

Schwannoma (Neurinoma) and Neurofibroma

The prevalence of these tumors in childhood is difficult to evaluate because in many series the term neurofibroma is used indiscriminately for both types of tumors. Considered together, they are quite rare, estimated at 4% of all intraspinal tumors (1,9). In children they are almost always associated with von Recklinghausen disease, and they can be multiple (2). These figures contrast with a 31% prevalence among the intraspinal tumors in adults (26).

Both tumors develop from the Schwann cells of the spinal nerves at any spinal level. Schwannomas tend to arise in the intradural space, originating on a posterior nerve root. The tumors can expand slowly in the intradural space until they protrude through the intervertebral foramina and exteriorize themselves, forming dumbbell tumors.

Microscopically, schwannomas hang from the nerve root, growing eccentrically in the nerve sheath, displacing it to one side. For this reason, the point of origin can always be identified. They are white, soft, and oval, with a fine and well-vascularized capsule. Histologically, there is a predominance of areas with elongated spindle-shaped bipolar cells, with elongated nuclei and scant cytoplasm. The cells are frequently arranged in fascicles and whorls and, less commonly, in parallel palisades. Edematous and xanthomatous types are uncommon in children (Fig. 4A).

The main differential diagnosis of spinal schwannoma is meningioma, from which it differs by its relation to a nerve. The meningioma is attached to the inner surface of the dura. Histological examination leaves no doubt.

On the other hand, neurofibromas, which also have their origin on a nerve, may appear anywhere along the nerve. For this reason, they are more often dumbbell-shaped than schwannomas, and they are encountered more frequently outside the spinal canal. Their prevalence is lower than that of schwannomas.

Macroscopically, they are poorly demarcated and produce diffuse thickening of the nerve. Instead of displacing the nerve, the tumor tissue dissects the nerve fibers that remain included in it. The cut surface of neurofibromas is white, more translucent than that of schwannomas, but often they are indistinguishable. They are practically always associated with von Recklinghausen disease. Micro-scopically, the image is similar, with elongated wavy bipolar cells. They are ar-ranged in an irregular plexus, mixing with collagenous and myelinated fibers. Neoplastic cells frequently attach themselves to adjacent collagen fibers or nerve bundles. Small vessels and thickened nerves may be seen inside the tumor mass (Fig. 4B).

The differential diagnosis of neurofibromas includes schwannomas and gan-glioneuromas. Schwannomas have a greater tendency to form whorls and fasci-cles, in contrast to the reticular pattern of neurofibromas. Attachment to a nerve is more common in schwannomas but is a less useful feature than for the differential

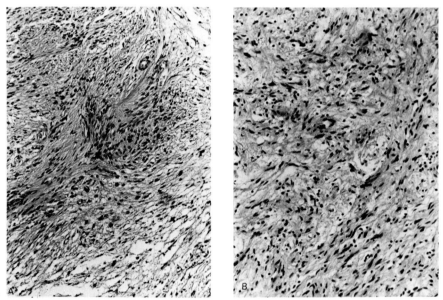

A,B

FIG. 4. A: Spinal neurinoma. Elongated cells with an oval nucleus and bipolar cytoplasm, tend-ing to form whorls in the center (A areas). *Below* and to the *right* there is an edematous type B zone (hematoxylin-eosin stain, 200×). **B:** Dumbbell neurofibroma. The cells have an elon-gated wavy shape with prominent nuclei and cytoplasm. The pattern is amorphous, with a ten-dency of the cells to join themselves to the collagenous fibers (hematoxylin-eosin stain, 400×).

diagnosis with meningiomas. The presence of nerve fibers within the tumor is in favor of neurofibroma. The differential diagnosis with ganglioneuroma arises in cases in which serial sections of the ganglioneuroma reveal no mature neurons and contain only interstitium. Owing to the similarity of the interstitium of these tumors to that of neurofibromas, the only valid method of diagnosis is the study of as many blocks as necessary until neurons are found or their presence is excluded.

Both tumors are benign. Malignant forms have not been observed in children. This may be because the process of malignant transformation of both tumors is very slow. In the adult, malignant transformation is common in cases associated with neurofibromatosis.

Vascular Tumors and Processes

The two more important processes are arteriovenous vascular malformations and hemangioblastomas. Both are rare.

Arteriovenous Vascular Malformation

Arteriovenous malformations of the spinal cord are rare in children (27). They tend to be located in the thoracolumbar region. In 15% of cases they coexist with a cutaneous angioma immediately superficial to the lesion. The association of spina bifida, cerebellar hemangioblastoma, and other intracranial arteriovenous malformations has been described.

Histologically, they are made up of tangles of blood vessels that are variably dilated. Some of these vessels are cavernous, whereas others are capillaries. They are always very irregular, with a wall of variable thickness. Sometimes they are constituted only of an endothelium lying over a thin layer of connective tissue, while others have a thick fibrous wall that can even at times contain variable amounts of smooth muscle and elastic tissue. Early arteriosclerotic changes are fairly common, as are hemorrhages and thromboses in various stages of organization.

These abnormal vessels are located within the arachnoid, lying over the surface of the spinal cord. They can assume three macroscopic appearances (28): (a) as one or two separate arteries that run along the surface of the cord, anastomosing with a single descending vein; (b) as a mass of anomalous vessels fed by several arteries and drained by one or two veins; and (c) as a large mass of malformed vessels extending over much of the spinal canal, fed by several arterial afferents. This last form is most frequent in children.

Hemangioblastoma

Spinal hemangioblastomas are rare at any age and exceptional in children. They are commonly located in the dorsal area of the spinal cord and are always attached to the arachnoid from which they originate. Some can be extramedullary, but never extradural. Histologically, the image is typical, consisting of anastomosed capillary vessels and a reticular stroma made up of cells more or less rich in intracytoplasmic lipid. Prognosis is good, although approximately one-third of cases coexist with von Hippel-Lindau syndrome, which worsens the prognosis.

Metastatic Tumors

Since the majority of the metastatic deposits in the nervous system arise from bronchopulmonary, prostatic, and mammary carcinomas, they are most common in the latter decades of life. Spinal metastatic tumors are exceptional in childhood. When they occur, they are usually due to dissemination of intracranial tumors such as medulloblastomas, or to hematologic malignancies, usually lymphomas or leukemias. These factors are responsible for differences between children and adults in the relative prevalence of spinal tumors.

Medulloblastoma

With the exception of very rare infiltration of the cervical spinal cord by an extension of a medulloblastoma of the vermis, the spinal cord is affected by arachnoid metastases, seeding in the CSF. These tumors, commonly seen in young children, tend to disseminate throughout the cranial and spinal subarachnoid spaces. This latter localization, which occurs in 35% of the cases (30), mandates prophylactic irradiation of the spine in children with medulloblastoma. Macroscopically, they appear as cotton-like masses or, less frequently, as white, soft, and friable, generally multiple nodules. They can also appear as massive diffuse infiltrations of the subarachnoid space, spinal cord roots, and the cauda equina. Microscopically, the appearance is that of a densely cellular tumor. Their cells have a round or oval hyperchromatic nucleus and scant cytoplasm. Mitoses are numerous and the tumor cells occur in sheets that fill the subarachnoid space. The picture is similar to that of lymphomas, but the differential diagnosis is obvious, since there is always a previous or simultaneous vermian tumor.

Lymphomas

Lymphomas and leukemias account for many of the spinal cord tumors in children. Metastatic disease of the central nervous system commonly coincides with both types of processes. Undifferentiated lymphomas, especially lymphoid leukemia, are the predominant form in children. In non-Hodgkin lymphomas the spine is affected in about 9% of cases (31,32). An estimated 8.2% of leukemias affect the spinal cord (33). The prevalence of each type of lymphoid malignancy influences the relative incidence of nervous system involvement in children and

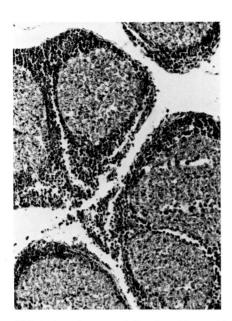 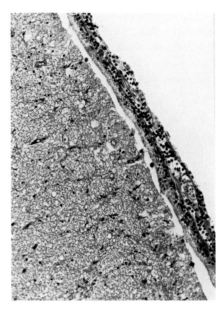

A,B

FIG. 5. Lymphomatous infiltration of the cord (both images are from the same case). **A:** Massive involvement of the spinal roots. The nerve coverings are occupied by neoplastic lymphoid cells. There is a tendency toward infiltration of the fascicles (hematoxylin-eosin stain, 200×). **B:** At the cord level, the arachnoid space is occupied by tumor cells, without parenchymal penetration (hematoxylin-eosin stain, 200×).

adults. Thus, acute lymphocytic leukemia comprises 23% of the childhood cases, whereas acute myeloblastic leukemia accounts for only 6%. A second factor is that, as survival increases, neurologic involvement occurs more frequently. The effect of modern treatment methods has increased survival rates from 4% in 1947 to 40% in 1960. Spinal cord involvement results from seeding of the subarachnoid space by tumor cells, which can be detected by cytologic examination of the CSF.

Lymphomas can affect the spinal cord through different mechanisms (34): (a) invasion of the spinal canal through the intervertebral foramina, from mediastinal or retroperitoneal nodes, whereby the low thoracic and lumbar regions are affected; (b) invasion of the spinal canal through affected vertebrae, which occurs less frequently; and (c) vertebral collapse and angulation of the vertebral column with involvement of the spinal cord.

Macroscopically, vertebral involvement by lymphoma and leukemia is established by infiltration of the bone marrow of the vertebra with destruction and secondary collapse. From there, the lymphocytic proliferation infiltrates the epidural space, affecting the correspondent spinal nerve in its extradural course. Infiltration of the spinal canal by tumor cells from retroperitoneal lymph nodes via the intervertebral foramina occurs through areas with loose tissues, including the nerve root, forming a dumbbell tumor of coarser morphology than tumors of the nerve sheaths.

Involvement of the epidural space, regardless of the type of tumor, consists of sheets of tissue that surround the external surface of the dura and, at times, extend along several spinal segments. The tumor cells massively infiltrate the epidural space and the nerve sheaths in their extradural course.

Finally, seeding of the subarachnoid space forms white, confluent, flat plaques or nodular masses situated over the surface of the spinal cord and involving the roots. When the cauda equina is affected, a nodule of greater size forms between the nerves or nodules appearing as small beaded thickenings occur along the course of nerve roots (Fig. 5A,B).

Neoplastic cells that fill the subarachnoid space tend to infiltrate the cord discretely through the pial perforating vessels and to surround the nerve roots, infiltrating them and dissecting the nerve fibers.

To the naked eye, the topographic distribution is always the same, irrespective of the type of leukemia or lymphoma, whereas the histologic picture varies with the type of tumor.

Prognosis is obviously unfavorable, but current therapeutic alternatives make long-term survival possible, especially in patients without nervous system involvement.

EXTRADURAL TUMORS

Under this heading a heterogeneous group of tumors are discussed, some of them described in other areas of this text. They can appear in more than one location. This chapter is limited to peripheral nerve tumors and osseous tumors capable of producing spinal cord symptomatology.

Peripheral Tumors

Tumors of neural origin are represented by a series of progressively undifferentiated and malignant tumors, from ganglioneuromas (differentiated and benign) to neuroblastomas (undifferentiated and malignant). Ganglioneuroblastomas are between these two extremes. These tumors account for 20% of spinal tumors. They predominate in females in a proportion of 3:2. Surprisingly, neuroblastomas occur most frequently (17%); the remaining 3% consisting of ganglioneuromas (1). Because of the slow growth of ganglioneuromas and ganglioneuroblastomas, it takes years for them to become symptomatic. Because the mediastinum and abdomen have an acceptable tolerance for these tumors, both can increase considerably in volume and often remain silent until neurologic symptoms develop.

These tumors originate from the sympathetic paravertebral ganglia and the adrenal medulla and grow into the mediastinum and the abdominal cavity of children and adults. In a small number of cases involving high thoracic and retroperitoneal regions, they grow into the spinal canal through the intervertebral foramina and form dumbbell tumors. Their association with von Recklinghausen disease is well established. Owing to their close relationship, these three types of tumors are dealt with together.

Ganglioneuroma

Ganglioneuromas are the most benign and differentiated of this group of tumors. They grow to considerable size, are lobulated and well circumscribed, though not encapsulated. The major part of the tumor lies outside the spine. Their penetration into the spinal canal is carried out through the intervertebral foramina, occupying the extradural space and never penetrating the dura. This fact does not decrease the importance of the process, as cord compression may be severe. Their cut surface is white, fibrous, and firm. If there is necrosis, the presence of malignant areas must be suspected.

Microscopically, they are characterized by the coexistence of two types of tissue. One consists of nests and scattered areas of large ganglionic cells, with central or peripheral nuclei with loose chromatin and prominent nucleoli. Their cytoplasm is abundant, containing Nissl substance, and it has expansions that can be demonstrated by silver staining. Between these groups of cells, there is a fibrous interstitium, usually abundant, traversed by collagenous fibers, vessels, and cells with Schwann-like characteristics. Areas of calcification are common in the extraspinal portion of the tumor (Fig. 6A).

Diagnosis is not difficult if neurons are found, but, in cases in which routine examination of the specimen does not demonstrate them, ganglioneuromas may be mistaken for neurofibromas because the interstitium is very similar to that of this neoplasm. In such cases, multiple blocks of the tumor must be studied. The tumor is almost always benign; nevertheless, in exceptional cases, focal areas of dedifferentiation or malignant degeneration may be found. In our opinion, these areas are most probably not areas of malignant transformation; rather, the tumor is a very differentiated ganglioneuroblastoma (see Ganglioneuroblastoma, below).

Neuroblastoma

Neuroblastomas represent the opposite extreme in the range of malignancy of neural tumors, constituting a very aggressive metastasizing neoplasm, usually found in children. Occasionally they may also appear in neonates. They are most common in the first 5 years of life. Forty to fifty percent of them originate in the adrenal medulla and 30% in the retroperitoneal space where they grow rapidly and are infiltrative. As in other tumors, some of them penetrate into the spinal canal through the intervertebral foramina and occupy the extradural space. Although they are very infiltrating, the dura is a barrier that is very rarely breached. Biochemically, the tumors produce catecholamines and vanillylmandelic acid (VMA), which is useful for establishing the diagnosis and in the control of eventual recurrences after remission.

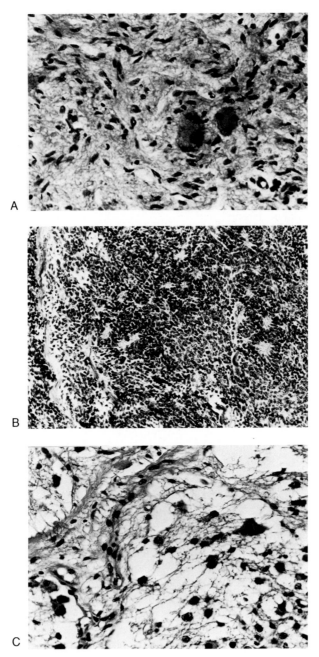

FIG. 6. A: Ganglioneuroma. The background tissue is loose, insinuating itself between two large neurons with a laterally placed nucleus and a well-defined cytoplasm. Observe the resemblance of the stroma to that of the neurofibroma in Fig. 4B (hematoxylin-eosin stain, 400 ×). **B:** Retroperitoneal neuroblastoma. A tumor of high cellular density with small cells with hyperchromatic nuclei that, at the *right*, tend to form Homer-Wright rosettes (hematoxylin-eosin stain, 200 ×). **C:** Ganglioneuroblastoma. The tumor has relatively large multipolar nerve cells intermixed with smaller and less well-differentiated cells. The stroma is formed by a plexiform neuropil. Fibrous tracts, like the one on the upper right quadrant, surround the lobules (hematoxylin-eosin stain, 440 ×).

Neuroblastomas present as large, pink, soft, sometimes lobulated masses with necrotic and, more frequently, hemorrhagic areas, divided by thin connective tissue tracts. They have a strong infiltrating capacity and poorly demarcated margins. Histologically, conventional techniques show neuroblastomas to be formed by cells with a round, oval, very hyperchromatic nucleus, and scant or invisible cytoplasm; the cells are densely packed with almost no stroma between them. Mitoses are very numerous. In the cell cords, there are circular structures formed of cells arranged radially around an acellular central space of reticular character formed by the processes of these cells. These are the rosettes of Homer-Wright. The true rosettes of Flexner never occur. Occasionally, there may be better differentiated areas with a neuropil and neuronal-like cells of somewhat larger size (Fig. 6B).

The most important differential diagnosis of neuroblastoma is lymphoma; and it is based on the immunohistochemical demonstration of immunoglobulin in lymphomas and by metallic impregnation of neuroblastomas. The presence of rosettes of Homer-Wright is another important differential feature. Tissue culture, despite its technical complexity, gives pathognomonic results, since neuroblastomas develop long divergent processes that grow out from the explant in the first two days of culture (35).

The prognosis of neuroblastomas is poor because of the frequency with which they metastasize. The distribution of metastases varies with age. In the first 6 months of life, the pattern observed is the Pepper type, in which the abdomen, and especially the liver, is affected. The route of dissemination in this case is transplacental, with subsequent hepatic seeding. After 6 months, the pattern observed is the Hutchinson type, with metastases to the orbits, cranial vault, and long bones, as well as to the lymph nodes. The reason for this change in the distribution pattern of metastases is the disappearance of the transplacental route after birth, and because the adult circulation pattern distributes metastases to the rest of the body. A mixture of both types of dissemination is common.

Paradoxically, the bad prognosis of neuroblastoma contrasts with the fact that it is one of the few tumors in which spontaneous maturation has been described (36,37). Even though the mortality from neuroblastomas is very high, death occurs in the first months. Therefore, should the patient survive the first 14 months, cure is almost certain (38). This rare phenomenon may either be due to tumor regression as a result of therapy or to spontaneous maturation.

Ganglioneuroblastoma

Between these two extremes in the spectrum of malignancy are the so-called ganglioneuroblastomas—neoplasms of intermediate maturity in which neuroblasts and young neurons make up a variable proportion of the tumor. Sometimes neuroblasts and young neurons are intermixed randomly in a loose neuropil, giving rise to the immature ganglioneuroblastoma. Other times, there are clusters of undifferentiated neuroblastoma cells and other more mature zones forming miniature ganglioneuroblastomas. Both types of ganglioneuroblastomas affect children between the ages of 0 and 5 years, in the same locations as neuroblastomas with the same disastrous prognosis. The importance of separating these subtypes lies in the fact that the immature tumors have a greater tendency to metastasize. In our experience, the ganglioneuroblastomas rarely affect the spinal canal (Fig. 6C).

Other tumors that must be included in this group, and that may also occupy the extradural region, are neurofibromas, lymphomas, and metastatic tumors.

Tumors of the Spine

The figures on the tumors of the spine that affect the spinal cord vary greatly for several reasons: (a) The relative prevalence of spinal tumors is different in children and adults. (b) General surgeons, orthopedists, and neurosurgeons all treat spinal tumors, and thus statistical data are difficult to collect. (c) Not all spinal tumors impinge on the spinal cord (40).

Spinal cord symptomatology usually reflects epidural compression or involvement of the intervertebral foramina, but occasionally it is vertebral collapse that affects the cord through vascular compromise.

The childhood tumors of the spine that most frequently are the cause of spinal cord symptomatology are osteoblastomas, aneurysmal bone cysts, and Ewing's tumor.

Osteoblastoma

The spine is a frequent site of osteoblastomas, in young adults as well as children, in whom they account for 5% of cases (41). They have a characteristic radiologic appearance and can compress the cord or the roots. Histologically, they are characterized by very active proliferation of osteoblasts that form a variable quantity of osteoid. The vessels are very abundant and frequently cavernous, and there is always a considerable number of multinucleated giant cells. They are always benign tumors, and the major problem is their differentiation from osteosarcomas (1).

Aneurysmal Bone Cyst

These tumors have been described occasionally in the spine of children (1). They may produce neurologic symptoms by compression by the tumor or by the collapse of the affected vertebra, as in the previous case. Histologically, wide vascular spaces are surrounded by bands of fibrous tissue, with plaques of linear calcification and with multiple cell types including fibroblasts, multinucleated giant cells, and a variable inflammatory component containing histiocytes loaded with red cell breakdown products. The lesion is usually benign.

Ewing's Tumor

Ewing's tumors commonly appear in the first two decades and account for 6% (42) or 9% (43) of bone tumors. They predominate in the long bones, whereas the vertebrae are affected in only 6% of cases. Of this low percentage, a small number infiltrate the spinal canal, growing diffusely until they reach the intradural space. Occasionally, they may grow in the form of dumbbell tumors, occupying the intervertebral foramina, the costovertebral angle, and the spinal canal.

They present as pinkish, friable, infiltrating masses that histologically offer the appearance of a small-cell sarcoma, with monotonous round or oval hyperchromatic nuclei. The tumors consist of tightly packed nuclei with barely visible or invisible cytoplasm. When the cytoplasm is fixed in alcohol, the Best carmine or PAS diastase technique demonstrates that it contains glycogen. Mitoses are abundant. The tumor cells are arranged in diffuse sheets traversed by fine capillaries and thin fibrous tracts.

Differential diagnosis must be made from other malignant tumors having small round cells, such as neuroblastomas, lymphomas, and with the less common metastases of medulloblastomas. The presence of glycogen in Ewing's sarcoma, the demonstration of immunoglobulins in lymphomas, and the subarachnoid seeding of the medulloblastomas of the cerebellum are the most reliable differential criteria.

Differential diagnosis with neuroblastoma can be very difficult, because Ewing's sarcoma can also take on a rosette-like appearance. The presence of glycogen is still the best way to differentiate them.

Chordomas, chondromas, chondrosarcomas, and fibrous dysplasia are bone tumors discussed in Chapter 9.

REFERENCES

1. Matson, DD. *Neurosurgery of infancy and childhood.* Springfield, Ill.: Charles C Thomas, 1969.
2. Milhoradt TH. *Pediatric neurosurgery.* Philadelphia: FA Davis, 1978.
3. Steinke CR. Spinal tumors: statistics on a series of 330 collected cases. *J Nerv Ment Dis* 1918; 47:418–426.
4. Kordas M, Balint K. Spinal tumors in children. 9th scientific meeting of the International Society of Pediatric Neurosurgeons (Abstr.). *Child's Brain* 1981;8:36.
5. Grant FC, Austin GM. The diagnosis, treatment and prognosis of tumors affecting the spinal cord in children. *J Neurosurg* 1956;13:535–545.
6. Jänisch W, Schreiber D, Gerlach H. *Tumoren des Zentralnervensystems bei Feten und Sauglingen.* Jena: VEB Gustav Fischer Verlag, 1980.
7. Alter M. Statistical aspects of spinal cord tumors. In: Vinken PJ, Bruyn GW, eds. *Handbook of clinical neurology,* vol. 19. Amsterdam: North-Holland, 1975;I:1–22.
8. Grote W. Tumores medulares y otros procesos espinales en la infancia. *Pract Pediatr (Madrid)* 1974;10:107–116.
9. Marsden HB, Steward JK. *Tumors in children.* Berlin: Springer Verlag, 1976;137–193.
10. Harwood-Nash DC. Spinal tumors in the child. In: Jeanmart L, ed. *Radiology of the spine tumors.* Berlin: Springer Verlag, 1986;65–71.
11. Till K. *Paediatric neurosurgery.* Oxford: Blackwell, 1975.
12. Ingraham FD, Matson DD. *Neurosurgery of infancy and childhood.* Springfield, Ill.: Charles C Thomas, 1954.

13. Arendt A. Spinal gliomas. In: Vinkin PJ, Bruyn GW, eds. *Handbook of clinical neurology*, vol. 20. Amsterdam: North-Holland, 1976; II.
14. Escalona-Zapata J. *Atlas de anatomia patológica de los tumores del sistema nervioso*. Madrid: Ed Complutense, 1986.
15. Zülch KJ. *Brain tumors: their biology and pathology*. Berlin: Springer Verlag, 1986.
16. Rubinstein LJ. *Tumors of the central nervous system*. Washington, DC: AFIP 2nd series, 1972.
17. Farwell JR, Dohrmann CJ, Flanery JT. Central nervous system in children. *Cancer* 1977;40:3123–3132.
18. Henschen F. Tumoren des Zentralnervensystems und seiner Hüllen. In: Henke-Lubarsch, ed. *Hand sprez Path Anat und Histol*, vol. 13. Berlin: Springer Verlag, 1955;III.
19. Fallon M, Gordon ARG, Lendrum AC. Mediastinal cysts of a foregut origin associated with vertebral abnormalities. *Br J Surg* 1954;41:520–533.
20. Bentley JFR, Smith JR. Developmental posterior enteric remnants and spinal malformations. *Arch Dis Child* 1960;35:76–78.
21. Salinero E, Escalona-Zapata J, Perez Calvo JM, Pedregal M. Quiste enterógeno medular. *Patologia (Madrid)* 1979;12:307–313.
22. Wilkins RH, Odom GL. Spinal epidural cysts. In: Vinkin PJ, Bruyn GW, eds. *Handbook of clinical neurology*, vol. 20. Amsterdam: North-Holland, 1976;II:55–102.
23. Gimeno Alava A. Arachnoid, neurenteric and other cysts. In: Vinkin PJ, Bruyn GW, eds. *Handbook of clinical neurology*, vol. 32. Amsterdam: North-Holland, 1978;393–446.
24. Burger PC, Vogel FS. *Surgical pathology of the nervous system and its coverings*. New York: John Wiley, 1976.
25. Mircewski M, Mircewska D, Bojadziew I, Basewska R. Surgical treatment of spinal lipomas in infancy and childhood. *Child's Brain* 1983;10:317–327.
26. Ross ER. Neural tumors of infancy and childhood. In: Minckler J, ed. *Pathology of the nervous system*, vol. 2. New York: McGraw-Hill, 1971;2196–2219.
27. Tada T, Sakamoto K, Kobayashi N, Tanaka Y. Arteriovenous malformation of the spinal cord in a 17 month old child. *Child's Nerv Syst* 1985;1:298–301.
28. Di Chiro G, Werner L. Angiography of the spinal cord. A review of contemporary techniques and applications. *J Neurosurg* 1973;39:1–12.
29. Browne TR, Adams RD, Robertson GH. Hemangioblastoma of the spinal cord. *Arch Neurol* 1976; 33:435–441.
30. Jänisch W, Guthert H, Schreiber D. *Pathologie der Tumoren des Zentralnervensystems*. Jena: VEB Gustav Fischer Verlag, 1976.
31. Currie S, Henson RA. Neurological syndromes in the reticulosis. *Brain* 1971;94:307–320.
32. Levitt LJ, Dawson DM, Rosenthal DS, Moloney WC. CNS involvement in the non-Hodgkin lymphomas. *Cancer* 1980;45:522–545.
33. Broder LE, Carter SK. *Meningeal leukemia*. New York: Plenum Press, 1972.
34. Ngan H, James KW. *Clinical radiology of the lymphomas*. London: Butterworths, 1973.
35. Murray MR, Stout AP. Distinctive characteristics of the sympathicoblastoma cultivated in vitro. *Am J Pathol* 1947;23:429–441.
36. Cushing H, Wolbach SB. Transformation of malignant paravertebral sympathicoblastoma into benign ganglioneuroma. *Am J Pathol* 1927;3:203–216.
37. Fox F, Davidson J, Thomas LB. Maturation of sympathicoblastoma into ganglioneuroblastoma. *Cancer* 1959;12:108–116.
38. Knox WE, Pillars EMK. Time of recurrence or cure of tumors in childhood. *Lancet* 1959;i:188–191.
39. Russell DS, Rubinstein LJ. *Pathology of tumors in the nervous system*. London: E Arnold, 1977.
40. Jeanmart L. *Radiology of the spine tumors*. Berlin: Springer Verlag, 1986.
41. Schajowicz F. *Tumors and tumorlike lesions of bone and joints*. New York: Springer Verlag, 1981.
42. Dahlin DC. *Bone tumors*, 3rd ed. Springfield, Ill.: Charles C Thomas, 1978.
43. Occhipintic E, Mastro Stefano R, Pompili A. Spinal chordomas in infancy. 8th scientific meeting of the International Society of Pediatric Neurosurgeons. *Child's Brain* 1981;8:67 (Abstr.).

3

Imaging of Pediatric Spinal Tumors

David G. Ashley, Marvin D. Nelson, Jr., and Hervey D. Segall

Numerous imaging modalities are now available for evaluation of the pediatric spine. The diagnostic algorithm depends on the clinical presentation, the location of the lesion, and the technological resources available. In children, it is always important to limit the dose of ionizing radiation.

In evaluation of the pediatric spine, a lesion may be anatomically localized to the vertebral body, the extradural soft tissues, extramedullary intradural space, spinal cord, or it may involve more than one compartment. Localizing a lesion to one of these sites enables one to narrow the differential diagnosis.

PLAIN FILMS

Plain film radiography remains a common modality in evaluation of the spine. All patients should be examined in at least two planes. X-rays are abnormal in 60 to 70% of children with intraspinal tumors, although findings may be subtle or nonspecific. As a general rule, a vertebral tumor will spare the disc space, and an infectious process will be centered in the disc with destruction of adjacent vertebral end plates (1). Kyphosis and scoliosis are frequent findings in children with slow-growing tumors.

The transverse and anterior-posterior diameters of the spinal canal are judged by the distance between the pedicles on the anteroposterior (AP) view and the distance between posterior vertebral body and the closest point on the spinous process on the lateral view. Long-standing cord widening may result in flattening or erosion of the medial aspects of the pedicles and widening of the AP diameter of the spinal canal. Enlargement of the spinal canal over several segments suggests the diagnosis of an intramedullary mass or syringohydromyelia. Posterior vertebral scalloping may be secondary to an intradural mass, connective tissue disorder, such as mesodermal dysplasia in association with neurofibromatosis, or to increased pressure (1,2).

Neuroforaminal widening is best seen on oblique views in the cervical spine. In the lumbar and thoracic spine, it is best seen on the lateral view. This type of widening is usually seen with neurofibroma, meningioma, and, rarely, dilated vessels related to an arteriovenous malformation. In addition, with neurofibromatosis, there may be multiple wide neuroforamina. These are most likely secondary to mesodermal dysplasia with lateral meningoceles rather than widening caused by multiple tumors (2). Apparent enlargement caused by hypoplasia of a pedicle should not be confused with true enlargement of a neuroforamen caused by a tumor (1).

The appearance of primary vertebral lesions on plain film may be diagnostic. An example is the waferlike collapse of the vertebral body seen in association with histiocytosis X. Osteoid osteoma is suggested when a small (<1.5 cm) sclerotic lesion, or lytic lesion with a sclerotic border, is seen in the lamina, pedicle, or transverse process. This lesion is commonly on the concave side of the scoliosis. The less common osteoblastomas may occur in the same location and have mixed osteosclerotic and osteolytic features; however, these tend to be larger than 1.5 cm, may be expansile, may involve the vertebral body, and have less associated pain. Aneurysmal bone cysts are lytic expansile lesions primarily involving the lamina. Giant cell tumor, Ewing's tumor, and osteosarcoma are also in the differential diagnosis. Vertebral osteosarcoma in children is almost always secondary to irradiation (3). Hemangioma of the vertebral body characteristically appears as prominent vertical trabeculations or honeycombing (4).

It may be difficult to define the level of a lesion specifically on clinical grounds. In such instances, plain X-rays may localize the abnormality for further study. Because of time constraints, it is important to restrict computerized tomography (CT) and magnetic resonance imaging (MRI) to one portion of the spine whenever possible.

MYELOGRAPHY

Myelography involves the injection of contrast into the subarachnoid space. Contrast agents have included air, oxygen, nitrous oxide, iophendylate (Pantopaque), water-soluble agents such as metrizamide, and the more recently introduced iopamidol and iohexol.

The gases, while being relatively inert, had the disadvantage of poor radiographic contrast. Iophendylate, a viscous oil-based contrast with extremely slow absorption, was the most widely used agent until the late 1970s. It fell out of use because of several disadvantages. The oil-based agent does not mix with cerebrospinal fluid (CSF). This prevents filling of nerve roots, results in clumping of contrast, and prevents passage of contrast around a lesion causing a high degree of block. Iophendylate was rarely associated with acute or subacute toxicity but did occasionally cause later arachnoiditis; this was especially true if subarachnoid blood was present. This complication necessitated complete removal of the iophendylate following completion of the examination. This removal was time consuming and painful for the patient, and, invariably, a few drops were left in the subarachnoid space. Owing to the high radiographic density of iophendylate, fine anatomic detail could be obscured. Residual droplets caused artifacts on later CT examinations of the spine or brain. Because of these disadvantages, this agent is now rarely used (1,5).

The water-soluble agents mix well with CSF. This allows identification of the entire diameter of the cord, since it may be completely surrounded by contrast material. Nerve roots are well filled. The contrast flows beyond areas that are nearly, but not completely, blocked. Rapid absorption makes removal unnecessary. Because of lower viscosity, a smaller needle may be used (22 gauge). This reduces the incidence of postmyelographic headaches thought to be secondary to CSF leakage (5). Because of some neurotoxic effects of metrizamide, it has been replaced by the less toxic nonionic-water soluble agents iohexol and iopamidol.

With the advent of MRI, the indications for myelography have decreased, but myelography with CT myelography remains superior to nonenhanced MRI in the detection of small intradural extramedullary lesions, such as subarachnoid metastatic disease (6). Such small lesions may be missed even after injection of gadolinium DTPA (Gd-DTPA). In the workup of children with suspected subarachnoid metastasis, we combine the lumbar puncture for CSF and myelographic study so the child is spared an additional interventional procedure.

Even with the new contrast agents, there are several disadvantages to standard myelography. It is invasive, and ionizing radiation is required. In the case of block, two punctures would be required and, even then, disease between two levels of block may not be identified. In patients with CSF block, lumbar puncture has the risk of clinical deterioration in approximately 20% of patients. Therefore, if lumbar puncture is performed, ideally no CSF should be removed. In the case of suspected block, puncture at the C1–C2 interspace is sometimes recommended. Puncture hematoma, postspinal puncture headaches, nerve root avulsion, spinal hemorrhage, and death are potential complications (7,8).

In intramedullary tumor, the myelogram shows widening of the cord demonstrated in two projections. This usually extends over several segments. The interpediculate distance may be widened and posterior aspects of vertebral bodies scalloped. Cord enlargement from syringohydromyelia cannot be distinguished from that caused by cord tumor without special manipulations to demonstrate cavity filling or by changing the patient's position to show the "collapsing cord" sign (9). In the pediatric population, astrocytomas constitute the majority of cord tumors (Fig. 1). Cord widening may be seen concomitantly with drop metastases. In this case, the enlarged cord may be secondary to a metastatic lesion growing into and expanding the cord. Other causes of cord enlargement are hematoma, abscess, infarction, myelitis, arteriovenous malformation, granuloma, and ependymal cyst (10).

Intradural extramedullary masses may appear as sharply defined defects with contralateral displacement of the spinal cord. There may be ipsilateral widening of the contrast column, and the site of dural attachment will usually be opposite the point of maximal displacement (Fig. 2).

With subarachnoid metastatic disease, tumor deposits may appear as discrete filling defects or may result in thickening of nerve roots. Drop metastases are often found in the caudal sac and lower spinal canal. In these patients it is imperative to obtain an upright lateral film to avoid missing small filling defects at the tip of the sac. Subarachnoid seeding may be from medulloblastoma, glioblastoma, ependymoma, pineal germinoma, choroid plexus papilloma, retinoblastoma,

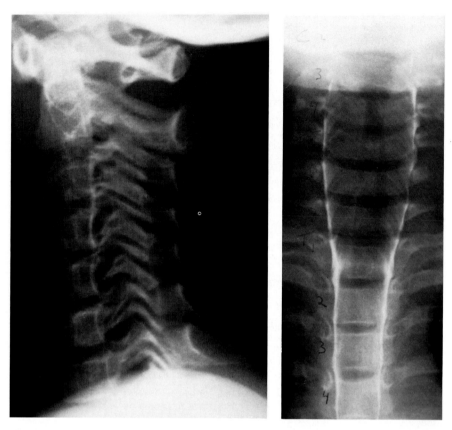

A,B

FIG. 1. Intramedullary tumor. This patient has a cord astrocytoma. **A:** The lateral X-ray of the cervical spine shows widening of the AP diameter of the spinal canal and posterior vertebral scalloping. **B:** In the same patient, the myelogram (PA projection) demonstrates marked widening of the cervical and upper thoracic cord.

brainstem glioma, or other tumors that have penetrated the dura. Differentiation of discrete subarachnoid filling defects also includes neurofibroma, dermoid, epidermoid, lipoma, arachnoid cyst, and air bubble. Benign tumors generally appear smooth with sharp margins, although there is overlap with the appearance of malignant tumors. Air bubbles will move from one side to another but are tenacious, so the patient must be moved often. Arachnoid cysts are usually posteriorly located, may show some movement fluoroscopically, and may or may not absorb water-soluble contrast on delayed myelographic images. Meningiomas, although uncommon, may also be seen in childhood and are dural based. Lipoma, dermoid, epidermoid, and teratoma may span the three anatomic compartments (extradural, intramedullary, and extramedullary) and may be associated with vertebral dysraphism (11).

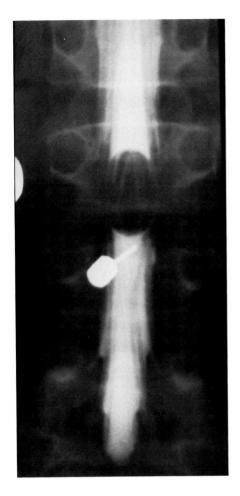

FIG. 2. Intradural extramedullary tumor. This patient has a neurofibroma. An intrathecal defect at the L3 level is seen with sharply defined margins.

Extradural masses result in displacement of the thecal sac and the spinal cord. Inward displacement of the thecal sac from the vertebral body and other osseous structures may result in tapering of the contrast column. When associated with complete block below the level of the conus, the nerve roots will result in a feathered appearance (1) (Fig. 3). The differential diagnosis includes metastatic neuroblastoma, lymphoma, sarcoma, Wilms tumor, hemangioma, aneursymal bone cyst, and nonneoplastic conditions such as epidural abscess, hematoma, arachnoid cyst, or herniated nucleus pulposus. Metastasis primarily involves the vertebral body and invades the epidural space secondarily. Epidural abscess will usually be associated with erosion of adjacent vertebral end plates. Herniated nucleus pulposus compression will be seen opposite the disc level. Subdural injection of contrast may produce an appearance suggesting cord enlargement or other abnormality not actually present. This should not cause confusion if two views are taken and there is scrutiny for poor delineation of subarachnoid structures.

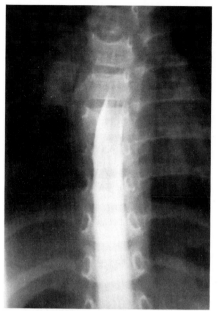 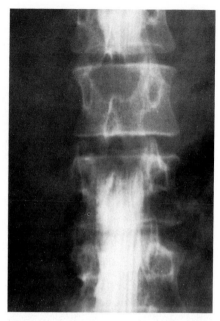

A,B

FIG. 3. Extradural masses. **A:** This patient with Wilms' tumor metastatic to the spine shows complete blockage of contrast. The thecal sac and cord are displaced away from the bony margins of the spinal canal to the left. **B:** This patient with lymphoma shows extradural compression of the spinal canal below the level of the conus. Note the contrast column is feathered in appearance inferiorly, and it shows some tapering superiorly.

COMPUTERIZED TOMOGRAPHY

A limitation of conventional radiography is its inability to distinguish and identify superimposed soft tissues. CT solves this by measuring the X-ray attenuation of an object from multiple projections and reconstructing the complex geometric relationships. The vertebral column, the paraspinal soft tissues, and the thecal sac are well demonstrated by CT. In addition to the cross-sectional imaging, computerized manipulation allows demonstration of the longitudinal extent of disease with sagittal or coronal reformatted images.

The demonstration of fat within a lesion may be diagnostic for a lipoma or teratoma. Vertebral body destruction and paraspinal masses are well shown. Small calcifications may be seen that are inapparent on conventional X-ray. Extradural compression on the thecal sac will be seen; however, intradural disease may be missed without addition of intrathecal contrast. In our workup of subarachnoid metastasis, we perform an abbreviated myelogram followed by CT myelography. CT myelography is especially valuable in detection of lesions at the craniovertebral junction. In the case of block, as shown on myelography, a small amount of water-soluble contrast often flows superior to the block, and this may be adequate

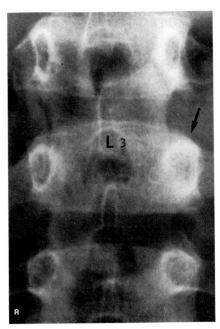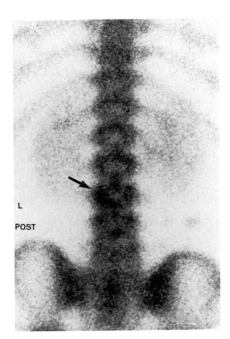

A,B

FIG. 4. This patient has an osteoid osteoma of the L3 vertebral body. **A:** X-ray shows subtle sclerosis (*arrow*) at the left pedicle of the L3 vertebral body. **B:** The radionuclide scan shows a definite area of increased activity at the left pedicle of the L3 vertebral body (*arrow*). POST, posterior.

for CT myelographic determination of the cephalad extent of the disease process. Previously, it was believed that contrast within a cord cavity on postmyelography CT was diagnostic of syringohydromyelia. However, contrast diffusing through the cord has subsequently been shown to enter tumor cavities (1,12).

NUCLEAR MEDICINE

Nuclear medicine has virtually no role in the evaluation of intradural disease. Bone scintigraphy is helpful in the evaluation of the child with back pain. Increased activity in a vertebral segment is nonspecific and does not distinguish between tumor, trauma, and infection. The positive nuclear scan will give a level of abnormality that may be examined with CT or MRI. The nuclear medicine examination may be positive when plain film findings are subtle or equivocal (Fig. 4).

ULTRASOUND

Ultrasound is a modality with no apparent biological hazard. Ultrasound may detect spina bifida or myelomeningocele *in utero*. In evaluating the pediatric

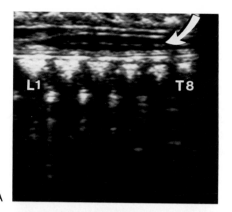

A

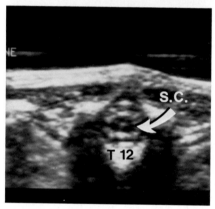

B

FIG. 5. Normal infant spinal ultrasound. **A:** Longitudinal image of the spinal cord (S.C.) shows the conus, filum terminale, vertebral bodies (T8, L1), and spinous processes. **B:** Axial image through the spinal cord shows cord with central echo complex, subarachnoid space, lamina, and vertebral body (T12).

spine, ultrasound is most valuable in the first year of life, prior to complete vertebral ossification. During this period, it is possible reliably to determine the level of the conus, the diameter of the cord, the filum terminale, and the presence of intradural mass, dysraphism, and syringohydromyelia. With absence of posterior elements from spinal dysraphism or laminectomy, the spinal contents may be noninvasively examined later in life. Intraoperative spinal ultrasound is a generally underutilized modality. The cystic and solid components of intrinsic cord tumor or syringomyelia can be well delineated at the time of surgery for precise determination of the site for biopsy and the extent of resection (13) (Fig. 5).

MAGNETIC RESONANCE IMAGING

Because the risk for ionizing radiation–induced malignancy increases with dose, MRI is preferable to CT in those patients who will require multiple follow-up examinations (14). MRI is noninvasive, and has no known significant biological risk at present magnet strengths (15). MRI is free of the bone-derived artifacts seen on CT. Images may be obtained in coronal and sagittal planes without loss of spatial resolution, as is the case with reformatted CT images. Soft tissue contrast and anatomic detail are displayed, which are unavailable with any other imaging modality (16,17).

Disadvantages of MRI are the long imaging times, which require sedation in small children. Motion artifacts are a major problem, resulting in image degradation. Since calcium produces no signal, even moderate-sized tumor calcifications (as seen on CT), may be invisible to MRI. Metallic devices may cause artifacts, resulting in uninterpretable images. Some, but not all, monitoring devices will cause image artifacts (18). There is danger with ferromagnetic neurovascular clips, a metallic foreign body in the eye, and cardiac pacemakers (19,20). Finally, claustrophobic patients may not tolerate enclosure within the magnet.

The physics of MRI is complex, and the reader is referred to textbooks on the subject. In clinical usage, spin-echo (SE) sequences are most commonly performed. Suffice it to say, an SE sequence with a short TR and short TE (e.g., SE

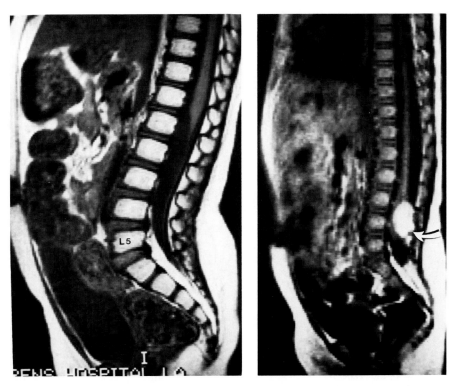

A,B

FIG. 6. A: Sagittal T1 weighted MRI of normal lumbar and sacral spine. Note clear definition of the cord, CSF, caudal sac, epidural fat, vertebral bodies, and discs. **B:** This T1 weighted image shows a low-positioned cord and lipoma (*arrow*). Note the lipoma's signal intensity matches that of subcutaneous fat.

500/30) will give a T1 weighted image. This sequence will give fat a bright signal, CSF a dark signal, and the cord an intermediate signal. The T1 weighted images have superior spatial resolution and best demonstrate anatomic detail. An SE sequence with a long TR and long TE (e.g., SE 2000/80) will give a T2 weighted image. On this sequence, CSF and many tumors become bright. Intradural pathology on T2 weighted images may be obscured by the bright signal of CSF. Rapidly flowing blood, cortical bone, calcium, and some collagen-rich or fibrous tissues will appear as a dark signal in T1 and T2 weighted SE sequences (21,22). Vascular malformations may be suspected by the appearance of a serpiginous signal void (23) (Fig. 6A,B).

Artifacts must be understood in order to avoid misdiagnosis. Some artifacts are unique to MRI. Like other imaging modalities, motion artifacts degrade image quality. Truncation artifacts are related to data sampling rates and abrupt signal intensity transition. These result in signal "overshoot" and "undershoot" around the interface. This may result in a thin band of low signal projected into the spinal cord simulating the appearance of a syringohydromyelia. A zero line artifact causes a linear artifact with a dashed pattern. This rarely interferes with image interpretation. Chemical shift artifact occurs as a high or low intensity band at the edge of a structure high in fat content. Metallic artifacts result in an area of low

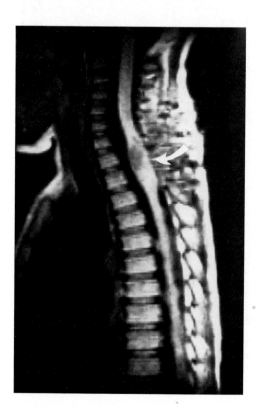

FIG. 7. Patient with cord astrocytoma. T1 weighted MRI demonstrates an expanded cord with areas of low signal intensity within the cord mass.

signal intensity surrounded by high intensity, or there may be a spectrum of appearances including spatial distortion, low signal intensity alone, or rings of high intensity (24).

DTPA is a paramagnetic agent that will shorten T1 relaxation times and, thereby, result in increased signal on T1 weighted images. Gd-DTPA is excreted by the kidneys and has no apparent serious side effects. Enhancement depends on an intact vascular supply and breakdown of the blood barrier. Contrast enhancement may be seen in tumor, necrotic tissue, infarction, infection, chronic arachnoiditis, and vascular lesions. There is no correlation between intensity of contrast enhancement and degree of malignancy. Even though contrast enhancement does not always correlate with tumor margins on pathologic examination, in practice, it is very helpful in localizing and defining the extent of a tumor, which otherwise would be impossible preoperatively (25–27).

In our experience, sagittal images are the most important plane for screening the spine. Any suspected abnormality is examined in at least one other plane, usually axially. If 1-cm-thick sagittal slices are obtained, small lesions may be missed

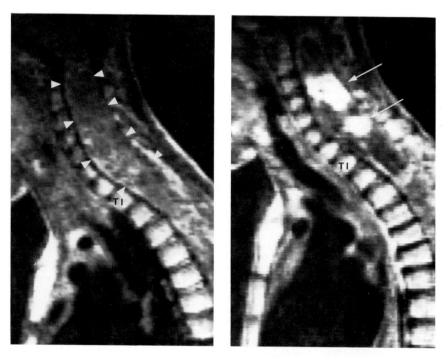

A,B

FIG. 8. Patient with cord astrocytoma. **A:** T1 weighted MRI shows an enlarged spinal canal (*arrowheads*) and spinal cord. Cord signal is heterogeneous. **B:** In the same patient, following Gd-DTPA, two areas of intense enhancement (*arrows*) are seen. At time of surgery, cystic and solid cord tumor was found from C1 to T1. In addition, cystic changes of the cord were noted inferiorly.

secondary to partial voluming effects. We do not recommend using greater than 5-mm-thick sagittal slices when examining for intradural tumor. If small intradural lesions are to be excluded, and time permits, we obtain 3-mm-thick sagittal T1 images with a small interslice gap. Images are obtained prior to and after the administration of Gd-DTPA. Following sagittal images, we obtain 5-mm-thick T1 weighted axial images and whatever further images that are thought likely to be beneficial. Images are examined prior to the patient's leaving the scanner. It is doubtful whether T2 weighted images will offer additional information in the case of intramedullary or intradural extramedullary tumor (28). It is possible to obscure a vertebral lesion if only post-Gd-DTPA images are obtained. This is because vertebral lesions are usually of relatively low intensity on T1 weighted images. By giving Gd-DTPA, the lesion may enhance to the point that it becomes isointense to the signal from fat in the vertebral marrow.

Cord enlargement and mass are usually well seen on sagittal T1 weighted images. Proteinaceous cord cysts associated with tumor, or intratumoral cysts may be indistinguishable from solid tumor owing to the high signal of proteinaceous fluid (29). In the series of Poser (30), 31% of intramedullary tumors were found to be associated with what he called syringomyelia. This term may be better used

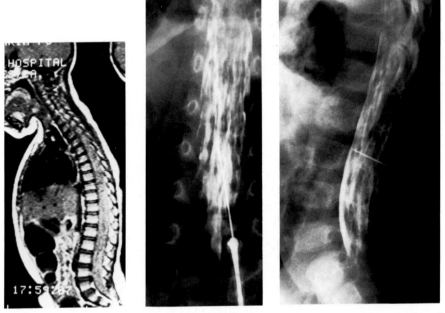

A-C

FIG. 9. Metastatic retinoblastoma. **A:** T1 weighted MRI shows obscuration of the normal cord and CSF signal. There was no change pre- and post-Gd-DTPA administration. **B,C:** Same patient (AP and LAT myelogram) shows multiple subarachnoid tumor deposits along nerve roots with filling of the caudal sac.

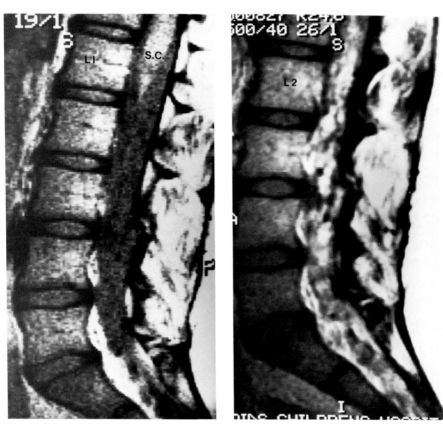

FIG. 10. Brainstem glioma with drop metastases. **A:** T1 weighted MRI shows subtle hetero-geneity of CSF signal. **B:** T1 weighted post-Gd-DTPA shows intense contrast enhancement of subarachnoid metastatic lesions throughout the lower spinal canal. S.C., spinal cord.

referring to cord cavitation by etiologies other than neoplasm. A cord cyst was found to be adjacent to, but not part of, the tumor in approximately 74% of his cases. Presently, the Gd-DTPA images may show an otherwise nonidentifiable nidus or rim of contrast enhancement, clarifying whether neoplasm is present, directing the site of biopsy, and helping in the determination of the extent of resection (3,27) (Figs. 7 and 8A,B).

Subarachnoid metastases causing high protein concentrations in the CSF may result in poor definition or obscuration of the cord (Fig. 9A–C). There may be a faint suggestion of heterogeneity of CSF signal within the canal. Following Gd-DTPA contrast, these suspected subarachnoid lesions become more conspicuous, and additional lesions are often seen. This often increases confidence in interpretation (Fig. 10A,B).

MRI is considered the imaging modality of choice to exclude intramedullary and extradural pathology. MRI is useful for the screening of children with intradural extramedullary disease. Myelography, for the present, remains superior in the detection of small intradural extramedullary lesions (6,28).

REFERENCES

1. Tievsky A, Davis OD. Radiology of spinal canal neoplasm. *Neurosurgery* 1985;124:1039–1046.
2. Yaghmai I. Spine changes in neurofibromatosis. *Radiographics* 1986;6(2):261–285.
3. Azouz EM, Kozlowski K, Marton D, et al. Osteoid osteoma and osteoblastoma of the spine in children. *Pediatr Radiol* 1986;16:25–31.
4. Ozonoff MB. *Pediatric orthopedic radiology*. Philadelphia: W.B. Saunders, 1979;1–69.
5. Benson JE, Han JS. Examination of the spine. In: Taveras JM, Ferrucci JT, eds. *Radiology—diagnosis, imaging, intervention*, vol. 3. Philadelphia: J.B. Lippincott, 1988;1–18.
6. Walker HS, Dietrich RB, Flannigan BD, et al. Magnetic resonance imaging of the pediatric spine. *Radiographics* 1987;7(6):1129–1152.
7. Smoker WRK, Godersky JC, Knutzon RK, et al. The role of MR imaging in evaluating metastatic spinal disease. *AJNR* 1987;8:901–910.
8. Walsh MN, Fischer GG, Anderson D, Mastri A. Fatal intracranial extention of spinal hemorrhage after lumbar puncture. *Arch Neurol* 1984;41:987–989.
9. Segall HD, Ahmadi J, Zee CS, Stanley P. Pathology of the craniovertebral junction. In: Taveras JM, Ferrucci JT, eds. *Radiology—diagnosis, imaging, intervention*, vol. 3. Philadelphia: J.B. Lippincott, 1988;1–27.
10. Epstein F, Epstein N. Intramedullary tumors of the spinal cord. In: *Pediatric neurosurgery*. New York: Grune & Stratton, 1982;529–541.
11. Baker RA. Spinal cord tumors: intramedullary and intradural/extramedullary. In: Taveras JM, Ferrucci JT, eds. *Radiology—diagnosis, imaging, intervention*, vol. 3, Philadelphia: J.B. Lippincott, 1988;1–12.
12. DiChiro G, Doppman JL, Dwyer AJ, et al. Tumors and arteriovenous malformations of the spinal cord: assessment using MR. *Radiology* 1985;156:689–697.
13. Rubin JM, Dohrmann GJ. The spine and spinal cord during neurosurgical operations: real-time ultrasonography. *Radiology* 1985;155:197–200.
14. Ron E, Modan B, Boice JD, et al. Tumors of the brain and nervous system after radiotherapy in childhood. *N Engl J Med* 1988;319(16):1033–1039.
15. Shellock FG, Crues JV. Temperature, heart rate, and blood pressure changes associated with clinical MR imagery at 1.5T. *Radiology* 1987;163:259–262.
16. Han JS, Kaufman B, Yousef SJE, et al. NMR imaging of the spine. *Am J Radiol* 1983;141:1137–1145.
17. Norman D, Mills CM, Brant-Zawadski M, et al. Magnetic resonance imaging of the spinal cord and canal: potentials and limitations. *Am J Radiol* 1983;141:1147–1152.
18. McArdle CM, Nicholas DA, Richardson CJ, et al. Monitoring of the neonate undergoing MR imaging: technical considerations. *Radiology* 1986;159:223–226.
19. Erlebacher JA, Cahill PT, Pannizzo F, et al. Effect of magnetic resonance imaging on DDD pacemakers. *Am J Cardiol* 1986;57:437–440.
20. Becker RL, Norfray JF, Teitelbaum GP, et al. MR imaging with intracranial aneurysm. *AJNR* 1988;9:885–889.
21. Aisen AM, Martel W, Braunstein EM, et al. MRI and CT evaluation of primary bone and soft tissue tumors. *Am J Radiol* 1986;146:749–756.
22. Fullerton GD, Cameron IL, Ord VA. Orientation of tendons in the magnetic field and its effect on T2 relaxation times. *Radiology* 1985;155:433–435.
23. Scotti G, Scialfa G, Colombo N, Landoni L. Magnetic resonance diagnosis of intramedullary tumors of the spinal cord. *Neuroradiology* 1987;29:130–135.
24. Pusey E, Lufkin RB, Brown RKJ, et al. Magnetic resonance imaging artifacts: mechanism and clinical significance. *Radiographics* 1986;6(5):891–911.
25. Dillon WP, Norman D, Newton TH. Intradural spinal cord lesions: Gd-DTPA enhanced MRI imaging. *Radiology* 1989;170:229–237.
26. Claussen C, Laniado M, Weinmann HJ, Schorner W. Paramagnetic contrast media in magnetic

resonance. In: Taveras JM, Ferrucci JT, eds. *Radiology—diagnosis, imaging, intervention*, vol. 3, Philadelphia: J.B. Lippincott, 1988;1–16.

27. Sze G, Krol G, Zimmerman RD, Deck MDF. Intramedullary disease of the spine: diagnosis using gadolinium-DTPA-enhanced MR imaging. *AJNR* 1988;9:847–858.
28. Sze G, Abramson A, Krol G, et al. Gadolinium-DTPA in the evaluation of intradural extramedullary spinal disease. *AJNR* 1988;9:153–163.
29. Goy AMC, Pinto RS, Raghavendra BN, et al. Intramedullary spinal cord tumors: MR imaging, with emphasis on associated cysts. *Radiology* 1986;161:381–386.
30. Poser CM. The relationship between syringomyelia and neoplasm. In: *American lecture series, no. 262, American lectures in neurology*. Springfield, Ill.: Charles C Thomas, 1956;28–32.

4

Surgical Treatment of Intramedullary Spinal Cord Tumors of Childhood

Fred J. Epstein

Intramedullary spinal cord tumors are relatively uncommon neoplasms, accounting for only 4% of central nervous system tumors of childhood (1,2). Because of their rarity, individual neurosurgeons and neurologists have relatively little experience with surgical management and long-term follow-up of afflicted patients. There has been little impetus to modify the traditional treatment of spinal cord neoplasms with radiation therapy, with or without biopsy, despite the recognition that, after a relatively short remission, serious disability or death ensues.

This is particularly tragic, since most intramedullary spinal cord tumors are low grade gliomas, ependymomas, lipomas, and, rarely, dermoids, all of which are amenable to surgical excision with long-term clinical remission and, hopefully, permanent cure. It was this perspective that encouraged the author to explore the technical feasibility of radical excision of spinal cord tumors. In this endeavor, 120 children have undergone gross total excision of spinal cord tumors over the past 9 years. This unusual series has provided a unique opportunity to study the biology of these tumors as well as their response to traditional, as well as recently introduced more radical, surgical techniques.

CLINICAL PRESENTATION

In most cases, signs and symptoms of spinal cord tumors are very slowly progressive, and parents become aware of a problem long before there are objective signs of neurologic dysfunction. In many cases, symptoms were present for months or years prior to definitive diagnosis.

The most common early symptom of an intramedullary tumor was local pain along the spinal axis. Other symptoms included motor disturbance, radicular pain, paresthesias, dysesthesias, and, rarely, sphincter dysfunction.

Seventy percent of patients experienced severe pain along the spinal axis, which was secondary to distension of the dural tube and was most acute in the bony segments, which were directly over the tumor. Characteristically, the pain was worse in the recumbent position as venous congestion further distended the dural tube and resulted in typical night pain. It was common to discover that the patients had been receiving analgesics, including narcotics, after a nondiagnostic orthopedic evaluation.

Weakness of the lower extremities was usually first manifest as an alteration of a previously normal gait. This was often extremely subtle, only obvious to parents who noted in their child a tendency to fall more frequently or walk on the heels or toes. In young children, there was commonly a history of being a "late walker," and, in the youngest (under 2 years), there was often a history of motor regression, that is, starting to crawl again instead of walking, or refusing to stand.

Painful dysesthesias occurred in 10% of the cases and were generally described as painful hot or cold sensations in one or more extremities. In rare circumstances, this was the primary symptom and not associated with objective signs of neurologic dysfunction.

Paresthesias were occasionally associated with the dysesthetic pain, and both of these symptoms were more common with neoplasms in the cervical than in the thoracic spinal cord.

Cervical Tumors

The most common early symptoms were nuchal pain and head tilt with torticollis. Mild upper extremity monoparesis was the next most common symptom and was often extremely subtle during the early stages of the illness. Very often in young children, the first manifestation of weakness was switching "handedness" in right- or left-handed patients. Neoplasms in the caudal cervical spinal cord commonly caused weakness and atrophy of the intrinsic muscles of the hand in contradistinction to tumors rostral to C5, which were less likely to cause significant weakness until relatively late in the clinical course. Interestingly, weakness of the lower extremities only evolved months or, rarely, 2 to 3 years after the first symptoms, and bowel and bladder dysfunction was rarely present at the time of primary diagnosis.

Secondary abnormalities were generally limited to one upper extremity, and a discrete sensory level was noted only very late in the course of the disease and, then, only in association with severe neurologic disability.

In most patients, there was increased reflex activity in the lower extremities with or without extensor plantar signs and clonus.

Thoracic Tumors

Mild scoliosis was the most common early sign of an intramedullary thoracic cord neoplasm. Pain and paraspinal muscle spasm commonly occurred before there were objective signs of neurologic dysfunction and were commonly assumed to be secondary to the evolving scoliosis. Insidious progressive motor weakness in the lower extremities was first manifest by "awkwardness" and, only later, by frequent falls and an obvious limp. Early sensory abnormalities were uncommon, although dysesthesias and paresthesias were occasionally present. Increased reflexes and extensor plantar signs, with or without clonus, occurred relatively early in the neurologic course.

A presenting complaint of bowel and bladder dysfunction was rare, and was diagnostic of solid neoplasm extending into the conus. In general, these symptoms evolved only late in the clinical course if the tumor was rostral to the conus medullaris.

NEURODIAGNOSTIC STUDIES

Astrocytomas

Spinal cord astrocytomas may be divided into two general categories: holocord and focal.

Holocord Astrocytomas

"Holocord" widening occurred in 60% of pediatric patients and was manifest by expansion of the entire spinal cord from the medulla or cervicomedullary junction to the conus.

These neoplasms were invariably cystic astrocytomas in which the solid component of the neoplasm spanned a variable length of the cord and was associated with huge non-neoplastic rostral and caudal cysts, which expanded the central canal above and below the tumor.

Plain spine X-rays commonly disclosed a diffusely widened spinal canal with relatively localized erosion or flattening of pedicles. Whereas the latter was secondary to long-standing expansion of the entire spinal cord, the former occurred only adjacent to the solid component of the neoplasm.

Although there were occasional early case reports of holocord widening, its relative frequency was probably not recognized because of the tendency to terminate the neurodiagnostic study when a lumbar myelogram disclosed a complete block secondary to an intramedullary neoplasm (2,3). In the first patients in this series, a cervical puncture was employed to identify the rostral extent of the cord widening. It was subsequently recognized that, although not apparent on the myelogram, a small amount of metrizamide almost invariably "trickles" past the block and is obvious on the immediate or delayed spinal computerized axial tomography (CAT) scan, which, therefore, defines the rostral extent of the expanded cord (4–8). It is for this reason that the availability of CAT of the spine is an invaluable adjunct to the neurodiagnostic evaluation of spinal cord tumors.

Holocord expansion caused by a spinal cord tumor may be confused with hydromyelia, and it is important that this differential diagnosis be firmly established prior to surgery. There are four major observations that will contribute to making the diagnosis.

1. Plain spine X-rays often disclose erosion of pedicles adjacent to a tumor,

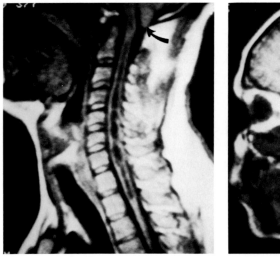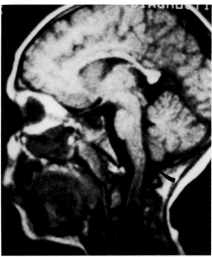

A,B

FIG. 1. A: MRI scan discloses cystic expansion of the cervical cord in the presence of a normal cervicomedullary junction in a patient with an intramedullary astrocytoma. **B:** MRI scan discloses cystic cervical cord in the presence of an Arnold-Chiari I malformation in a patient with hydromyelia.

while this is rarely present in hydromyelia. Both of these entities may be associated with a diffusely widened spinal canal.

2. Hydromyelia is almost invariably associated with an Arnold-Chiari I malformation, and thus it is essential that, in the presence of any diagnostic uncertainty, the contrast study include the cervicomedullary junction (Fig. 1A,B).

3. While 95% of spinal cord astrocytomas are associated with a complete subarachnoid block, there is, very rarely, an obstruction to the flow of metrizamide in the presence of hydromyelia. Even in the rare absence of a complete myelographic block, a spinal cord astrocytoma is associated with some distinct focal widening, whereas hydromyelia usually causes diffuse widening of the spinal cord without one area being significantly more widened than another.

4. In the presence of hydromyelia, the delayed metrizamide spinal CAT scan discloses homogeneous enhancement of the entire hydromyelic cavity, while cystic tumors have relatively localized collections of intracyst contrast.

Focal Astrocytoma

Focal spinal cord astrocytomas were generally four to eight segments in length and are commonly associated with flattening of pedicles immediately adjacent to the neoplasm. In some cases, plain film changes were as precise as the myelogram for tumor localization (though obviously never a substitute).

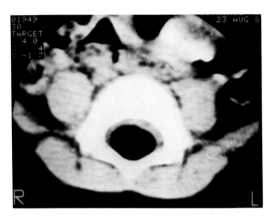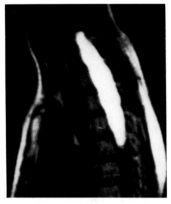

A,B

FIG. 2. A: CAT scan discloses hypodense mass, which is pathognomonic of lipoma. **B:** MRI scan discloses bright signal, which is diagnostic of lipoma (the signal is identical on T1 and T2 image).

Focal astrocytomas were associated with a total subarachnoid block in 90% of the cases, and, for this reason, an immediate and delayed CAT scan was necessary to define the rostral extent of cord expansion. Intratumor cysts were rarely present in the previously unoperated and nonradiated patient.

Lipoma

Spinal cord lipomas accounted for 2% of intramedullary tumors in the authors' series of patients. While the clinical manifestations were identical to the other intra-axial tumors, the radiologic studies were very specific. The spinal CAT scan with or without subarachnoid contrast disclosed fat within the spinal cord. The MRI scan was even more specific, disclosing a bright signal on both the T1 and T2 images, which was diagnostic of an intramedullary spinal cord lipoma (Fig. 2A,B).

Ependymoma

Spinal cord ependymomas were often identical to spinal cord astrocytomas, as demonstrated on neurodiagnostic studies. However, in the presence of a very focal expansion of the spinal cord (one to two segments), the tumor was more likely to be an ependymoma than an astrocytoma. In patients with very diffuse spinal cord widening with or without associated cysts, astrocytoma was present in 90% of the cases and ependymoma in 10%. It is important to recognize that, in children under 15 years of age, an intramedullary spinal cord tumor has an 80% likelihood of being an astrocytoma and only a 20% likelihood of being an ependymoma, which is in contradistinction to patients over 20 years of age, in whom there is approximately a 50/50 distribution of these tumors.

Congenital Tumors

Occasional congenital tumors include dermoids, epidermoids, as well as hamartomas. These generally appear as relatively localized tumors with focal expansion of the spinal cord. Although it seems likely that the MRI scan will contribute to a specific pathologic diagnosis, our experience to date is not of sufficient volume to describe diagnostic radiologic characteristics.

MRI Scan

It has become evident that MRI scanning will relegate most invasive neurodiagnostic studies to history. The MRI scan provides an excellent image of intramedullary neoplasms, and it is often unnecessary to carry out additional studies if the scan is satisfactory.

Radiologic Indicators of Tumor Location in the Presence of Holocord Expansion

While the entire spinal canal may be widened in the presence of a holocord astrocytoma, erosion of pedicles occurs only immediately adjacent to the midportion of the neoplasm (most commonly associated with total subarachnoid block). Finally, the delayed metrizamide spinal CAT scan may disclose the rostral and caudal tumor-cyst junction as the contrast diffuses into the latter.

Clinical Indicators of Tumor Location in the Presence of Holocord Expansion

In the presence of holocord widening associated with a cystic astrocytoma, it is the solid component of the neoplasm that is responsible for primary neurologic dysfunction, while the rostral and caudal cysts, which expand the remainder of the spinal cord, remain asymptomatic in the early stages of the disease. Therefore, neurologic symptoms in one or both upper extremities in the presence of holocord widening suggest that the solid component of the neoplasm is within the cervical cord.

Conversely, progressive scoliosis and/or neurologic dysfunction limited to the lower extremities are strongly suggestive of solid neoplasm within the thoracic cord, while bowel and bladder dysfunction indicates extension of neoplasm into the conus. In the presence of normal bowel and bladder function, an expanded conus, in our experience, is invariably associated with a cyst.

Spinal cord ependymomas do not adhere to this clinical pattern, as they may expand any length of the spinal cord with a relative paucity of signs and symptoms referable to the segmental involvement. It is tempting to speculate that this is directly related to the primary anatomic location of the tumor in the region of the central canal, which causes very gradual compression of adjacent neural structures as the tumor increases in volume. This may be analogous to the rostral and caudal cystic component of the spinal cord astrocytomas, which are also in the region of the central canal and asymptomatic at the time of primary diagnosis. The origin of the solid component of the astrocytomas is probably relatively asymmetric and may cause symptoms as a result of both compression and infiltration of adjacent neural tissues.

Surgical Technique

Spinal cord astrocytomas are firm, often contain microscopic foci of calcium, and only rarely have a cleavage plane to facilitate an "en bloc" resection. In the overwhelming majority of cases, it is necessary to remove the tumor from inside-out until the almost invariably present "glia–tumor interface" is recognized as a change in color and consistency between the tumor and adjacent normal neural tissue.

In the past, neurosurgeons were extremely limited in terms of available techniques for the removal of spinal cord tumors. The major surgical hazard was the infliction of severe neurologic dysfunction as a result of injury to the normal neural tissue, which was in close proximity to the neoplasm.

The development and application of ultrasonic and laser instrument systems were a significant improvement over the conventional systems and made a major contribution to spinal cord surgery (11,12).

The ultrasonic dissecting system is capable of discrete removal of a broad range of tissue. It is the ideal instrument to "debulk" rapidly and remove all but residual fragments of a spinal cord neoplasm. The neurologic laser is equally ideal to remove the residual fragments, because it can be employed with great precision along the length of the glia–tumor interface.

In patients who have not previously undergone surgery, an osteoplastic laminectomy is carried out. This permits replacement of the bone, which is a nidus for subsequent osteogenesis and posterior fusion. Replacement of the bone does not prevent the postsurgical evolution of spinal deformity but offers protection against further local trauma.

Even following careful consideration of the clinical and neuroradiologic examination, it is not possible to be certain that the laminectomy is of sufficient length to expose the entirety of the solid component of the neoplasm. For this reason, transdural ultrasonography is utilized to define further the location of the tumor vis-à-vis the bone removal.

Therefore, after laminectomy is carried out, the wound is filled with saline and the head of the instrument is placed into gentle contact with the dura. Utilizing this technique, the spinal cord is viewed in both sagittal and transverse section. The rostral and caudal limits of the tumor, as well as the presence or absence of associated cysts, are immediately obvious. Occasionally, an echogenic tumor provides a striking ultrasound image, though most commonly the solid component of the neoplasm is only manifest as a widened spinal cord. If the laminectomy is not sufficiently long to expose the entirety of the solid component of the neoplasm, it is lengthened, segment by segment, until the ultrasound discloses that the entire tumor mass is exposed. Only at this juncture is the dura opened, and this is limited to the portion overlying the expanded spinal cord—it is not necessary to open the dura widely over the rostral or caudal cyst, as these are easily drained as the solid component of the neoplasm is excised.

The carbon dioxide laser utilized at 6 to 8 watts is an ideal instrument for carrying out the myelotomy, as the cord is incised and hemostasis is obtained simultaneously. After the cyst is entered, inspection of the cavity will localize the rostral or caudal neoplasm which extends into it. It is not necessary, in most cases, to extend the myelotomy over the cyst, since it is easily drained as either pole of the neoplasm is identified and removed. Because the cyst fluid is produced by the tumor, it is unlikely to reaccumulate following gross total excision of the neoplasm.

After identifying the rostral and caudal cyst-tumor junction, the myelotomy is continued over the midline of the cord between the previously placed incision.

In the presence of cystic holocord neoplasm, tumor removal is initiated either at the rostral or caudal pole of the neoplasm in the region of the tumor-cyst junction.

The excision of the solid noncystic neoplasm is initiated in the midportion, rather than at the rostral or caudal poles of the tumor. In addition, the poles of the neoplasm are the least voluminous, and, for this reason, removal of the part of the neoplasm may be the most hazardous, as normal neural tissue may be easily disrupted.

The ultrasonic system is utilized to remove the bulk of the neoplasm, following which the carbon dioxide laser is employed to vaporize the visible remaining fragments (Figs. 3–5). The dura is closed primarily, as it is unnecessary to utilize a dural substitute for decompression if tumor excision has been grossly complete.

Ependymoma

Intramedullary

Intra-axial ependymomas are very similar to astrocytomas, as disclosed by the neuroradiologic examination. At surgery, however, the ependymoma is a fleshy, relatively vascular neoplasm that is often dark red in appearance and easily differentiated from adjacent neural tissues. In addition, there is a cleavage plane between the tumor and adjacent spinal cord with relative adherence of the tumor to the anterior median raphe. It is almost possible to obtain a gross total excision of

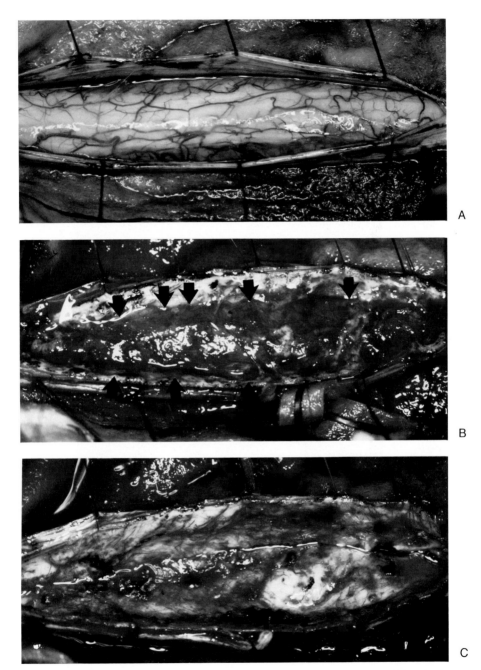

FIG. 3. A: External appearance of expanded cervical spinal cord. **B:** Following myelotomy, the intramedullary tumor is visualized (*arrows*). Note the difference in color between the tumor and the adjacent white matter. **C:** Tumor removed. Note that normal-appearing white matter lines the residual intramedullary cavity.

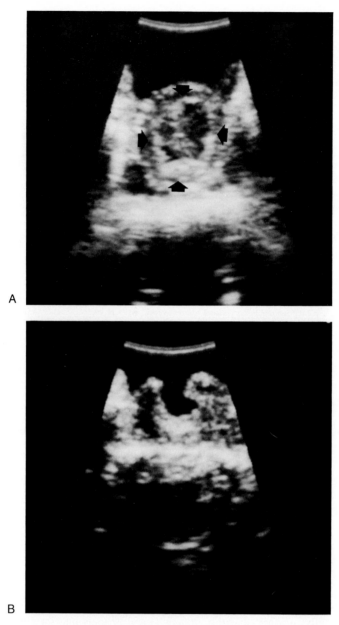

FIG. 4. A: Transdural ultrasonogram in cross section discloses expanded spinal cord. **B:** Following tumor removal, the residual cavity is obvious on ultrasonogram.

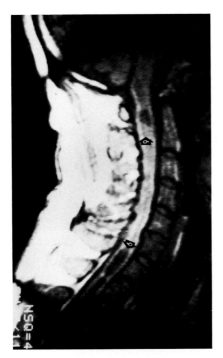 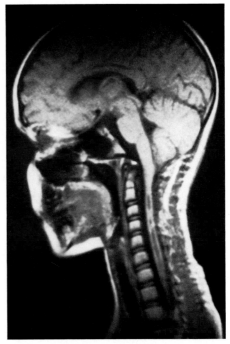

A,B

FIG. 5. A: Preoperative MRI scan discloses solid tumor and rostral and caudal cysts (*arrows*). **B:** Postoperative MRI scan discloses normal diameter of cord and residual intramedullary cavity.

the tumor; the surgical technique is not very different from that employed for astrocytomas, as it is necessary to debulk the neoplastic tissue with the ultrasonic dissecting system or the laser prior to developing the interface.

Following excision of an ependymoma, the residual tumor cavity is lined by normal-appearing white matter (Fig. 6A,B).

Conus, Filum Terminale, and Cauda Equina

While intramedullary neoplasms of childhood are more often astrocytomas than ependymomas, this is not the case when the tumor is within the conus or caudal to it. In the latter circumstances, the most likely diagnosis is ependymoma, which, very commonly, originated within the conus and extends into the filum terminale or cauda equina. It is quite common to discover an ependymoma that is confined to the conus without significant rostral or caudal extension.

The caudal extension of the ependymoma has one of two appearances. In the most common case, the tumor expands the filum terminale, which appears much like a sausage-shaped mass that displaces the normal nerve elements of the cauda

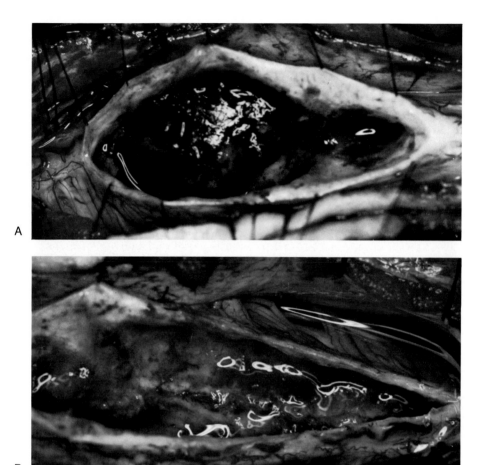

FIG. 6. A: Spinal cord ependymoma is a relatively discrete intramedullary mass (following myelotomy). **B:** After tumor removal, there is normal-appearing white matter around the margins of the residual cavity.

equina circumferentially around it. In these cases, it is relatively simple to remove the tumor "en bloc" by dividing the distal filum terminale caudal to the tumor, then displacing the entire mass out of the cauda equina and incising the remainder of the tumor just below the conus. In many cases, the entire mass is within the filum, and it is not necessary to pursue tumor fragments rostrally into the conus. However, in occasional situations, this may be mandatory in an effort to obtain a surgical cure, but it is essential that no neural tissue in the conus be manipulated in any way and that the tumor fragments be "extracted" from below (Fig. 7A–C).

A few ependymomas of the cauda equina seem to have grown from the region of the conus and to have erupted out of the filum, with tumor tissue filling the

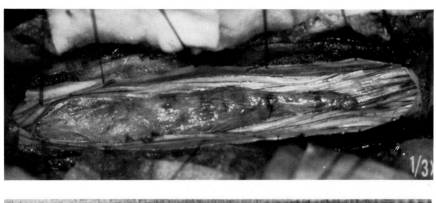

A

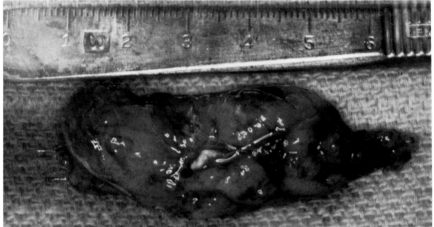

B

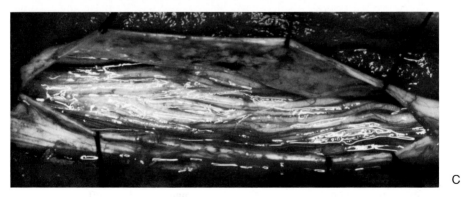

C

FIG. 7. A: Sausage-shaped mass expanding the filum terminale. **B:** After mass is removed, it is often obvious that it was part of the filum. **C:** Appearance of cauda equina, which has returned to normal anatomic position.

entire thecal sac below the conus. In these cases, the normal neural elements of the cauda equina are not displaced circumferentially around the mass but, rather, run through the tumor tissue. In these cases, it is necessary to remove the tumor bit by bit by working between and around the neural elements until all of the neoplastic tissue is removed. In these cases, it is also commonly necessary to extract remaining tumor fragments from the conus. It is again important that the neural tissue be undisturbed and that tumor fragments be removed by working through the area through which the tumor has grown into the thecal sac.

Lipoma

Intramedullary lipomas are obvious immediately beneath the pial surface of the spinal cord (Fig. 8). These tumors are not true neoplasms, and it is important to emphasize that the goal of surgery is to reduce the volume of the mass but not to make any effort to remove it completely. The lipoma is an ideal tumor to be removed with the laser, inasmuch as the high water content of the mass is easily vaporized as it is "stroked" with this instrument. It has been my general experience that removal of only approximately 50% of the volume of the mass is necessary to achieve a symptomatic remission and it is unnecessary to be more ambitious surgically. In most cases, a dural graft is utilized further to decompress the spinal cord.

Congenital Tumors

Epidermoid and dermoid tumors are quite rare compared to the other intramedullary neoplasms. In all these congenital tumors, the primary goal of surgery is to remove the centrum of the mass, but it is not wise to make any vigorous effort to remove the capsule of the tumor. This is because of its close adherence to

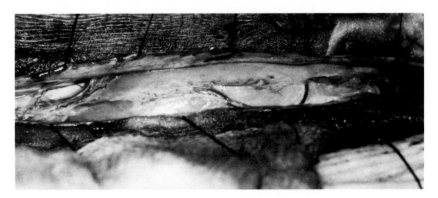

FIG. 8. External appearance of intramedullary lipoma of thoracic cord.

normal surrounding neural tissue structures and the likelihood of inflicting a neurologic injury as a result of a vigorous surgical endeavor to excise the capsule
completely. Interestingly, these tumors rarely recur if the contents have been completely removed.

Evoked Potential Monitoring

The conventional averaging systems such as the Tracor or Nicolet are only
capable of updating information every 1 to 2 min and require an evoked-potential
(EP) amplitude in the order of 0.25 mV. Since EP from a spinal cord compressed
by a tumor are often less than 0.10 mV in amplitude, these instruments are not
helpful surgical adjuncts for intramedullary spinal cord surgery.

This is quite a different situation from scoliosis surgery or spinal cord angiography, in which more conventional monitoring systems may provide valuable information, inasmuch as, after the straightening of the spine or injection of the contrast media, the surgeon may pause to be updated on the status of the spinal cord.
The hiatus in time is not important, as the event and its place in time are well
established. Since neither of these procedures is expected to affect electrical conductivity adversely, if electrical changes are observed, it may be advisable for the
orthopedist to release the instrumentation to correct the scoliosis or for the an-
giographer to delay further instillation of contrast material until there is electrical
recovery.

In our early experience, 24 patients were monitored via the traditional EP instrument system. In no situation was this either prospectively or retrospectively
helpful, and, in fact, we temporarily abandoned monitoring utilizing the conventional averaging technique.

In our last 91 consecutive patients, monitoring has been performed with the
Cordis Brain State Analyzer, which utilizes a new technique known as optimized
digital filtering for averaging the EP. This is a highly sensitive instrument that can
update information as fast as every 5 to 10 sec and can detect an EP as small
as the 0.10 μV. For this reason, there is a continuous stream of information in
realtime, and it is simple to relate this to the ongoing surgical procedure. Both
brainstem (far field) and somatosensory (near field) EPs are used for intraoperative
monitoring. Only the near field potentials are effective when the cord is very
compressed.

Several clinical correlations have been made utilizing the Cordis Brain State
Analyzer. Placement of pial traction sutures commonly results in transient decre-
ments in the amplitude of potentials that probably occur as a result of movement
of the posterior columns. Usually, the potential recovers within a few minutes. If
not, the suture is removed and placed in another location under less tension.

If the dissection is inadvertently extended beyond the poles of the tumor, as is
possible when there are no rostral or caudal cysts, there is a dramatic decrease in
amplitude and increase in latency of the evoked potential. This is most likely

secondary to manipulation of the posterior columns, which are in their normal anatomic position, and indicates a normal cord is being disrupted.

In some cases, there is deterioration of EPs as the dissection is directed toward tumor removal in specific locations. When this occurs, the manipulation is temporarily interrupted, and the electrical activity permitted to recover. It is very common to start and stop the procedure many times during the course of tumor removal.

Improved electrical conductivity following tumor removal is invariably associated with a benign postoperative course. Impaired activity, as compared with the preoperative baseline, is not rare and is not necessarily associated with neurologic morbidity. Nevertheless, the majority of patients with deteriorated activity have had transiently greater neurologic dysfunction although, in most circumstances, this has ultimately recovered. In one patient, all electrical activity was lost, and, postoperatively, there was complete absence of position sense in the lower extemities.

Postoperative Neurologic Morbidity Related to Segmental Location of Neoplasm

Postoperative neurologic morbidity may be correlated with segments of spinal cord that are involved with neoplasm. Whereas an extensive dissection may be carried out with little risk in those segments of spinal cord that are largely white matter, this does not seem to be the case in the lower segments, where gray matter is most abundant.

Dissections within the cervical spinal cord are associated with little morbidity, but it is not uncommon to note some anterior horn cell dysfunction as manifested by atrophy of one or more muscle groups of an upper extremity. When this has occurred, it has been permanent.

Dissections extending from the junction of the cervical and thoracic regions to T9 are associated with remarkably little neurologic morbidity.

Tumors that are located in the lower cord segments from T9 to S3 have a greater incidence of significant postoperative neurologic morbidity. This is because neoplasms in the conus or just above it compress or infiltrate gray matter, while tumors that occur in more rostral regions of the spinal cord compress white matter tracts; therefore, the resultant signs and symptoms are based on pathologic anatomy and pathophysiology, which are specific to the segmental location of the neoplasm.

Whereas an extensive intramedullary dissection may be carried out with relative impunity in white matter in the rostral cord, this is not the case in the gray matter in the region of the conus, and the surgeon must be aware of these technical limitations.

Significant preoperative sphincteric dysfunction suggests that the tumor is caudal to T12. Conversely, the absence of bowel and bladder problems suggest that

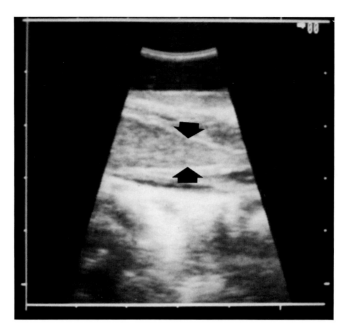

FIG. 9. Transdural ultrasonogram discloses location of conus medullaris (*arrows*).

the tumor does not extend into the conus, which may be asymptomatically expanded by a caudal cyst.

If there is no preoperative bowel and bladder dysfunction, it will occur postoperatively if the conus is disrupted. It is, therefore, essential that the myelotomy not be extended over the conus, as this will invariably result in sphincter dysfunction that may be permanent.

Intraoperative ultrasound is invaluable (10), since it clearly discloses the location of the conus, which may not be obvious to the surgeon as a result of distortion and rotation, as well as superimposed neural elements (Fig. 9).

It is important that the patient be advised that at least a temporary increase in neurologic dysfunction is to be expected with surgery in this area, and that long-term or permanent morbidity will also be significant.

Hydrocephalus

Twelve patients developed hydrocephalus, and it was occasionally fulminating in its presentation (13). In each of these cases, the tumor extended into the cervical cord, and we noted that there was obvious thickening of the leptomeninges overlying the cervicomedullary junction. It seems likely that this caused obstruction of the outlets of the fourth ventricle.

DISCUSSION

Astrocytoma

There are a number of important features that are clearly relevant in terms of understanding the biology of this group of neoplasms, as well as recommending proper surgical management. It has been a consistent observation that, in the presence of holocord expansion, the solid component of the astrocytoma is often not as extensive as myelography suggests; indeed, the actual location of the neoplasm may be in those segments of the spinal cord that correspond to the neurologic dysfunction. This dysfunction corresponds to spinal segments distended by the cyst within the center of the cord, as compared with the solid component of the neoplasm, which is relatively diffuse.

The presence of cysts that are similar in appearance to those associated with the cystic astrocytomas of the cerebellum suggests that the neoplasms are congenital tumors that have their inception sometime during gestation. The fluid produced by the tumor extends up and down the spinal cord in the region of least resistance, that is, the central canal.

One might also speculate that, in some cases, the classical symptoms of syringomyelia may in fact be a late manifestation of such a cyst, in which the tumor either has involuted or is not anatomically obvious. Perhaps the centrally located cyst may gradually expand over many years and compress the surrounding cord. In this regard, it is significant that a few patients with holocord widening had exceedingly small neoplasms, between 1.5 and 3 cm, and were mistakenly diagnosed as syringomyelia or hydromyelia. Our experience suggests that the presence of xanthochromic cyst fluid is pathognomonic of an associated neoplasm, while clear fluid is diagnostic of hydromyelia.

It is our opinion that the presence of a widened spinal cord from the cervicomedullary junction to the conus, which is associated with a relatively slowly evolving neurologic deficit, is indicative of a very slowly growing and perhaps even hamartomatous type of lesion, which has a good long-term prognosis and should be treated aggressively.

Nevertheless, it must be emphasized that despite a "gross" total tumor excision, it would be naive to assume that residual tumor fragments were not commonly left *in situ*. We have hypothesized that these remaining fragments may remain dormant, or involute, in a way similar to what has been noted to occur in many astrocytomas of the cerebellum (14,15). However, whether this is reality or wish-fulfillment will only be known many years from now, following long-term follow-up and retrospective analysis.

In most cases of holocord tumor, the initial complaint was a weak arm, or a mildly weak leg, and associated pain somewhere along the spinal axis. The signs and symptoms were consistently relatively minor when compared with the apparently diffuse nature of the pathologic process. It is perfectly understandable why neurosurgeons faced with this clinical dilemma have been most concerned about inflicting a greater neurologic deficit as a result of extensive dissection within a rather well-functioning spinal cord. This rationale has been used for a temporizing surgical approach consisting of a limited laminectomy and biopsy and relying on radiation therapy to control tumor growth. Unfortunately, the natural history of these tumors, with radiation therapy, is slow deterioration and eventual severe neurologic disability and death.

The outcome following radical resection of these tumors was directly related to the preoperative neurologic status. Although a transient increase in weakness or sensory loss was commonly present in the immediate postoperative period, only one patient had a significant permanent increase in neurologic deficit following operation. Patients with paraparesis or quadriparesis, who were ambulatory before surgery, had neurologic improvement over several weeks. The group with severe deficits preoperatively rarely made any significant improvement, although their downhill course abated.

There is no evidence that radiation will cure benign astrocytomas of the spinal cord, and there is abundant evidence that it has a deleterious effect on the immature developing nervous system. Spinal cord astrocytomas should be recognized as potentially excisable lesions, with radiation therapy reserved for possible adjunctive use if there is a recurrence. At that time, it might be employed following a second radical surgical resection.[1]

Other Tumors

Ependymomas and congenital tumors have long been recognized as being potentially surgically curable. There is no justification for carrying out a biopsy or a limited excision of the tumor. This is because most of these neoplasms are benign and, with proper surgical attention, may not recur. It is essential, however, that the operation be carried out by an experienced neurosurgeon, as spinal cord surgery is very exacting in terms of margin of error and the surgical result will be directly related to the experience of the operator.

Malignant Tumors

Seven percent of spinal cord gliomas were Grade IV astrocytomas. In each of these cases, the tumor recurred locally and disseminated over the entire neuraxis within 6 to 12 months of surgery, and there has been no patient who survived more than 18 months after surgery. For this reason, all patients with malignant neoplasms now receive neuraxis radiation and chemotherapy after the primary surgery.

---

[1]See following chapter for an alternative opinion.

SUMMARY

The author has carried out gross total excisions of intramedullary spinal cord tumors in 180 consecutive patients. This experience has led to the following conclusions:

1. Holocord widening occurs in 60% of cases, and is diagnostic of a cystic tumor—most commonly an astrocytoma and, occasionally, an ependymoma.
2. Despite the absence of a surgical plane of dissection, astrocytomas may be removed from inside-out until a glia–tumor interface is recognized. Ependymomas almost invariably have a clear cleavage plane and may be totally removed.
3. Radical tumor excision is compatible with partial or total recovery of neurologic function.
4. The success of surgery is directly related to the preoperative neurologic status of the patient. Those with minimal or moderate neurologic dysfunction commonly recovered, but paralysis or near paralysis was never improved.

While this experience has established the efficacy of radical surgery, there is no information regarding the duration of remission or the likelihood of permanent cure. This will only become known at the time of retrospective analysis many years from now.

REFERENCES

1. Anderson FM, Carson MU. Spinal cord tumors in children. A review of the subject and representation of twenty-one cases. *J Pediatr* 1953;43:190–207.
2. Arseni C, Norvath L, Illiescu D. Intraspinal tumors in children. *Psychiatr Neurol Neurochir* 1967;70:123–133.
3. Coxe WS. Tumors of the spinal canal in children. *Am Surg* 1961;27:62–73.
4. Epstein F. The cavitron ultrasonic aspirator in tumor surgery. *Clin Neurosurg* 1984;31:497–505.
5. Epstein F, Epstein N. In: McLaurin R, et al., eds. *Pediatric neurosurgery: surgery of the developing nervous system.* New York: Grune & Stratton, 1982;529–539.
6. Epstein F, Epstein N. Surgical management of extensive intramedullary spinal cord astrocytomas in children. *Concepts Pediatr Neurosurg* 1981;2:29–44.
7. Epstein F, Epstein N. Surgical management of "holo-cord" intramedullary spinal cord astrocytomas in children. Report of three cases. *J Neurosurg* 1981;54:829–832.
8. Epstein F, Epstein N. Surgical treatment of spinal cord astrocytomas of childhood: a series of 19 patients. *J Neurosurg* 1983;57:685–689.
9. Braun IF, Raghavendra BN, Kricheff II. Spinal cord imaging using real-time resolution ultrasound. *Radiology* 1983;147:459–465.
10. Raghavendra BN, Epstein FJ, McLeary L. Intramedullary spinal cord tumors in children: localization by intraoperative sonography. *Am J Neuroradiol* 1984;5:395–397.
11. Epstein F, Raghavendra BN, John ER, Pritchett L. Spinal cord astrocytomas of childhood: surgical adjuncts and pitfalls. *Concepts Pediatr Neurosurg* 1985;5:224–237.
12. Flamm ES, Ransohoff J, Wachinich D, Broadwin A. A preliminary experience with ultrasonic aspiration in neurosurgery. *Neurosurg* 1984;2:240–243.
13. Schijam E, Zuccaro G, Monges JA. Spinal tumors and hydrocephalus. *Child's Brain* 1981;8:401–403.
14. Bucy BC, Theiman PW. Astrocytomas of the cerebellum. A study of a series of patients operated on over 18 years ago. *Arch Neurol* 1968;18:14–19.
15. Geissinger JD, Bucy PC. Astrocytomas of the cerebellum in children. Long-term study. *Arch Neurol* 1971;24:125–135.

5

Nonsurgical Management of Spinal Tumors

Walter J. Curran, Jr., and Giulio J. D'Angio

Neoplasms involving the spinal canal and its contained neural structures are significantly less common in childhood than intracranial tumors, and their rarity often contributes to delay in diagnosis. For the purpose of this discussion, intraspinal neoplasms will be classified according to their relationship to the dura and the spinal cord. These categories of tumor location will be (a) intramedullary, (b) intradural extramedullary, and (c) extradural.

INTRAMEDULLARY TUMORS

Intramedullary tumors develop within the spinal cord itself, and afflicted patients frequently present a prolonged history of signs and symptoms, beginning with a segmental sensory loss and progressing to reflex abnormalities, motor dysfunction, and incontinence. Delay in diagnosis is frequent, and symptoms can be present for years prior to diagnosis. The most common intramedullary tumors among children and adults are ependymomas and astrocytomas. Ependymomas are derived from the ependymal cells that line the ventricular system and are particularly common in the region of the conus medullaris and filum terminale, possibly because of the large number of ependymal cells lining the terminal ventricle of the conus and the core of the filum terminale. Astrocytomas arising in the spinal cord are histologically similar to those arising in the brain and can be classified according to the same grading systems.

Ependymomas

Clinical Features

Primary ependymomas of the spinal cord, cauda equina, conus medullaris, and/ or filum terminale are uncommon and represent less than 2% of all primary neoplasms of the central nervous system. Ependymal neoplasms also originate in the fourth ventricle and in the lateral ventricles of the brain. The distribution of ependymomas above and below the foramen magnum varies from series to series according to the age distribution of patients. Among children, the cranial location predominates over spinal or caudal locations in a ratio of approximately 10:1, and, among adults, cranial and spinal ependymomas are often equal in frequency. In 12 published series of spinal/caudal equina ependymomas (1–12), 40 of 208 patients (19%) were less than 20 years old. This compares with 102 children in 144 cases of cranial ependymomas or 71% of those reported in several large institutional series (1,2,4,5,9,13–16).

Pathology

According to their degree of anaplasia, ependymal tumors can be classified into typical ependymomas, anaplastic ependymomas, and ependymoblastomas. Typical ependymomas include the papillary and cellular types as well as the myxopapillary form commonly seen in cauda equina tumors. Anaplastic ependymomas are primarily reported among cranial tumors, and no case of ependymoblastoma meeting the criteria defined by Mork and Rubinstein (17) has been described in the spine.

Diagnosis and Treatment

Following the clinical evaluation and radiographic demonstration of an intramedullary mass, a surgical procedure must establish the histologic diagnosis and extent of disease. An attempt to remove as much of the tumor as possible without contributing to further neurologic decline is generally undertaken. Of the 231 spinal/caudal ependymomas on which surgical information was available, 102 (44%) were judged by the surgeon to have been totally removed (1–15). While several neurosurgeons describe a greater ability to excise totally ependymomas located in the cauda equina than in the spinal cord, no difference in the rate of gross total removal is apparent among these reported patients.

The treatment results in spinal ependymomas are available in a number of retrospective reports in which patient accrual occurred over long time intervals. In the 15 reports evaluated (1–15), the average number of patients per study was 17 retrospectively collected over an average period of 24 years. Such studies span periods of significant technical advancement in the diagnostic, surgical, and radiotherapeutic approach to spinal neoplasms, making results of varied treatment approaches difficult to compare.

Follow-up information is available on 127 patients with spinal/cauda ependymoma, and 102 (80%) have no evidence of disease (NED) with a minimal follow-up of 4 years. Among those with cauda equina tumors, 40 of 42 (95%) have NED compared with 22 of 35 (63%) with spinal ependymomas. The majority who failed did so locally and did not disseminate throughout the craniospinal axis. Only two cases (less than 2%) are reported to have disseminated intracranially, and both occurred within the posterior fossa.

Radiation Therapy

Postoperative local field radiation therapy (RT) was given to 93 of 118 patients on whom treatment details are available, and an additional 18 patients received craniospinal axis irradiation. Attempts have been made to analyze patient outcome in terms of the radiation dose and the volume irradiated. Barone and Elvidge (1) reported 27 patients, 11 of whom received "adequate" postoperative irradiation, defined as three or more radiation treatments. While they found no difference in median survival overall between the irradiated and nonirradiated patients, a longer median survival was present in the irradiated group if their surgical resection was incomplete. Mork and Loken (2) described no difference in 10-year survival between 9 irradiated and 17 nonirradiated patients with spinal ependymoma, but they gave no surgical or radiotherapeutic details.

Garcia (3) noted that both the two patients who received less than 40 Gy in 1.7 to 2.0 Gy/day fractionation had local tumor regrowth, while only 2 of 13 who received 40 Gy or more failed locally. Garrett and Simpson (4) reported on 41 patients, 23 of whom received local spine irradiation, and 18 of whom were given craniospinal RT. Survival was superior in the locally irradiated group vs. the craniospinal group (91% vs. 72%). Only one patient failed outside the region of the primary tumor, and that patient had a thoracic anaplastic ependymoma, which recurred in the posterior fossa. No dose response was noted above and below 45.0 Gy in that study.

Shuman et al. (5) reported on seven children with cauda equina ependymomas, four of whom received local RT and remain NED and three of whom received no RT and failed locally. Kopelson et al. (6) also reported that two of three nonirradiated patients failed locally compared with two of nine given RT. In a group of 22 irradiated patients recently reported, Shaw et al. (7) stated that prognostic factor most closely associated with local failure was the length of spinal cord involvement. Four of eight patients with "extensive" lesions occupying six or more vertebral segments regrew locally, compared with 3 of 14 less extensive tumors. When patient outcome was evaluated for a RT dose response, a higher failure rate (6/17) occurred in those receiving less than 50 Gy compared with those with a dose over 50 Gy (1/5).

In summary, 80% of the reported spinal/caudal ependymomas have been controlled using a treatment approach typically involving partial or total resection followed by local spinal irradiation. We find no support for the use of craniospinal irradiation, since, in its absence, the cranial relapse rate among 127 patients was less than 2%. Assuming that the patient's radiologic workup includes a total spinal myelogram and a computerized tomography (CT) scan of the brain, the postoperative radiation field should include the involved spinal segments and two vertebral levels above and below the abnormality seen on myelogram and at the time of surgery. Since most failures seem to occur at the primary site, only patients with extensive or multifocal lesions would require irradiation of the majority of the spinal cord.

Glioma

Clinical Features

Primary gliomas of the spinal cord are more commonly seen than spinal ependymomas in children. Forty-one of the 110 patients (37%) from 10 collected series

(3,6,8,12,14,18–22) were children, compared with 19% for spinal ependymomas. While the clinical and radiographic picture may be indistinguishable between these entities, neurosurgeons describe gliomas as typically more infiltrating and less well defined than ependymal tumors. It is no surprise that only 23 of 143 glioma cases (16%) were reported as total excisions compared with 44% of ependymomas. Both tumors can produce widening of the spinal cord on myelography similar to the abnormality seen with syringomyelia. At least 30% of intramedullary gliomas have associated fluid-filled cavities, which can only be distinguished from a benign syrinx at the time of surgery.

Treatment Results

Follow-up information is available on 132 patients with spinal gliomas (3,6,8,12,14,18–23). Of the 112 patients with Grade I or II gliomas, 55 (49%) were alive for 4 years or more, but there was only one long-term survivor among 20 patients with Grade III or IV gliomas. No patient with a Grade IV spinal glioma has been reported to survive more than 2 years.

Radiation Therapy

Postoperative local radiation therapy was given to 103 of these 132 glioma patients (78%). While a wide range of doses of treatment and retreatment were described in the earlier papers, the studies published since 1960 describe doses ranging from 36 to 55 Gy. Among 87 irradiated patients with reported follow-up, 50 (57%) survived 4 or more years. This compares with a 4-year survival of 5 of 29 (17%) among glioma patients who receive no postoperative RT (3,8,12,19,23). While these studies do not contain important data regarding extent of surgical resection, tumor grade, and neurologic status on all patients, this difference in outcome between irradiated and nonirradiated patients (57% vs. 17%) lends support to the use of postoperative irradiation.[1]

There are at least five reported cases of spinal gliomas with subsequent dissemination intracranially (24–26). Three were reported prior to the introduction of computed tomography, making the pretreatment screening for an occult cranial glioma less reliable, and four were glioblastoma mutiforme. Because of the rarity of dissemination and because of the dismal outcome of high grade spinal gliomas with or without intracranial seeding, we find no support for extended field or craniospinal irradiation for localized spinal gliomas.

Secondary Irradiation Effects

The radiation dose recommended by most authors for spinal ependymomas and gliomas is 40 to 55 Gy. Garcia (3) found that none of the 5 glioma patients

---

[1]See previous chapter for a dissenting opinion.

receiving less than 40 Gy was controlled and that 8 of 10 receiving more than 40 Gy were free of disease. While the optimal dose is unknown, many radiation therapists attempt to deliver the highest dose tolerated by the spinal cord without an unacceptably high risk of radiation myelopathy. The generally accepted spinal cord tolerance level (the dose that produces less than a 5% incidence of radiation myelopathy by 5 years) is 50.0 Gy in 25 fractions over 5 weeks. Kopelson (27) reported no cases of radiation myelopathy among 24 patients irradiated post-operatively for spinal cord tumors, and this series included several patients in whom doses equaled or exceeded 50.0 Gy. Kopelson found no support in his series for the theory that spinal cord tolerance of radiation is reduced by prior spinal cord damage from tumor or surgery.

It is unknown whether children have a lower threshold for radiation myelopathy than adults, but it is well known that children are at risk for bone growth arrest and growth retardation subsequent to total or partial spinal irradiation. Probert et al. (28) reported that 10 of 22 children (45%) receiving total spinal irradiation for medulloblastoma, leukemia, or lymphoma had a sitting height (a measurement more reflective of impaired spinal growth length than standing height) more than 2 standard deviations below the mean for their age. This occurred at dose levels of 20 to 49 Gy and appeared to be most pronounced when radiation was delivered prior to age 6 or at puberty. It would be expected that the growth arrest would be less severe when partial spinal irradiation is given for a spinal tumor. The neuro-muscular and skeletal abnormalities seen in some of the long-term survivors can be attributed to the tumor itself, to surgery, to irradiation, or to their various and several combinations (see Neuroblastoma section, below). Other potential side effects of high dose spinal irradiation relate to the inadvertent delivery of radiation to vital structures anterior to the spinal cord. These include the thyroid gland, the upper aerodigestive tract, the lungs, and the heart. One method of reducing the radiation dose to these structures is to deliver treatment using a three-field tech-nique (one posterior and two posterior oblique fields) rather than a posterior-only field.

Chemotherapy

Systemic chemotherapy has been used for intramedullary tumors predominantly as salvage therapy for those who relapse after surgery and irradiation. Two cir-cumstances in which chemotherapy might be appropriately integrated into initial therapy are in the treatment of high grade spinal gliomas and of low grade spinal tumors in very young children. The Children's Cancer Study Group (CCSG) re-ported a survival advantage for children with high grade cranial gliomas ran-domized to receive CCNU, vincristine, and prednisone and irradiation vs. irradia-tion alone (29). It is unknown whether this would hold true in high grade spinal gliomas, but the dismal results with current therapy certainly justify such a study. Chemotherapy could also be used postoperatively in children under 4 years of age with low grade gliomas as a means of delaying radiation until further vertebral growth and neurologic maturation have occurred. This approach has currently been adopted by CCSG and the Pediatric Oncology Group for brain tumors in children under 3 and has typically allowed the interval between surgery and radiation to extend to 1 year.

INTRADURAL EXTRAMEDULLARY TUMORS

The most common tumors in the intradural extramedullary space in the adult population are meningiomas and neurofibromas. The former are extremely rare in childhood, and the latter, when present, are usually associated with von Recklinghausen's disease. More prominent in childhood are tumors that metastasize via the cerebrospinal fluid (CSF), and developmental tumors.

CSF metastases most commonly arise from medulloblastomas, posterior fossa ependymomas, or pineal tumors. The incidence of metastatic involvement of the spinal cord in medulloblastoma at presentation varies from 3 of 43 (7%) as reported by Kopelson et al. (30) to 7 of 16 (43%) as reported by Deutsch and Reigel (31). These metastases typically appear as discrete nodules on myelography with displacement of the spinal cord. Curative treatment of such medulloblastoma patients usually consists of resection of the posterior fossa tumor, craniospinal irradiation to 30 to 60 Gy, supplemental posterior fossa radiation to 50 to 55 Gy total, and a "boost" to the spinal nodules to a total of 45 to 50 Gy. With such an approach, the Intergroup Medulloblastoma Trial reports a 2-year relapse-free survival rate of 43% for patients with spinal metastases. This compares with a 2-year relapse-free survival rate of 72% in patients without metastases (32). Comparable differences in outcome have been reported between cranial ependymomas and pineal tumor patients with and without spinal metastases.

Developmental tumors in the extramedullary space are primarily found in the lumbosacral region in association with a soft tissue cutaneous abnormality or a developmental bony abnormality. They can be found in the intradural or extradural space, or both. These tumors include epidermoid tumors, dermoid tumors, and lipomas and are usually successfully managed with surgery alone.

EXTRADURAL TUMORS

The distribution of all intraspinal tumors by level affected was reviewed by DiLorenzo and colleagues (33). They found that more arise in the thoracic region, but, as they point out, this is the longest segment of the vertebral column. That is, each segment of the spinal column is roughly equally at risk. An exception is the sacral region, which has a disproportionately lower frequency of tumors, presumably for the reason that is obvious when one considers the content of the spinal canal at that level.

Extradural tumors were the most common among the 1,234 spinal tumors of

TABLE 1. *Distribution of 789 intraspinal childhood tumors by site of origin[a]*

Site	No.	(%)
Extradural	340	(43)
Intradural + C.E.[b]	193	(25)
Extra-intradural	8	(1)
Intramedullary	248	(31)
Total	789	

[a] Adapted from ref. 33.
[b] C.E., cauda equina.

childhood collected by them and accounted for 43% of the total (Table 1) (33).

Compression of the spinal cord can occur because of primary or secondary tumors (a) within the spinal canal or (b) the adjacent vertebral bodies; or (c) from tumor growth into the spinal canal from the adjacent soft tissues. Typical examples are non-Hodgkin's lymphoma (NHL), rhabdomyosarcoma, and neuroblastoma, respectively. Sarcomas, primary and secondary, are the most common offenders (33).

Pain is the usual presenting sign, found in perhaps three of four patients. Extremity weakness, sphincter impairment, and the other signs of cord and radicular compromise are frequent concomitants (34).

It should be emphasized that recovery of function is often possible in children despite severe paresis and even paralysis present for 24 hr or more (35). We have seen return of lower extremity function in a child paraplegic for several days. "Rules" applicable to adults concerning the irreversibility of neurologic damage present for more than a few hours should not be applied to children whose tissues are surprisingly resilient.

Intraspinal Tumors

Lymphoma

Diagnosis

Epidural compression of the cord by intraspinal growth of NHL, with or without bone disease, can sometimes be seen in patients with that diagnosis at some time during the course of the illness, especially in those with NHL of Burkitt's type. The presenting signs are usually those of a cord block; it is imperative that a myelogram be performed outlining the entire spinal canal both above and below the level of the block, because the lesions can be multiple.

Management

RT is preferable to surgery (36). The fields include the obviously involved vertebral segments with at least one vertebral body above and below the lesion as "margins." When this complication occurs relatively late in the course of the disease, the cells tend to be radiation unresponsive in the authors' experience, unlike those found earlier in the illness. Therefore, we agree with those who give doses higher than the 2,400 cGy used in meningeal leukemia. We prefer doses in the 3,000 cGy range, e.g., 300 cGy/day × 10, which seems appropriate for both these reasons. (Corticosteroid coverage is advisable in these patients and all those who receive RT without surgical decompression.)

Hodgkin's disease (HD) rarely causes cord compression, but it is approached in the same way.

Aggressive multiple agent chemotherapy is added to the treatment of all patients with NHL and HD who demonstrate this constellation of findings. Commonly used drug regimens include LSA_2L_2 combination for NHL, MOPP for HD, and their derivatives. The interested reader is referred to standard texts for details of these complex regimens (37–39).

Vertebral Body Lesions

Compression of the cord can occur because of lesions expanding from the vertebral body.

Malignant Conditions, Secondary

Secondary cord compression is more commonly seen in children with those cancers that tend to metastasize to bone, such as neuroblastoma (NBL), embryonal rhabdomyosarcoma (ERMS), clear cell sarcoma of the kidney (CCSK), and, rarely, renal cell carcinoma (RCC). Wilms tumor (WT) itself can, on occasion, infiltrate an adjoining vertebra and, from there, protrude into the spinal canal.

Management

RT for the radioresponsive tumors (NBL, ERMS, CCSK, WT) is preferable to laminectomy because of their poor prognosis. Should there be rapidly developing neurologic signs, three daily doses of 400 cGy for a total of 1,200 cGy can be given on each of three successive days, with steroid coverage (40). Thereafter, the daily dose is reduced to 200 cGy for 4 or 9 fractions for a total of 2,000 or 3,000 cGy, the higher dose being used for children with more massive disease. Laminectomy is preferable for the unresponsive lesions, such as the RCC.

Malignant Conditions, Primary

These are uncommon and include osteogenic sarcoma (OS), Ewing's tumor (ET), and, rarely, chondrosarcoma (CS).

Management

ET is treated with combination chemotherapy and RT. A regimen in common use includes vincristine, actinomycin D, cyclophosphamide, and Adriamycin (41). Irradiation is given in daily doses of 150 to 180 cGy to totals ranging from 4,500 cGy to 5,580 cGy, depending on whether the lesion is above or below the conus medullaris. However, even the 4,500-cGy dose is approaching the limit of cord tolerance, especially when the radiation enhancers and reactivators actinomycin D and Adriamycin are also given. Parents and comprehending patients should be advised accordingly before RT is initiated.

The other primary neoplasms (OS and CS) are not radioresponsive, and laminectomy is the mainstay of management when there are cord signs. Combination chemotherapy is not of proven value for CS; it is added for OS. A randomized trial reported by Link et al. (42) found the 2-year relapse-free survival for patients with nonmetastatic extremity OS was 66% vs. 17% for those treated with surgery only. It seems reasonable to extrapolate these results to this desperate clinical situation.

Benign Conditions

Aneurysmal bone cysts and hemangiomas of the vertebral bodies can grow to protrude into the spinal canal. RT (200 cGy/day × 10) is the treatment of choice with a high likelihood of success. Steroids in higher doses have been used to shrink large soft-tissue hemangiomas and could, perhaps, be tried. There is an insufficient clinical experience to indicate its efficacy under these circumstances, however. RT, long known to be effective, remains the recommendation, especially when time is a factor (43). Giant cell tumors also are radioresponsive, but higher doses (e.g., 4,000 cGy) are used. Neurofibromas, whether as part of von Recklinghausen's disease or not, can extend through intervertebral foramina, like the neuroblastomas. These lesions are not amenable to RT and require surgery, as does the rare meningioma, which constitutes less than 5% of the childhood intraspinal neoplasms. Meningiomas may be either extradural or intradural in location, as are many dermoids, teratomas, or lipomas. When the latter neoplasm is extradural, the thoracic level seems more commonly affected (33). Surgical removal suffices for all these tumor types.

Langerhans' cell histiocytosis (previously histiocytosis X), a self-limiting process, often affects the vertebral bodies but seldom causes cord compression. Then RT doses of 600 cGy (200 cGy/day × 3) suffice to control the lesion (44). Chemotherapy is not used unless there is systemic disease.

Paravertebral Tumors

Neuroblastoma

This is the most frequent single entity listed by DiLorenzo et al. (33) in their excellent review of childhood spinal tumors. The majority are extradural, although, rarely, intradural neuroblastoma can occur. Fifty of the sixty-two cases collected by DiLorenzo et al. were of the dumbbell type (v.i.).

Diagnosis

A characteristic presentation of a paravertebral NBL, especially in the thoracic region, is the so-called dumbbell tumor. This is found in about 10% of NBL patients. The lesion grows in the posterior paravertebral soft tissues and extends through one or more intervertebral foramina to impinge on the spinal cord. The X-ray films are virtually diagnostic of the condition when it develops in the thorax. There is widening of the intercostal space(s), at the level(s) of involvement with concomitant widening of the intervertebral foramina (45). The intraspinal component can sometimes assume a very large size without any neurologic signs or symptoms. Therefore, preliminary workup of all patients with tumors of this type, who tend to be under 5 years of age, should include evaluation of the spinal cord either by traditional myelography using Pantopaque or by CT with metrizamide outlining the subarachnoid space.

Management

The choice of treatment is colored by the long-term sequelae associated with these and other tumors affecting the spinal axis. These sequelae can be profound (34,35,38,46) and are correlated with the signs found at the time of diagnosis. Return of function is governed by the amount of neurologic, vascular, and osseous damage caused by the tumor itself, by the surgical procedure, or both. While return of function is surprisingly good, even in children with relatively prolonged cord signs (more than 48 hr), residual neurologic deficits are often seen in these patients, and appropriate continuing orthopedic, neurologic, and physiotherapeutic supervision is necessary.

The orthopedic problems are caused by the tumor itself, by its removal, and by postoperative radiation therapy. Some tumors are so large as to erode and destroy the articular apophyses, which can be further damaged during surgery; and, occasionally, apophyseal growth can be impaired by aggressive laminectomy. Tumor involvement and postoperative changes lead to lumbar lordoses and to thoracic kyphoscolioses that can be quite deforming, if not disabling. Certain surgical techniques are said to reduce the severity of postoperative curvatures. Hemilaminectomy is one such method. Another is advocated by Udvarhelyi and Winfield (34) when several adjoining segments need to be decompressed. The posterior bony structures are removed as a single unit, which is then returned to the original site at the end of the operation and wired in place.

By contrast, RT produces a more uniform growth suppression if the entire vertebral bodies are included in the field and are irradiated uniformly (47). Other late irradiation complications have been discussed above. Therefore, there continues to be considerable controversy regarding the best form of management, because of the late effects associated with both surgery and RT. Surgery, nonetheless, remains the most rapid and definitive means of handling the problem (35,46). RT alone has been advocated, especially when several levels are affected, and there are no associated neurologic signs and symptoms. The field includes at least one vertebral body above and below the myelographic defect. The long-term deleterious effects of irradiation can be minimized if doses in the 2,000-cGy range are not exceeded (47). Thus, 10 daily doses of 200 cGy would seem appropriate, the dose being reduced to 1,400 cGy in children under 2 years of age. Follow-up films 3 to 4 weeks after irradiation can be used to assess the result, and additional irradiation, not exceeding 1,000 cGy, can be added if there is not an adequate response. The difficulty, of course, lies in the fact that many of these tumor lesions have a ganglioneuromatous component, so that the tumor may not show an appreciable change after irradiation. The objective is to prevent proliferation of the neuroblastomatous portion, however.

Whether postoperative RT should be given is also in doubt. We do not irradiate if tumor excision has been complete or nearly so. Otherwise, RT is given as detailed above.

The role of chemotherapy remains unclear. It has not been shown to be of value in children with Stage I, II, or IV-S disease and is not ordinarily given at this institution. Children with Stage III or IV disease have chemotherapy added to prolong the relapse-free interval, even though better survival rates have not been proven to be produced by adjuvant drugs (48). Several combinations are in common use. Among the more effective regimens are vincristine + cyclophosphamide + DTIC, and cisplatin + VP-16 or VM-26.

Teratomas

Rarely, presacral malignant teratomas have been associated with extradural and even intradural masses at one or more levels. Direct tumor extension through sacral foramina can impinge on the distal cauda equina. Such direct extension is readily explicable, but it is difficult to understand the manner of apparently discontinuous tumor spread to higher levels seen in some patients. A careful neurologic evaluation in patients with these neoplasms is warranted. Should there be neurologic signs, workup is as for lymphomas, and the same RT and surgical principles apply. The lymphoma dose (3,000 cGy) seems reasonable with supplements of 1,000 cGy to areas of bulky tissue.

The chemotherapy is different, however. Since the malignant component often is of germ cell origin, drugs useful for that class of neoplasm seem indicated. Ablin et al. (49) have reported favorable results using six chemotherapeutic agents given to children with germ cell tumors. Those initial observations have been confirmed here by our team. The drugs employed are actinomycin, vincristine, cyclophosphamide, Adriamycin, bleomycin, and cisplatin.

REFERENCES

1. Barone BM, Elvidge AR. Ependymomas, a clinical survey. *J Neurosurg* 1970;33:428–438.
2. Mork SJ, Loken AC. Ependymoma, a follow-up study of 101 cases. *Cancer* 1977;40:907–915.
3. Garcia DM. Primary spinal cord tumors treated with surgery and postoperative irradiation. *Int J Radiat Oncol Biol Phys* 1985;11:1933–1939.
4. Garrett PG, Simpson WJK. Ependymomas: results of radiation treatment. *Int J Radiat Oncol Biol Phys* 1983;9:1121–1124.
5. Shuman RM, Ellsworth CA Jr, Leech RW. The biology of childhood ependymomas. *Arch Neurol* 1975;32:731–739.
6. Kopelson G, Linggood RM, Kleinman GM, et al. Management of intramedullary spinal cord tumors. *Radiology* 1980;135:473–479.
7. Shaw EG, Evans RG, Scheithauer BW, et al. Radiographic management of adult intraspinal ependymomas. *Int J Radiat Oncol Biol Phys* 1986;12:323–327.
8. DeSousa AL, Kalsbeck JE, Mealey J, et al. Intraspinal tumors in children. A review of 81 cases. *J Neurosurg* 1979;51:437–445.
9. Dohrmann GJ, Farwell FR, Flannery JT. Ependymomas and ependymoblastomas in children. *J Neurosurg* 1976;45:273–282.
10. Peschel RE, Kapp DS, Cardinale F, Manuelidis EE. Ependymomas of the spinal cord. *Int J Radiat Oncol Biol Phys* 1983;9:1093–1096.
11. Sagerman RH, Bagshaw MA, Hanbery J. Considerations in the treatment of ependymoma. *Radiology* 1965;84:401–408.
12. Wood EH, Berne AS, Taveras JM. The value of radiation therapy in the management of intrinsic tumors of the spinal cord. *Radiology* 1954;63:11–22.
13. Greenwood J. Surgical removal of intramedullary tumors. *J Neurosurg* 1967;26:276–282.
14. Malis LI. Intramedullary spinal cord tumors. *Clin Neurosurg* 1978;25:512–539.
15. Scott M. Infiltrating ependymomas of the cauda equina. *J Neurosurg* 1974;41:446–448.
16. Wallner KE, Wara WM, Sheline GE, Davis RL. Intracranial ependymomas: results of treatment with partial or whole brain irradiation with spinal irradiation. *Int J Radiat Oncol Biol Phys* 1986;12:1937–1941.
17. Mork SJ, Rubinstein LJ. Ependymoblastoma. *Cancer* 1985;55:1536–1542.
18. Farwell JR, Dohrmann GJ, Flannery JT. Central nervous system tumors in children. *Cancer* 1977;40:3123–3132.
19. Levy LF, Elvidge AR. Astrocytoma of the brain and spinal cord. *J Neurosurg* 1956;13:413–443.
20. Schwade JG, Wara WM, Sheline GE, et al. Management of primary spinal cord tumors. *Int J Radiat Oncol Biol Phys* 1978;4:389–393.
21. Stein BM. Intramedullary spinal cord tumors. *Clin Neurosurg* 1983;30:717–741.
22. Woltman HW, Kerwohan JW, Adson AW, Craig WM. Intramedullary tumors of the spinal cord and gliomas of intraductal portion of filum terminale. *Arch Neurol Psychiatry* 1951;65:387–393.
23. Anderson FM, Carson MJ. Spinal cord tumors in children. A review of the subject and presentation of twenty-one cases. *J Pediatr* 1953;43:190–207.
24. Renudin A, Enriques J, Tomiyasu A. Spinal intramedullary glioblastoma with intracranial seeding. *Arch Neurol* 1978;35:244–245.
25. Eden KC. Dissemination of a glioma of the spinal cord in the leptomeninges. *Brain* 1938;61:298–310.
26. O'Connell J. The subarachnoid dissemination of spinal tumors. *J Neurol Neurosurg Psychiatry* 1956;9:55–62.
27. Kopelson G. Radiation tolerance of the spinal cord previously damaged by tumor and operation:

long-term neurological improvement and time-dose-volume relationships of intraspinal gliomas. *Int J Radiat Oncol Biol Phys* 1982;8:925–929.

28. Probert JC, Parker BR, Kaplan, HS. Growth retardation in children after megavoltage irradiation of the spine. *Cancer* 1973;32:634–639.
29. Allen JC, Bloom J, Ertel I, et al. Brain tumors in children: current cooperative and institutional chemotherapy trials in newly diagnosed and recurrent disease. *Semin Oncol* 1986;13:110–122.
30. Kopelson G, Linggood RM, Kleinman GM. Medulloblastoma. The identification of prognostic subgroups and implications for multimodality management. *Cancer* 1983;51:312–319.
31. Deutsch M, Reigel DH. The value of myelography in the management of childhood medulloblastoma. *Cancer* 1980;45:2194–2197.
32. Evans AE, Anderson J, Chang C, et al. Adjuvant chemotherapy for medulloblastoma and ependymoma. In: Paoletti P, Walker MD, Butti G, Knerich R, eds. *Multidisciplinary aspects of brain tumor therapy.* Amsterdam, New York, Oxford: Elsevier/North-Holland, 1975;219–222.
33. DiLorenzo N, Giuffre R, Fortuna A. Primary spinal neoplasms in childhood: analysis of 1234 published cases (including 56 personal cases) by pathology, sex, age, and site. Differences from the situation in adults. *Neurochirurgia* 1982;25:153–164.
34. Udvarhelyi GB, Winfield JA. Tumors of the brain and spinal cord. In: Welch KJ, Randolph JG, Ravitch MM, et al., eds. *Pediatric surgery,* 4th ed. Chicago: Year Book Medical Publishers, 1986;338–341.
35. Traggis DG, Filler RM, Druckman H, et al. Prognosis for children with neuroblastoma presenting with paralysis. *J Pediatr Surg* 1977;12:419–425.
36. White L, Siegel SE. Non-Hodgkin's lymphoma in childhood. In: Sutow WW, Fernbach DJ, Vietti TJ, eds. *Clinical pediatric oncology,* 3rd ed. St. Louis: C.V. Mosby, 1984;452–497.
37. Sutow WW, Fernbach DJ, Vietti TJ, eds. *Clinical pediatric oncology,* 3rd ed. St. Louis: C.V. Mosby, 1984.
38. Schweisguth O. *Solid tumors in children.* New York: John Wiley, 1982.
39. Voute PA, Barrett A, Bloom HJG, et al., eds. *Cancer in children: clinical management,* 2nd ed. New York: Springer Verlag, 1986.
40. Tefft M, Mitus A, Schultz MD. Initial high dose irradiation for metastases causing spinal cord compression in children. *Am J Roentgenol* 1969;106:385–389.
41. Nesbit ME, Perez CA, Tefft M, et al. Multimodal therapy for the management of non-metastatic Ewing's sarcoma of bone: an intergroup study. *Natl Cancer Inst Mongr* 1981;56:255–262.
42. Link MP, Goorin AM, Miser AW, et al. The effect of adjuvant chemotherapy on relapse-free survival in patients with osteosarcoma of the extremity. *N Engl J Med* 1986;314:1600–1606.
43. Ferber L, Lampe I. Hemangioma of vertebra associated with compression of cord. Response to radiation therapy. *Arch Neurol* 1942;47:19–29.
44. Smith DG, Nesbit ME, D'Angio GJ, Levitt SH. Histiocytosis X: role of radiation therapy in management with special reference to dose levels employed. *Radiology* 1973;106:419–422.
45. Fagan CJ, Swischuk LE. Dumbbell neuroblastoma or ganglioneuroma of the spinal canal. *Am J Roentgenol* 1974;120:453–460.
46. Punt J, Pritchard J, Pincott JR, Till K. Neuroblastoma: a review of 21 cases present with spinal cord compression. *Cancer* 1980;45:3095–3101.
47. Neuhauser EBD, Wittenborg MH, Berman CZ, Cohen J. Irradiation effects of roentgen therapy on the growing spine. *Radiology* 1952;59:637–650.
48. Evans AE, D'Angio GJ, Propert KJ, et al. Prognostic factors in neuroblastoma. *Cancer* 1987; 59:1853–1859.
49. Ablin A, Ramsay N, Krailo M, et al. Effective therapy for malignant germ cell tumors in children. A study by the Children's Cancer Study Group. *Proc Am Soc Clin Oncol* 1982;1:108 (Abstr.).

6

Tumors of Neural or Glial Origin

Ignacio Pascual-Castroviejo

EPENDYMOMAS AND EPENDYMOBLASTOMA

Generalities

Spinal ependymomas are intramedullary tumors. More than 42% of all ependymomas are located in the spinal canal (1). Twenty-seven percent of all ependymomas occur below 20 years of age and only 19.6% occur at less than 15 years of age (1). Although spinal ependymoma is said to be twice as frequent as astrocytoma in adults (1,2), this is not the case for children who present four times more astrocytomas than ependymomas in some series (3); in other series, both entities show a similar frequency (4–6). Ependymomas are the most common tumors of the cauda equina after the first year of life, exceeded only by lipomas. According to some authors (7,8), 2 to 10% of presacral tumors are extradural extramedullary ependymomas. In children and adolescents the prevalence of ependymomas is twice as high in males as in females. They occurred in patients of all ages (from 8 months to 72 years) in a series of 102 cases (1).

Extension of ependymomas into the spinal cord is very variable. The majority of tumors are well demarcated, although not encapsulated. Usually they occupy a few segments of the spinal cord. Ependymomas grow very slowly, and some, especially those located in the cauda equina or the filum terminale, may slowly increase in size and extend through many segments. Giant spinal ependymomas extending more than ten vertebral segments occur occasionally. When the tumor extends from the high cervical spine to the conus, it may be considered "panmedullary." Panmedullary tumors, as well as giant ependymomas, have been reported most often in adult patients (5), but do occur on occasion in children (9) or teenagers (10). Some ependymomas originate in the fourth ventricle and extend to the upper cervical spinal cord, accounting for about 25% of the ependymomas of the posterior fossa (1).

Several types of ependymomas may be distinguished. Some are entirely intramedullary, and others are both intra- and extramedullary. This latter location is exceptional; a tumor of this type may reach a giant size (11), the greater part of the tumor being extramedullary. Ependymomas of the conus and the cauda equina are intramedullary without an extramedullary component. They are, in fact, ependymomas of the filum that have displaced the conus either by stretching it or by invaginating it (1). Ependymomas located in the sacrum or pre- or retro-sacral spaces have their origin in the intradural portion of the filum terminale and have spread into the sacrum (1). These tumors may destroy a portion of the sacrum and may spread into the retroperitoneal or retrorectal zones. Ectopic cells occur near the spine occasionally. Tumors arising from these cells are called "ectopic ependymomas," or presacral and postsacral extraspinal ependymomas. They may arise in the spine below the dermis, in dermal sinuses, etc. Tumors of this type are quite rare in children (1,11–17). Ependymomas can metastasize into surrounding tissues or to distant parts of the body.

Primary ependymomas of the spinal leptomeninges are extremely rare. We know only of the description of Wada et al. (18) concerning a 17-year-old girl who suffered from a primary leptomeningeal ependymoblastoma with diffuse thickening and small nodules on the spinal cord and on the roots of the cauda equina.

Clinical Findings

Symptoms and signs consist of pain, motor and sensory signs, subarachnoid bleeding, and sphincter and genital disturbances. Back pain is the first symptom. It may be local or diffuse, with a sudden or an insidious onset, and an unpredictable course. It is resistant to nonsurgical treatment. Its intensity can increase or decrease unpredictably, but there is often a zone of lancinating pain. Pain is made worse in the recumbent position and during the latter part of the night. Its character varies depending on the location of the tumor. Cervical ependymomas produce muscle spasms in the neck, often with torticollis and arm pain. Ependymomas of the thoracic cord commonly present with excruciating pain localized to the level of the tumor. Ependymomas of the cauda equina and filum terminale may show chronic low back pain, coccydynia, or diffuse pain irradiating to the pelvis, hips, and lower limbs, often presenting as unilateral or bilateral sciatica. Quite often patients complain of low back pain or coccydynia for several years before the diagnosis of ependymoma in the lower spinal cord is made (19–21).

Sphincter and genital disturbances consist of urinary and/or fecal incontinence, and priapism or impotence. Subarachnoid hemorrhage, frequently associated with impairment of consciousness (22–25), is a fairly common complication of the ependymomas located in the cauda equina. Bleeding can occur in patients of any age (26). Spinal tumors causing subarachnoid bleeding are located mainly in the cauda equina, filum terminale, and lumbar cord. In children, subarachnoid hemorrhage has been reported when ependymoma was in the cauda equina (24) as well as in the cervical cord (25) or any other region. Sixty-four percent of the subarachnoid hemorrhages caused by spinal tumors is due to ependymoma (27). Astrocytomas, neurinomas, meningiomas, and hemangioblastomas may produce subarachnoid hemorrhage even when they are located about or in the spinal canal. Ninety percent of spinal tumors causing subarachnoid hemorrhage are benign (28). The spinal subarachnoid hemorrhage may be mistaken for a ruptured intracranial aneurysm or bacterial meningitis (23), especially if it is the first episode of bleeding and there were no previous clinical symptoms or signs involving the lower limbs or sphincters. Trauma (26) and strenuous exercise may trigger subarachnoid bleeding. Bayley (26) describes the case of a 9-year-old girl whose symptoms began suddenly after her father threw her roughly over his shoulder. Bleeding may recur if an ependymoma is only partially removed (25). Acute and violent back pain, which precedes the headache, and more or less localized root pain and arreflexia in the lower limbs suggest a spinal origin of the subarachnoid hemorrhage (27). Signs of meningeal irritation may be delayed for several days or weeks after a bleed, and in some patients the diagnosis of ependymoma was not made until they sustained severe subarachnoid hemorrhage (29).

Increased intracranial pressure with papilledema is an occasional complication of spinal cord tumors. Ependymomas are responsible in 54% of such cases (22). Papilledema is easily explained by obstruction of the spinal fluid pathways if the tumor is located in the cervical cord, but in the majority of cases the tumor is located in the lumbar or thoracolumbar regions (22). The diagnosis of spinal cord tumor is very difficult when papilledema is the first sign of the disease, since it is such a rare occurrence. However, all neurologists must remember to consider a spinal cord tumor when a patient presents with true papilledema or subarachnoid hemorrhage and no intracranial tumor or vascular malformation is found. Moreover, such tumors have been associated not only with papilledema as a sign of increased intracranial pressure, but also with several other symptoms and signs, such as nystagmus, oculomotor palsy (especially of one or both sixth nerves), diplopia, tinnitus, blurred vision, headache, paracentral scotoma, enlarged blind spot, etc. Although several mechanisms have been proposed to explain the raised intracranial pressure, it remains unexplained.

The duration of symptoms in spinal cord ependymomas may range from months to many years. For example, Sonneland et al. (30), in a series of 77 myxopapillary ependymomas of the spinal cord in patients of various ages seen over 60 years at the Mayo Clinic, found that low back pain was the most frequent complaint, with a duration of symptoms ranging from 1 month to 30 years. This variant of ependymoma is, with few exceptions, limited to the filum terminale, conus, and surrounding areas.

Laboratory Tests

The cerebrospinal fluid (CSF) is often, but not always, xanthochromic with albumino-cytologic dissociation. Protein levels are highest in patients with ependymomas of the cauda equina, who also may show Froin's syndrome with a total block of the spinal canal. It is obvious that, in subarachnoid bleeding, the CSF is hemorrhagic. Tumor cells in the CSF have been found only occasionally; they are more often found in children with widespread ependymoma having intratumoral necrotic areas, and in ependymoblastoma (1).

Radiology

Plain films are usually unremarkable (30), especially in very young infants. However, pedicle erosion, widened interpedicular distance, vertebral body erosion and, occasionally, laminar erosion may be seen, especially in slow growing tumors.

Myelography demonstrates total or partial block in more than 90% of cases (30).

Arteriography of the spinal cord can reveal ependymomas of the spinal cord and filum terminale. This procedure used to be used (31) because ependymoma can mimic an arteriovenous malformation (32); arteriography is not currently used for the diagnosis of spinal ependymomas.

Magnetic resonance (MR) demonstrates the tumor's exact location, size, extension, and intratumoral cavities (33). In some cases, a residual surgical cavity in the cord has been detectable weeks and even several months after removal of the tumor (33).

Histology

Ependymomas derive from differentiated ependymal cells. Histologically, the most characteristic features are the presence of ependymal rosettes and the formation of perivascular pseudorosettes. Blepharoplasts are also always found, and cilia may often be seen. Several variants of ependymoma have been described. Subependymomas, also known as subependymal astrocytoma and subependymal glomerate astrocytoma (34), have occasionally been detected in the cervical cord in adults.

Myxopapillary ependymomas involve the filum terminale or the lumbosacral spinal cord in 95% of the cases, and only 5% are located in the cervicothoracic cord (30). These have very rarely been described intracranially (35). They seem to be a distinct clinicopathologic variant, easily recognizable histologically. The term myxopapillary is based on the tendency of this variant of ependymoma to produce mucin and to form papillae. Immunocytochemistry may aid in its identification. Neuron-specific enolase, S-100 protein, neurofilament protein, and glial fibrillary acid protein have been used to characterize this tumor (30). Although its occurrence in children is rare, Ciraldo et al. (36) reported five cases, four of which were infants in the first year of life, and found 13 cases previously published in the literature. These lesions arise from a coccygeal vestige of the primitive spinal cord which corresponds to the original site of the final closure of the posterior neuropore. The presence of ependymal rests in many patients with sacral dimples suggests that the prevalence of this lesion should be greater. Bale (15) examined the coccygeal region in 15 random necropsies of infants aged 1 day to 1 year and observed a small, deep dermal and subcutaneous myxopapillary ependymal island in 10 of them. This lesion has a potential for lymph node and pulmonary metastases (8,14,16). Systemic metastases of myxopapillary ependymoma of the conus and filum terminale, although rare, have been well documented (37–39).

Occasionally, ependymomas can present malignant features, including invasive characteristics, foci of necrosis, increased cellularity, mitotic figures, multinucleated cells, and giant cell formation (34). Such tumors receive the name ependymoblastoma or malignant ependymoma. They almost never occur in the spinal cord. The majority of ependymomas, including the variants subependymoma and myxopapillary ependymoma, may be considered benign Grade I gliomas. Intraneural or extraneural metastases from spinal ependymoma are uncommon, especially in children and adolescents.

Treatment and Prognosis

Complete removal of the ependymoma is indicated whenever feasible. Among very extensive spinal tumors, ependymomas are those most likely to be removable in their entirety. Incomplete resection may be followed by serious complications after a relatively short time (25). Patients who undergo radical operations commonly show rapid, often surprising, clinical improvement, which is permanent in many cases (1). This occurs in giant ependymomas (10,11), and even in pan-intramedullary ependymomas (5). Incomplete recovery after late removal (5,40) and after recurrence is quite common. Theoretically, radiotherapy should have very little effect on the ependymoma and its benign variants. However, Sonneland et al. (30) believe that radiotherapy may be beneficial to patients whose tumors are not amenable to total removal. Dorhrmann et al. (41) report that 100% of their patients with spinal ependymoma were alive 5 years after the diagnosis, regardless of whether they were treated only by removal of the tumor or with radiotherapy as well. In cases with malignant histologic features, radiotherapy is always advisable. However, in Fischer's series (1), the only patient with malignant ependymoma who survived 10 years had not received radiotherapy. Chemotherapy may have the same indications and problems as radiotherapy.

Encapsulated myxopapillary ependymomas have a lower recurrence rate (10%) because they may be easily reached and totally removed, whereas those that are removed either piecemeal or subtotally have a higher recurrence rate (19%), based on the series of Sonneland et al. (30). Survival was most closely related to residual disease; total removal of the tumor, whether intact and encapsulated or piecemeal, resulted in longer survival (19 years) than did subtotal resection (14 years) (30). Similar results have been reported in other series involving all ages (42) and in infants below one year of age who did not suffer recurrence for several years after complete tumor removal (36).

SPINAL ASTROCYTOMA AND GLIOBLASTOMA

Generalities and Histology

In children, astrocytomas are the most frequent gliomas of the spinal cord (6,43–46). The term spinal glioma includes all types of tumors that originate from glial cells, that is, astrocytomas, ependymomas, and oligodendrogliomas. Astrocytomas have a clear predominance in males, ranging between 63.6% (43,44) and 82% (45) in various series.

They occur most commonly in the cervical and thoracic segments. With MR, detection of the spread of bulbar astrocytomas to the upper segments of the cervical spinal cord is now possible. Holocord astrocytoma is the term applied to astrocytomas extending down from the lower brainstem or upper cervical cord to the conus (47), an occurrence which is quite common [14 of the 19 patients in the series of Epstein and Epstein (47)]. Histologically, astrocytomas are subdivided into three groups: fibrillary, protoplasmic, and gemistocytic tumors, all of Grade II malignancy. Astrocytoma Grade I is characterized by fusiform cells, Rosenthal fibers, and granular bodies, and it has a more benign biological behavior. The term pilocytic astrocytoma refers to a special subtype, which corresponds to the older term polar spongioblastoma.

Clinical Findings

Symptoms and signs are the same as those of other spinal masses: gait disturbance, pain with stiffness; tilted head, paralysis of one, two, three, or four limbs, usually progressively; hyperreflexia; Babinski response; sensory deficits with a sensory level; sphincter dysfunction; priapism in males; and paravertebral muscle spasm. The duration of symptoms prior to definitive diagnosis varies from days to several years, the average being 2 years.

Torticollis and scoliosis are often the first signs of a spinal mass in the cervical segments, and, less frequently, in other spinal regions (48–51). The neurologic disability may not be apparent until long after the deformity is present. Neurologists must be aware of these facts, lest they make a tardy diagnosis. The duration of the interval between the onset of the scoliosis and the appearance of the neurologic signs may range from 1 month to 11 years (49), or even longer in some cases (52). The adage is that tumors in the cervical region present as a stiff neck, in the thoracic region as a cautious gait, and in the lumbar region as a change in the normal lumbar lordosis (51).

Intracranial hypertension, sometimes with papilledema and hydrocephalus, is a complication that may be the first sign of the disease. It results occasionally from seeding by intraspinal astrocytomas, more frequently by malignant tumors (glioblastomas) but also by other tumors, such as ependymomas, schwannomas, meningiomas, or vascular tumors. Spontaneous subarachnoid hemorrhage has been associated with astrocytoma (25,48,53). Cystic degeneration or syringomyelia is quite frequent in astrocytoma (49–51). Although these cavities are more common at the rostral and caudal end of the lesion, multiple cysts (51) or syringomyelia extending from the medulla to the conus (49) may also be found. The CSF has increased protein with cells.

Glioblastomas of the spinal cord, which are rare in adults, are more common in infancy and childhood (54). However, it is difficult to obtain adequate information about them because they have been given many names, including glioblastoma, glioblastoma multiforme, isomorphic glioblastoma, spongioblastoma multiforme, undifferentiated malignant glioma, Grade IV astrocytoma, malignant glioma of mixed type, and cellular glioma (mostly small cells). Glioblastomas are poorly differentiated tumors. They have a heterogeneous appearance with areas of necrosis, pseudopalissading, fistulous vessels, vascular endothelial proliferation, and old and fresh hemorrhage (55). A clear preponderance of females over males (3:1) is seen before 14 years of age, but the ratio is reversed in adult life (54). Most tumors are located in the cervical, cervicothoracic, and thoracic segments. As occurs with astrocytomas, glioblastomas also present intramedullary cavitation, sometimes of intratumoral necrotic type, and other times of syringomyelic or hydromyelic type.

The clinical history is short and duration of the symptoms, which are similar to those of astrocytomas, is between a few days and 1 year. The CSF protein is markedly elevated. Dissemination to the spinal subarachnoid space, basal cisterns, and ventricles is quite common (56).

Radiology

Spine X-ray films show abnormalities in about 60% of patients with astrocytomas (43). The most common findings are increased interpedicular distance at the level of the tumor, the eroding of pedicles, kyphoscoliosis, kyphosis, or scoliosis (49–52). Intraspinal calcifications may also be seen in some cases (Fig. 1).

Myelography shows complete or incomplete block of the contrast medium with the appearance of an intramedullary tumor. Computerized tomography (CT) scanning of the spine, enhanced with intrathecal metrizamide or intravenous contrast material, may reveal not only enlargement of the cord caused by the mass but also its solid and cystic components (57). All our patients with spinal astrocytoma had intratumoral hyperdensities (Fig. 2).

MR with the use of a surface coil has proven to be the most informative neuroimaging method (58). Especially in the sagittal plane, MR provides visualization of the whole extent of the tumor in the cord (Fig. 3A,B) and even into the brainstem. Sagittal MR also allows one to visualize a kyphosis and the appearance of the vertebrae, as well as areas of intratumoral cystic degeneration (33). However, MR imaging characteristics of low-grade astrocytomas of the spinal cord are

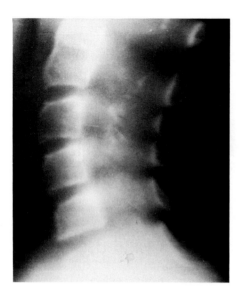

FIG. 1. Twelve-year-old girl with a cervical astrocytoma. The sagittal X-ray tomogram shows a widened spinal canal and intraspinal calcifications.

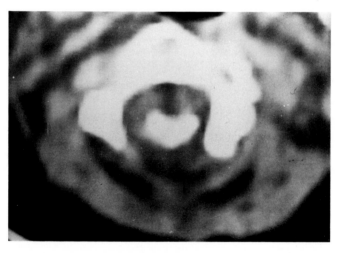

FIG. 2. Computerized tomography after surgical biopsy showing intratumoral calcification within the spinal cord.

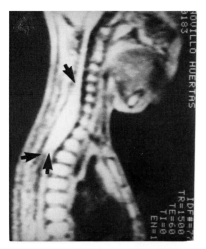
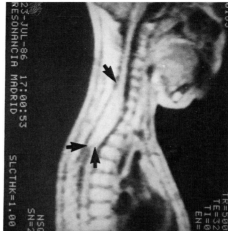

A

B

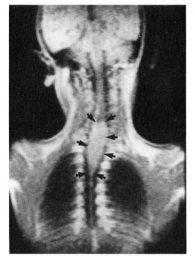

FIG. 3. **A:** Five-year-old boy with an astrocytoma invading the cervicothoracic region. The sagittal magnetic resonance (MR) view clearly shows the extension of the tumor (*arrows*) in T2 (*left*) and T1 (*right*). **B:** Frontal view of the same case showing the tumor in T1 (*arrows*). Scoliosis is also evident.

sometimes ambiguous (59). The use of gadolinium to enhance the tumoral images may be necessary.

Treatment

Radical removal of the tumor should be performed when feasible. The use of the Cavitron ultrasonic surgical aspirator, permitting nontraumatic aspiration of all of the visible tumor without lesioning the surrounding normal spinal cord, considerably improves the surgical results (17). There are a significant number of patients in whom only decompression and biopsy, or subtotal or partial removal, can be performed (43). The mean survival period after radical removal is much higher (66.6 months) than after incomplete resection (43).

Postoperative radiotherapy for spinal cord astrocytomas is controversial because of the unpredictable biological behavior of these tumors. Long-term survival seems to be related to tumor grade (60). Radical removal of the tumor can make postoperative radiation unnecessary, whereas radiation may be reasonable after simple biopsy or partial extirpation (47). A commonly used dose is 5,000 rad in 25 treatments. The risk of radiation therapy to the spinal cord is not well defined (61).

Postlaminectomy spinal deformity, especially in children, is a common complication, and orthopedic treatment is recommended after surgery in most cases.

OLIGODENDROGLIOMA

Primary spinal cord oligodendrogliomas are the rarest of the spinal gliomas. Only 38 cases were collected in a recent review of the literature (62), 12 of whom were under 20 years of age. Spinal oligodendrogliomas account for about 0.45% of all spinal tumors, 1.80% of intramedullary tumors, and 1.59% of all oligo-dendrogliomas (62). Boys and girls and adolescents are equally affected. Tumors are found more frequently in the thoracic region, followed by the cervical and lumbar regions. The filum terminale is a less common location.

Clinical signs and symptoms are no different from those of other spinal tumors. Back pain is the first symptom in more than two-thirds of the patients, followed by motor deficit, twitching, or contracture, and, occasionally, by paresthesias. Later, depending on the level of the tumor, quadriparesis, spastic paraparesis, complete cord transsection, sensory deficits, sphincter disturbances, flaccid paresis of a limb (63), radicular syndromes in the upper or lower limbs, and, sometimes, sciatica or cauda equina syndrome may appear. Length of history ranges from 1 month (64) to 3 years (63) in children and adolescents. Hyperreflexia below the lesion is common, although hyporeflexia or areflexia may be found in cases of radicular involvement. A meningeal syndrome is observed in patients with leptomeningeal oligodendrogliomatosis. Unilateral deficit of the pontine cranial nerves was reported in a case with a spinal tumor and spread to the parenchyma of the brainstem (65). As occurs with other spinal tumors (ependymoma, neurilemmoma, neurofibroma, glioma), symptoms of raised intracranial pressure may appear in cases of oligodendrogliomas located anywhere along the spine, although most often in low dorsal and dorsolumbar regions. This has been described in 31% of spinal oligodendrogliomas, always shortly before death. Increased intracranial pressure may become manifest before the spinal disease (66), after the spinal disease (65,67), or after removal of the tumor (67,68). In two cases, the cause of the intracranial hypertension was overlooked until necropsy showed an oligodendroglioma in the cervical region with spinal and intracranial oligodendrogliomatosis (69,70). Secondary spinal dissemination from intracranial oligodendrogliomas occurs occasionally in children (71,72). In the case of a

27-year-old woman there were multiple metastases from a malignant cerebral oligodendroglioma seeding diffusely in the subarachnoid space with small tumor nodules among the roots of the cauda equina (73). All metastases were gelatinous and mucin-positive.

Laboratory

The CSF protein is usually very elevated, seldom normal. Some patients present a moderate pleocytosis with granulocytes, and also tumor cells in the case of oligodendrogliomatosis. The Queckenstedt test has shown total or partial block in most patients who were examined but is no longer indicated with modern neuroimaging.

Radiology

Plain X-rays show signs of a spinal mass in less than 50% of cases. Kyphoscoliosis has occasionally been observed. Myelography showed an intramedullary tumor in all patients but one who presented spinal and intracranial oligodendrogliomatosis and hydrocephalus. MR images, especially in the sagittal plane, provide a clear depiction of the tumor's appearance and extent; it sometimes invades essentially the entire cord and extends upwards to involve the medulla oblongata (33). MR can also reveal cavities within the tumor (33).

Histology

Oligodendrogliomas are white or grayish-pink in color. Although sometimes they are circumscribed, most cases are infiltrating, soft, and gelatinous. Intratumoral hemorrhages and intra- or peritumoral cysts are sometimes observed (33). The diagnosis of oligodendroglioma using standard microscopic methods is difficult. Some of the most consistent characteristics of this tumor include (63) cells of uniform size and shape, with each cell displaying a clear halo around the nucleus; the virtual absence of glial fibrils; rarity of coagulation necrosis; and a paucity of nuclear abnormalities. Astrocytic cells can always be identified when gold sublimate impregnation techniques are used or ultrastructural study is performed (63). Garcia and Lemmi (63) studied the ultrastructure of spinal cord oligodendrogliomas. They observed that the dominant cell type possesses relatively electron-dense scanty cytoplasm with very few short cell processes. Its perikaryon contains many microtubules with an average diameter of 200 Å, as well as abundant ribosomes.

Therapy and Prognosis

Total removal of the tumor is sometimes possible. Usually the neurosurgeon can achieve only partial removal or biopsy. Radiotherapy after operation may prolong survival somewhat. The mean survival of operated patients with spinal cord oligodendrogliomas is 2.4 years (62).

GANGLIOGLIOMA

Clinical Findings and Histology

Ganglioglioma is a tumor with Grades I and II malignancy, which contains mature ganglion cells, such as the gangliocytoma, and neoplastic cells (55). Clusters of ganglion cells resembling mature neurons are surrounded by loose glial tissue. Occasionally, binucleated and multinucleated cells are seen, as well as cells with hyperchromatic nuclei. Foci of calcification and small cysts are frequent. Ganglioglioma was thought to be a hamartomatous lesion until recently. Today, it is accepted as a true neoplasm (55,75).

There are rare anaplastic gangliogliomas (Grades II to IV) with anaplastic cell or tissue architecture. These constitute about 1% of spinal neoplasms. Sixty percent of gangliogliomas appear before age 30 (76).

This tumor is an infiltrating intramedullary mass located anywhere within the spinal cord between the upper cervical segments and the conus medullaris. Gangliogliomas tend to be slow growing and infiltrative, rather than compressive, and to extend over a long region of the cord. They tend to be sharply demarcated from surrounding tissues (76). The development of neurologic signs may be gradual and symmetrical or asymmetrical. Spastic paraparesis and scoliosis are the main clinical findings. We observed two children, a boy and a girl, both presenting slowly progressive spastic paraparesis and moderate scoliosis, with the ganglioglioma extending from C7 to the conus in one case and from T7 to the conus in the other. Most cases reported in the literature were located in the cervical cord. Ganglioglioma has occasionally been observed in the conus medullaris (77). Tumors extending through the entire length of the spinal cord have also been described (78). The CSF protein is elevated (51).

Radiology

Plain X-ray films usually show pronounced widening of the spinal canal in the region of the tumor, advanced erosion of pedicles, scalloping of the vertebral bodies, and scoliosis. Myelography, sometimes requiring the uses of both suboccipital and lumbar injection of contrast, shows a voluminous intramedullary tumor (Fig. 4). MR shows the extent of the intramedullary mass which has increased signal intensity in T2-weighted images (Fig. 5).

Treatment

Excision of the tumor is considered the treatment of choice. Although successful removal of intramedullary ganglioglioma has been achieved (51,77,78), it is

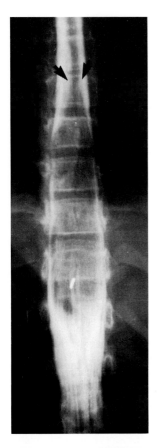

FIG. 4. Ganglioglioma. Metrizamide myelography shows an intramedullary mass extending from T7 (*arrows*) to L1 with a widened spinal canal with eroded pedicles.

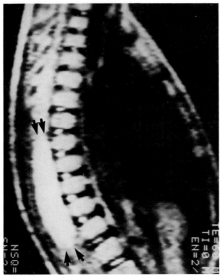

FIG. 5. Magnetic resonance T2 weighted study in the same case as Fig. 4. The bright image in the spinal cord depicts the extent of the tumor (between *arrows*).

very difficult and depends on the anatomic characteristics of the tumor. Total removal was possible in only one case of four spinal gangliogliomas in the largest series (79). Our patients were submitted only to biopsy or partial excision of the tumor. There is no experience in the use of postoperative radiotherapy in spinal cord gangliogliomas.

In summary, histologically, spinal ganglioglioma is usually a benign tumor, but it has a malignant behavior because of its usual intramedullary location, its size, and the difficulty of its removal.

REFERENCES

1. Fischer G. Les épendymomes intra-rachidiens. *Neurochirurgia* 1977;23(Suppl. 1):149–236.
2. Sloof JL, Kernohan JW, McCarty CS. *Primary intramedullary tumors of the spinal cord and filum terminale.* Philadelphia, London: W.B. Saunders, 1964;255.
3. Matson DD. *Neurosurgery of infancy and childhood.* Springfield, Ill.: Charles C Thomas, 1969; 934.
4. Dodge HW, Keith HM, Campagna MJ. Intraspinal tumors in infants and children. *J Int Coll Surg* 1956;26:199–215.
5. Fischer G, Pierluca P, Sindou M, Pialat J. L'épendymome pan-médullaire. A propos de deux cas d'exérèse complète. *Neurchirurgie* 1975;21:5–20.
6. Koos W, Laubichler W, Sorgo G. Statistische Untersuchungen bei spinalen Tumoren im Kindes und Jungendalter. *Neuropediatrie* 1973;4:273–303.
7. Morantz RA, Kepes JJ, Batnitzky S, Masterson BJ. Extraspinal ependymomas: report of three cases. *J Neurosurg* 1979;51:383–391.
8. Vagaiwala MR, Robinson JS, Galicish JH, et al. Metastasizing extradural ependymoma of the sacrococcygeal region. *Cancer* 1974;44:326–333.
9. Cushing H. The intracranial tumors of preadolescence. *Am J Dis Child* 1927;33:551–584.
10. Corriero G, Maiuri F, Colella G, Venvenuti D. Giant spinal ependymoma. A case report. *Neurochirurgia* 1985;28:232–234.
11. Gonzalez Feria L, Fernandez Martín F, Ginoves Sierra M, Galera Davidson H. Ependimoma extramedullar dorsal gigante. *Arch Neurobiol* 1971;34:325–332.
12. Prabhaker V, Rao D, Subrahmanian MV, Indira C. Extraspinal ependymoma. *Neurol Ind* 1969;17:82–84.
13. Scharr VE, Heiming E. Trabekulär-papilläres Ependymoma über der Sakrokokzgealregion. *Zentralbt Neurochir* 1974;35:131–136.
14. Hendren TH, Hardin CA. Extradural metastatic ependymoma. *Surgery* 1963;54:880–882.
15. Bale PM. Ependymal rests and subcutaneous sacrococcygeal ependymoma. *Pathology* 1980; 12:237–243.
16. Wolff M, Santiago H, Dubby MM. Delayed distant metastasis from a subcutaneous sacrococcygeal ependymoma. *Cancer* 1972;30:1046–1072.
17. Sanjuan Rodriguez S. Castejón Casado J, Pimentel Leo JJ, et al. Ependimoblastoma presacro extramedular. *An Esp Pediat* 1986;24:333–335.
18. Wada C, Kurate A, Hirose R, et al. Primary leptomeningeal ependymoblastoma. Case report. *J Neurosurg* 1986;64:968–973.
19. Houlding RN, Matheson AT. Intrathecal spinal tumour as a cause of coccydynia. Report of a case. *J Bone Joint Surg* 1961;43B:344–345.
20. Chateau R, De Rougemont J, Bonneville B, et al. Coccygodynie révélatrice d'une tumeur géante de le queue de cheval. *J Méd Lyon* 1967;48:573–578.
21. Charpentier J, Messimy R, Da Lage C. Coccygodine révélatrice d'un épendymome du filum terminale. Ablation complète sans séquelles. *Rev Neurol (Paris)* 1968;118:160–162.
22. Iob I, Andrioli GC, Rigobello L, Salar G. An unusual onset of a spinal cord tumour: subarachnoid bleeding and papilloedema. Case report. *Neurochirurgia* 1980;23:112–116.
23. Okawara S. Ruptured spinal ependymoma simulating bacterial meningitis. *Arch Neurol* 1983; 40:54–55.

24. Payne NS, McDonald JV. Rupture of spinal cord ependymoma. Case report. *J Neurosurg* 1973; 39:662–665.
25. Ucar S, Florez G, García J. Increased intracranial pressure associated with spinal cord tumours. *Neurochirurgia* 1976;19:265–268.
26. Bayley P. Ependymoma of the cauda equina. *Arch Neurol Psychiat* 1935;33:902–904.
27. Djindjian M, Djindjian R, Hurth M, et al. Les hémorrhagies méningées spinales tumorales. A propos de 5 cas artériographiés. *Rev Neurol (Paris)* 1978;134:658–692.
28. Neau JP, Lefèvre JP, Gil R, et al. Hémorrhagies méningées spinales d'origine tumorale. *Semin Hôp Paris* 1983;59:5–11.
29. Perel Y, Got M, Dufillot D, Fontan D, Guillard J-M. Hémorrhagie méningée symptome révélateur d'une tumeur spinale chez l'enfant. *Pediatrie* 1985;40:645–651.
30. Sonneland PRL, Scheithauer BW, Onofrio BM. Myxopapillary ependymoma. A clinicopathologic and immunochemical study of 77 cases. *Cancer* 1985;56:883–893.
31. Di Chiro G, Wener L. Angiography of ependymomas of the spinal cord and filum terminale. *Am J Roentgenol* 1974;122:628–633.
32. Yuhl ET, Bentson JR. Rapid arteriovenous shunting in a spinal cord ependymoma. Case report. *J Neurosurg* 1976;44:744–747.
33. Di Chiro G, Doppman JL, Dwyer AJ, et al. Tumors and arteriovenous malformations of the spinal cord: assessment using MR. *Radiology* 1985;689–697.
34. Rubinstein LJ. Tumors of the central nervous system. In: Armed Forces Institute of Pathology, eds. *Atlas of tumor pathology*, vol. 6. Washington, DC: Armed Forces Institute of Pathology, 1972;104–126.
35. Sato H, Ohmura K, Mizushima M, et al. Myxopapillary ependymoma of the lateral ventricles: a study on the mechanism of its stromal myxoid change. *Acta Pathol Jpn* 1983;33:1017–1025.
36. Ciraldo AV, Platt MS, Agamanolis DP, Boekman CR. Sacrococcygeal myxopapillary ependymomas and ependymal rests in infants and children. *J Pediatr Surg* 1986;21:49–52.
37. Rubinstein LJ, Logan WJ. Extraneural metastases in ependymoma of the cauda equina. *J Neurol Neurosurg Psychiatry* 1970;33:763–770.
38. Wight DGD, Holley KJ, Finbow JAH. Metastasizing ependymoma of the cauda equina. Case report. *J Clin Pathol* 1973;26:929–935.
39. Mavroudis C, Townsend JJ, Wilson CB. A metastasizing ependymoma. A case report. *J Neurosurg* 1977;47:771–775.
40. De Divitiis E, Spaziante R, Stella L. Giant intramedullary ependymoma. A case report. *Neurochirurgia* 1978;21:69–72.
41. Dohrmann G, Farwell JR, Flannery JT. Ependymomas and ependymoblastomas in children. *J Neurosurg* 1976;45:273–283.
42. Fearnside MR, Adams CBT. Tumours of the cauda equina. *J Neurol Neurosurg Psychiatry* 1978;41:24–31.
43. Reimer R, Onofrio BM. Astrocytomas of the spinal cord in children and adolescents. *J Neurosurg* 1985;63:669–675.
44. Di Lorenzo N, Giuffre R, Fortuna A. Primary spinal neoplasms in childhood: analysis of 1,234 published cases (including 56 personal cases) by pathology, sex, age and site. Differences from the situation in adults. *Neurochirurgia* 1982;25:153–164.
45. De Sousa AL, Kalsback JE, Mealey J Jr, et al. Intraspinal tumors in children. A review of 81 cases. *J Neurosurg* 1979;51:437–445.
46. García Tigera J, Hernandez Zayas H, Galarraga Inza J, et al. Tumores intrarraquiedos en el niño. Estudio clínico de 30 casos. *Rev Cub Pediatr* 1979;51:549–558.
47. Epstein F, Epstein N. Surgical treatment of spinal cord astrocytomas of childhood. A series of 19 patients. *J Neurosurg* 1982;57:685–689.
48. Bhandari YS. Subarachnoid haemorrhage due to cervical cord tumor in a child. *J Neurosurg* 1969;30:749–751.
49. Kiwak K, Deray MJ, Shields D. Torticollis in three children with syringomyelia and spinal cord tumor. *Neurology* 1983;33:946–948.
50. Banna M, Pearce GM, Uldall R. Scoliosis: a rare manifestation of intrinsic tumours of the spinal cord in children. *J Neurol Neurosurg Psychiatry* 1971;34:637–641.
51. Citron N, Edgar MA, Sheehy J, Thomas DGT. Intramedullary spinal cord tumours presenting as scoliosis. *J Bone Joint Surg* 1984;66:513–517.
52. Dalloz JC, Queneau P, Canlorbe P, Rubin S. Modifications de la statique rachidienne au cours des compressions médullaires par tumeur chez l'enfant. *Arch Franç Pediatr* 1963;20:309–319.

53. Runnels JB, Hanbery JW. Spontaneous subarachnoid hemorrhage associated with spinal cord tumor. *J Neurosurg* 1974;40:252–254.
54. Fortuna A, Giuffré R. Intramedullary glioblastomas. *Neurochirurgia* 1971;14:14–23.
55. Zülch KJ. Principles of the new World Health Organization (WHO) classification of brain tumors. *Neuroradiology* 1980;19:59–66.
56. Andrews AA, Enriques L, Renaudin J, Tomiyasu U. Spinal intramedullary glioblastoma with intracranial seeding. Report of a case. *Arch Neurol* 1978;35:244–245.
57. Handel S, Grossman R, Sarwar M. Computed tomography in the diagnosis of spinal cord astrocytoma. *J Comput Assist Tomogr* 1978;2:226–228.
58. Masaryk TJ, Modic MT, Geisinger MA, et al. Cervical myelography: a comparison of magnetic resonance and myelography. *J Comput Assist Tomogr* 1986;10:184–194.
59. Rubin JM, Aisen AM, Di Pietro MA. Ambiguities in MR imaging of tumoral cysts in the spinal cord. *J Comput Assist Tomogr* 1986;10:395–398.
60. Kopelson G, Linggood RM. Intramedullary spinal cord astrocytoma versus glioblastoma. The prognostic importance of histologic grade. *Cancer* 1982;50:732–735.
61. Patterson RH Jr. Metastatic disease of the spine: surgical risk versus radiation therapy. *Clin Neurosurg* 1980;27:641–644.
62. Fortuna A, Celli P, Palma L. Oligodendrogliomas of the spinal cord. *Acta Neurochir* 1980; 52:305–329.
63. García JH, Lemmi H. Ultrastructure of oligodendroglioma of spinal cord. *Am J Clin Pathol* 1970;54:757–765.
64. Brahe-Pedersen C. Gliomer medulla spinalis. *Ugeskr Laeger* 1969;131:1837–1843.
65. Wöber G, Jellinger K. Intramedulläres Oligodendrogliom mit meningozerebraler Aussaat. *Acta Neurochir* 1976;35:261–269.
66. Ridsdale L, Moseley I. Thoracolumbar intraspinal tumours presenting features of raised intracranial pressure. *J Neurol Neurosurg Psychiatr* 1978;41:737–745.
67. Michel D, Lemercier G, Beau G, et al. Gliomatose méningée et ventriculaire diffuse secondaire à un oligodendrogliome intramédullaire. A propos d'une observation. *Lyon Méd* 1975;234:37–41.
68. Maurice-Williams RS, Lucey JJ. Raised intracranial pressure due to spinal tumours: 3 rare cases with a probable common mechanism. *Br J Surg* 1975;62:92–95.
69. Russell JR, Bucy PC. Oligodendroglioma of the spinal cord. *J Neurosurg* 1949;6:433–437.
70. Toso V. Diffusione metastiche alle leptomeningi. *Acta Neurol (Napoli)* 1967;22:366–376.
71. Spataro J, Sacks O. Oligodendroglioma with remote metastases. Case Report. *J Neurosurg* 1968;28:373–379.
72. Arseni C, Horvath L, Carp N, et al. Spinal dissemination following operation on cerebral oligodendroglioma. *Acta Neurochir* 1977;37:125–137.
73. Voldby B. Disseminated, mucin-producing oligodendroglioma. Report of two cases. *Acta Neurochir* 1974;30:299–307.
74. O'Brien CP, Lehrer HZ. Extensive oligodendrogliomas of the spinal cord with assoicated bone change. *Neurology* 1968;18:887–890.
75. Johannson JH, Rekate HL, Roessmann U. Gangliomas: pathological and clinical correlation. *J Neurosurg* 1981;54:58–63.
76. Russell DS, Rubinstein LJ. Ganglioma: a case with long history and malignant evolution. *J Neuropathol Exp Neurol* 1962;21:185–193.
77. Wald U, Levy PJ, Rappaport ZH, et al. Conus ganglioglioma in a two-and-one-half-year-old boy. Case report. *J Neurosurg* 1985;62:142–144.
78. Albright L, Byrd RP. Ganglioglioma of entire spinal cord. *Child's Brain* 1980;6:274–280.
79. Garrido E, Becker LF, Hoffman HJ, et al. Gangliogliomas in children. A clinicopathological study. *Child's Brain* 1978;4:339–346.

7

Tumors of the Meninges and Roots

Ignacio Pascual-Castroviejo

MENINGIOMAS

Clinical Findings

Spinal meningiomas are uncommon during childhood and adolescence. The incidence of spinal meningiomas during the first two decades of life has been estimated at 2.2% (1), 3.7% (2), and 5.5% (3), with nearly all cases appearing in children over 12 years of age. The prevalence of spinal meningiomas is 5% of all childhood meningiomas (4). There was not a single meningioma in our series of more than 100 children under the age of twelve with spinal cord masses. Meningiomas account for 22.0% (5) to 25.5% (6) of all intradural spinal tumors in adults. They may occur anywhere along the spinal canal, though they are most frequent in the thoracic region [80% of spinal meningiomas in adults (5)]. The thoracic region is also the most common location for intradural meningiomas in children, although with a lesser predilection, and the cervical and lumbar regions may be affected as well (7). Meningiomas may sometimes be found in the foramen magnum in adults, a location that is extremely rare in children. In about 20% of patients, meningioma are a manifestation of von Recklinghausen's disease (7). The female to male ratio is 1:1 in children, with 1:3 in our series (3), in contrast to the usual female preponderance of 4:1 seen in adults (8,9). Spinal meningiomas tend to be more invasive in young male patients, spreading to the epidural space (10).

The proportion of extradural meningiomas, as compared to intradural meningiomas, is said by some (10) to be higher in children than in adults. However, there were no extradural tumors in a large series of spinal meningiomas in children and adolescents (15). The first case of spinal extradural meningioma in a child was reported by Ingraham (16) in a 10-year-old boy who had von Recklinghausen's disease. A few cases have been described later (3,10–14,17,18). These tumors are contained within the spinal canal, although ectopic extraspinal meningiomas have also been reported in adults (19,20).

Presenting symptoms are appropriate to the location of the tumor. Local or radicular pain, sphincter problems, increased tendon reflexes, sometimes uni- or bilateral clonus, and Babinski signs are common findings. Quadriparesis, paraparesis, neck pain, leg pain, or sensory disturbances can occur, depending on the level of the tumor. Duration of symptoms before diagnosis ranges from 1 week

(11,12) to a few weeks or months (13,14) in children. The cerebrospinal fluid (CSF) is usually slightly xanthochromic and has an elevated protein content.

Histology

Among the several histologic types of meningiomas, the meningocytic is the most common (59%), followed by the psammomatous (21%), the nonspecific (12%), and isolated cases of fibrous, angiomatous, and transitional types (9). Several different histologic types may be found in a single meningioma (9). When a meningioma has a prominent vascular component, it may be named an angiomatous meningioma, which is sometimes almost indistinguishable from a hemangioblastoma, although it differs by its encapsulated and noninvasive aspect (21). It may be termed the hemangioblastic variant. All types mentioned are Grade I tumors and usually have a favorable prognosis. The hemangiopericytic subgroup is indistinguishable from a hemangiopericytoma; although it is encapsulated and noninvasive, it has a poorer prognosis. Papillary meningioma is a rare form with a worse prognosis (22). Typical anaplastic changes may occur in several of the subgroups. Meningeal sarcomas are invasive, but malignant meningiomas are exceptional.

Radiology

Plain X-ray films may show widening of the interpedicular distances and flattening of the pedicles in the area occupied by the tumor. Myelography demonstrates a partial or complete block, although it was normal in two of three patients studied by Scotti et al. (23), with meningiomas located at the C1–C2 level. Computerized tomography (CT) scans show a high density homogeneous mass, which is enhanced with the intravenous injection of contrast material. Magnetic resonance (MR) may delineate the location and size of the tumor as well as its relationship with and mass effect on the adjacent spinal cord. Meningiomas tend to have relaxation times close to those of the normal parenchyma (24); in multiple echo sequences, their signal tends to decay in a way similar to that of the spinal cord (23). As a result, MR studies may not provide a definite diagnosis, and myelography may be required (23).

Treatment

Removal of the tumor is necessary as soon as the diagnosis is made. Some authors believe that, together with removal of the tumor mass, an ample excision of the epidural fat should be carried out in order to reduce the probability of recurrence (13). Residual neurologic deficits in patients in whom complete resection is possible, which includes almost all patients, depend on the location, the size, and, especially, the anatomic and functional alterations of the spinal cord present before surgery. Although there seems to be no histologic difference in meningiomas related to age, children seem to have a worse prognosis than adults (10,18). Regarding histology, 80% of papillary meningiomas recur, whatever their location, as compared with 35% for the more benign histologic subtypes (15). Spinal meningiomas seem to have a lower recurrence rate (20%) (15). However, postoperative recurrences after many years, even decades, have been reported (9,25,26).

Cutaneous Meningioma

Extraspinal meningiomas are called cutaneous meningiomas (27) or primary cutaneous extravertebral meningiomas (28). They are among the rarest tumors of the skin, and very few cases have been described. They occur in children, are asymptomatic, and are present at birth as a paravertebral mass that can be mistaken for a myelomeningocele, a lipoma, or a dermoid or epidermoid cyst. The mass does not change with time. Plain radiographs of the spine commonly show underlying bifid vertebrae.

A primary cutaneous extravertebral meningioma can be an isolated finding without any relation to the intraspinal space, although a meningocele and a cutaneous meningioma may be associated. The extraspinal meningioma is better defined as a malformation than a true tumor. The lesion may be the result of a developmental defect. Meningeal cells become trapped or sequestered in the skin when the neural crest closes and form either a cutaneous meningioma or a meningocele. There may be a fibrous stalk instead of a meningocele connecting the cutaneous mass to the intraspinal dura mater through defects of the posterior arches of the vertebrae. Thus the extraspinal meningioma can be interpreted as a spontaneously obliterated meningocele (27).

Treatment is surgical, with resection of the mass, which is usually curative.

NEURILEMMOMAS AND NEUROFIBROMAS

Generalities

Neurilemmoma, neurinoma, schwannoma, and perineural fibroblastoma are the terms used to designate the tumors derived from the Schwann cells that envelop the axons of the peripheral nerve roots.

Most spinal neurilemmomas are intradural, some cases are intramedullary, some are intradural-extradural, and the remainder are entirely extradural in location. Most cases present in the third and fourth decades of life.

Histology

The tumors derived from nerve sheaths are (21,29,30) (a) the neurilemmoma or schwannoma, which is composed of Schwann cells (Grade I); (b) the neurofibroma, which may be localized or diffuse, consisting of a mixture of Schwann cells and fibroblasts with abundant collagen fibers, and which is usually associated with von Recklinghausen's disease; (c) the anaplastic neurilemmoma (Grade III), which is rare; and (d) the anaplastic malignant neurofibroma (Grades III and IV), which is the malignant transformation of the neurofibroma and is also referred to as neurosarcoma.

The term neuroma is incorrect when applied to the above entities, because it designates a non-neoplastic overgrowth of nerve fibers, Schwann cells, and other components of scar tissue.

Malignant deterioration of neurilemmoma is estimated to occur in about 3% (31) to 13% (32), half or possibly more of these cases being associated with von Recklinghausen's disease (32–34). Malignancy occurs more frequently in children than in adults (7).

The neurilemmoma is a benign and usually solitary encapsulated soft tissue tumor. It rarely presents malignant changes. Its growth rate is very slow. It compresses but does not infiltrate the surrounding tissues, although it may have adhesions that make its complete enucleation difficult. Intratumoral cysts and hemorrhage can occur. It can take either of two histologic types. Both may be seen in the same tumor. Antoni type A tumors are composed of dense fibrous masses of undulating cell bundles. Antoni type B tumors consist of a much coarser reticular web with a widespread cell population and a looser structure. Electron microscopically, neurilemmomas are constituted of Schwann cells separated by collagen.

Clinical Findings

Extramedullary Neurilemmomas

Extramedullary neurilemmomas, either intradural or extradural, are among the more frequent spinal tumors [9.6% (3) to 10.9% (7)] in children. They are only half as frequent as in adults (5). Their distribution along the spine is quite uniform, although two-thirds of them are located in the cervical and lumbar regions. The tumor is usually a smooth, encapsulated ovoid mass that slowly causes cord compression. Extension of the intraspinal nerve root neurilemmoma outside the spinal cord in a dumbbell manner through the intervertebral foramina is more frequent in children between the ages of 9 and 15 years (48.0%) than in adults (26.9%) (7). More than 25% of these tumors occur in patients with von Recklinghausen's disease. Their clinical history is shorter in children than in adults.

The extravertebral mass may attain a considerable volume. Intratumoral cystic formation is more frequent in spinal than in intracranial neurilemmomas. Their focal symptomatology includes uni- or bilateral radicular pain, monoparesis, paraparesis, a sensory level, and muscular atrophy in the distribution of a specific nerve root. General symptoms and signs are stiff neck and spine, bladder dysfunction, and spinal tenderness. These symptoms are more intense, occur earlier, and are more frequent in children than in adults.

Spinal subarachnoid hemorrhage with papilledema, vertigo, and diplopia is seen occasionally. Spontaneous spinal subarachnoid hemorrhage may be the first and abrupt manifestation of a neurilemmoma or neurofibroma in a child or adolescent (35–37), although other tumors such as ependymomas, meningiomas, astrocytomas, vascular malformations, and some other processes can present in the same way. Occasionally, thoracic neurofibromas present with spinal subarachnoid hemorrhage (37). Neurilemmomas of the cauda equina may mimic a prolapsed lumbar intervertebral disk with sciatic pain occurring for several years before correct diagnosis (38). Neurilemmomas are very rarely found in the foramen magnum in children. In a series of 57 tumors located in this region, there was only one child, 12 years of age, who had a neurofibroma associated with neurofibromatosis (39).

Plexiform neurofibromas may sometimes be located in the lumbar or cervical region, but without penetrating into the spinal canal through the intervertebral foramina. This form of the disease is observed in adults as well as in children (40), and most often it occurs without neurologic problems.

Intramedullary Neurilemmomas

Neurilemmomas are rarely intramedullary. Less than 20 patients, between the ages of 12 and 68 years, have been described in the literature (41,42). Children (43) and young adults (42,44) are not often affected. The tumor is most frequently located in the cervical region, followed by the thoracic and lumbosacral segments. The tumor starts to develop in the posterior or lateroposterior portion of the spinal cord and usually grows to one side. Pardatscher et al. (45) described a 41-year-old man with multiple intramedullary neurinomas extending along the spinal cord without any external sign of neurofibromatosis. Clinical signs are motor weakness, diminished sensitivity, loss of bladder or bowel control, pain, paresthesias, and amyothrophy. Muscular fasciculations have sometimes been observed (42). The time interval between appearance of symptoms and surgical treatment ranges from a few weeks to several or many years. The symptomatology develops gradually, and there are asymptomatic periods. The intramedullary location of a neurilemmoma is a paradox since nerve fibers of the CNS do not have Schwann cell sheaths. Various hypotheses have been advanced to explain this paradoxical occurrence.

Intraosseous Neurilemmomas

Only 6 cases of neurilemmomas were encountered in a large series of 3,987 primary bone tumors (46). A review of the literature on intraosseous neurilemmomas came up with only 31 cases, 4 of them affecting the spine (47). Three of these were in the sacrum and one at L3 (48). A single case with a thoracic location has been reported recently (49). For a neurilemmoma to arise within bone, it is necessary that nerves be present in the bone. Although these nerves are not numerous, they are detectable and are unmyelinated (50). It is believed that these tumors enter the spinal canal via one of the neurovascular foramina. Once the tumor is in the bone, it enlarges, eroding the vertebrae and ribs.

Radiology

Plain films of the spine usually show abnormalities that include a widened canal, eroding of the pedicles, scalloping of the posterior margins of the vertebral bodies, and thinning of the laminae. Extradural neurofibromas usually cause widening of the intervertebral foramina and of the intercostal space, and erosion and sometimes luxation of the ribs (Fig. 1). However, more than 30% of plain spine films show no abnormality (7). Findings on myelography, CT scan, and MR dif-

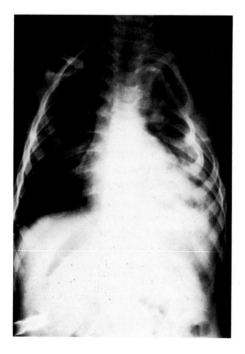

FIG. 1. A six-year-old boy with neurofibromatosis and spinal neurofibroma. The X-ray film in frontal view shows the location of the tumor in the left thoracic region (T3–T4) with displacement of the third rib upward and the fourth rib downward.

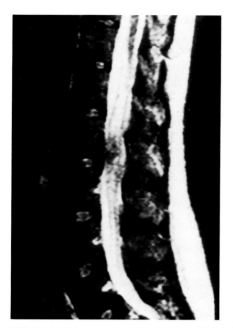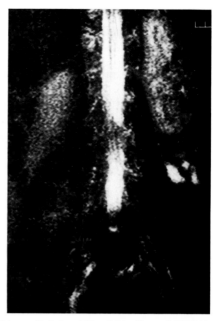

A,B

FIG. 2. A: Schwannoma of the cauda equina. MR in sagittal view (T2 weighted image). TE 200, TR 1500. Image of an intradural mass at the level of L2–L3. (Courtesy of Dr. Luis Lopez-Ibor.) **B:** Same case as (A). MR in frontal view (T2-weighted image). TE 300, TR 1000. Obstruction of the spinal canal by the tumor. (Courtesy of Dr. Luis Lopez-Ibor.)

fer, depending on the location of the tumor with respect to the spinal cord and the intervertebral foramina. A positive contrast myelogram commonly shows characteristic intradural or extradural defects, providing definite confirmation of the lesion. CT and MR are more informative because they reveal the exact location and extent of the tumor, even in difficult locations, through the use of multiplane tomographic cuts (51). However, intradural cervical neurofibromas smaller than 4 mm in diameter, which were clearly demonstrated by myelography, were missed by MR (23). Schwannomas and neurofibromas produce less predictable images by MR than other tumors of the nervous system; their T2 relaxation time may be slightly longer than that of the spinal cord and the tumor may display a more intense signal in T2 weighted images (23) (Fig. 2A,B).

Treatment

Neurilemmomas are usually benign, encapsulated, and located in the posterior aspect of the spinal canal, which makes them surgically accessible for complete removal. However, removal is not easy because damage to the surrounding structures must be avoided. Incomplete removal is commonly followed by later recurrence. Although the survival rate is very high, the quality of the patients' lives depends on timely removal of the tumors. Only two of the seven patients with a long clinical history in the series of Nayernouri (38) were free of symptoms after operation. Radiotherapy has been used for intramedullary neurofibromas (52), and is indicated as an adjunctive therapy in pathologically proven cases showing malignant changes (42,53).

REFERENCES

1. Matson DD. Intraspinal tumors in children. In: *Neurosurgery of infancy and childhood*, 2nd ed. Springfield, Ill.: Charles C Thomas, 1969.
2. De Sousa AL, Kalsbeck JE, Mealey J Jr, et al. Intraspinal tumors in children. A review of 81 cases. *J Neurosurg* 1979;51:437–445.
3. Koos W, Laubichler W, Sorgo G. Statistische Untersuchungen bein spinalen Tumoren im Kindes und Jugendalter. *Neuropadiatrie* 1973;4:273–303.
4. Merten DF, Gooding CA, Newton TH, Malamud N. Meningiomas of childhood and adolescence. *J Pediatr* 1974;84:696–700.
5. Nittner K. Spinal meningiomas, neurinomas and neurofibromas and hourglass tumours. In: Winked PJ, Bruyn GW, eds. *Handbook of clinical neurology*, vol. 20, chapter 7. Amsterdam: North-Holland, 1976.
6. Sloof JL, Kernohan JW, McCarty CS. *Primary intramedullary tumors of the spinal cord and filum terminale*. Philadelphia, London: W.B. Saunders, 1964.
7. Fortuna A, Nolletti A, Nardi P, Caruso R. Spinal neurinomas and meningiomas in children. *Acta Neurochir* 1981;55:329–341.
8. Rubinstein LJ. Tumours of the central nervous system. In: Armed Forces Institute of Pathology, eds. *Atlas of tumor pathology*, series 2, fascile 6. Washington, DC: Armed Forces Institute of Pathology, 1972;169.
9. Levy WJ Jr, Bay J, Dohn D. Spinal cord meningioma. *J Neurosurg* 1982;57:804–812.
10. Calogero JA, Moossy J. Extradural spinal meningiomas: report of four cases. *J Neurosurg* 1972;37:442–447.
11. Rand RW, Rand CW. *Intraspinal tumors of childhood*. Springfield, Ill.: Charles C Thomas, 1960;560.
12. Haft H, Shenkin HA. Spinal epidural meningioma. Case report. *J Neurosurg* 1963;20:801–804.
13. Early CB, Sayers MP. Spinal epidural meningioma. Case report. *J Neurosurg* 1966;25:571–573.
14. Kaya U, Ozden B, Turantan I, et al. Spinal epidural meningioma in children: a case report. *Neurosurgery* 1982;10:746–747.
15. Deen HG Jr, Scheithauer BW, Ebersold MJ. Clinical and pathological study of meningiomas of the first two decades of life. *J Neurosurg* 1982;56:317–322.
16. Ingraham FD. Intraspinal tumors in infancy and childhood. *Am J Surg* 1932;39:342–376.
17. Stern J, Whelan MA, Correll JW. Spinal extradural meningiomas. *Surg Neurol* 1980;14:155–159.
18. Motomochi M, Makita Y, Nebeshima S, Aoyama I. Spinal epidural meningioma in childhood. *Surg Neurol* 1980;13:5–7.
19. Hallpike JF, Stanley P. A case of extradural spinal meningioma. *J Neurol Neurosurg Psychiatry* 1968;31:195–197.
20. Ibrahim AW, Satti MB, Ibrahim EM. Extraspinal meningioma. Case report. *J Neurosurg* 1986;64:328–330.
21. Zülch KJ. Principles of the new World Health Organization (WHO) classification of brain tumors. *Neuroradiology* 1980;19:59–66.
22. Ludwin SK, Rubinstein LJ, Russell DS. Papillary meningioma: a malignant variant of meningioma. *Cancer* 1975;36:1363–1373.
23. Scotti G, Scialfa G, Colombo N, Landoni L. MR imaging of intradural extramedullary tumors of the cervical spine. *J Comput Assist Tomogr* 1985;9:1037–1041.
24. Aichner F, Poewe W, Rogalsky W, et al. Magnetic resonance imaging in the diagnosing of spinal cord diseases. *J Neurol Neurosurg Psychiatry* 1985;48:1220–1229.
25. Svien HJ, Wood MW. Recurrence of a meningioma of the spinal cord after 23 years. *Proc Mayo Clin* 1957;32:573–578.

26. Feiring EH, Barron K. Late recurrence of spinal-cord meningioma. *J Neurosurg* 1962;19:652–656.
27. Lopez DA, Silvers DN, Helwig EB. Cutaneous meningiomas—a clinical study. *Cancer* 1974; 34:728–744.
28. Zaaroor M, Borovich B, Bassan L, et al. Primary cutaneous extravertebral meningioma. Case report. *J Neurosurg* 1984;60:1097–1098.
29. del Rio-Hortega P. *The macroscopic anatomy of tumors of the central and peripheral nervous system.* Springfield, Ill.: Charles C Thomas, 1953;114–145.
30. Russell DS, Rubinstein LJ. *Pathology of tumours of the nervous system. Tumours of the nerve roots and peripheral nerves.* London: Edward Arnold, 1963;242–257.
31. Canale D, Bebin J, Knighton RS. Neurologic manifestations of von Recklinghausen's disease of the nervous system. *Confin Neurol* 1964;24:359–403.
32. Hosoi K. Multiple neurofibromatosis (von Recklinghausen's disease) with special reference to malignant transformation. *Arch Surg* 1931;22:258–281.
33. Stout AP. Tumors of the peripheral nervous system. In: Armed Forces Institute of Pathology, eds. *Atlas of tumor pathology,* section 2, fascicle 6. Washington, DC: Armed Forces Institute of Pathology, 1949;28.
34. D'Agostino AN, Soule EH, Miller RH. Sarcomas of the peripheral nerves and somatic soft tissues associated with multiple neurofibromatosis (von Recklinghausen's disease). *Cancer* 1963; 16:1015–1027.
35. Halpern J, Feldman S, Peysere E. Subarachnoid hemorrhage with papilledema due to spinal neurofibroma. *Arch Neurol Psychiatry* 1958;79:138–141.
36. Prieto A Jr, Cantu RC. Spinal subarachnoid hemorrhage associated with neurofibroma of the cauda equina. *J Neurosurg* 1967;27:63–69.
37. Grollmus J. Spinal subarachnoid hemorrhage with schwannoma. *Acta Neurochir* 1975;31:253–256.
38. Nayernouri T. Neurilemmomas of the cauda equina presenting as prolapsed lumbar intervertebral disks. *Surg Neurol* 1985;23:187–188.
39. Yasuoka S, Okazki H, Daube JR, McCarty CS. Foramen magnum tumors. Analysis of 57 cases of benign extramedullary tumors. *J Neurosurg* 1978;49:828–838.
40. Gruszkiewiez J, Doron Y, Gellei B. Plexiform neurofibromatosis of spine. *Neurochirurgie* 1972;3:99–106.
41. Cantore C, Ciapetta P, Delfini R, et al. Intramedullary spinal neurinomas. Report of two cases. *J Neurosurg* 1982;57:143–147.
42. Lesoin F, Delandsheer E, Krivosic I, et al. Solitary intramedullary schwannomas. *Surg Neurol* 1983;19:51–56.
43. Sloof JL, Kernohan JW, McCarty CS. *Primary intramedullary tumors of the spinal cord and filum terminale.* Philadelphia, London: W.B. Saunders, 1964;132–138.
44. Shalit MN, Sandbank U. Cervical intramedullary schwannoma. *Surg Neurol* 1981;16:61–64.
45. Pardatscher K, Iraci G, Cappellotto P, et al. Multiple intramedullary neurinomas of the spinal cord. Case report. *J Neurosurg* 1979;50:817–822.
46. Fawcett KJ, Dahlin DC. Neurilemmoma of bone. *Am J Clin Pathol* 1967;47:758–766.
47. Wirth WA, Bray CB Jr. Intraosseous neurilemmoma. Case report and review of thirty-one cases from the literature. *J Bone Joint Surg* 1977;59A:252–255.
48. Dickson JH, Waltz TA. Intra-osseous neurilemmoma of the third lumbar vertebra. *J Bone Joint Surg* 1971;53A:349–355.
49. Wells F, Thomas TL, Matthewson MH, Holmes AE. Neurilemmoma of the thoracic spine. A case report. *Spine* 1982;7:66–70.
50. Sherman M. The nerves of bone. *J Bone Joint Surg* 1963;45A:522–528.
51. Yang WC, Zappulla R, Malis L. Neurilemmoma in lumbar intervertebral foramen. *J Comput Assist Tomogr* 1981;5:904–906.
52. Wood WG, Rothman LM, Nussbaum BE. Intramedullary neurilemmoma of the spinal cord. Case report. *J Neurosurg* 1975;42:465–468.
53. Thommeer RTWM, Bots GTAM, Van Dulken H, et al. Neurofibrosarcoma of the cauda equina. Case report. *J Neurosurg* 1981;54:409–411.

8

Tumors of the Neural Crest

Ignacio Pascual-Castroviejo

NEUROBLASTOMAS

Generalities

Neuroblastoma is one of the neural crest tumors. It is the most common extracranial malignant solid tumor in infancy and childhood. One in 18,900 Japanese infants screened in a program to detect neuroblastoma showed the tumor (1). Neuroblastomas account for approximately 15 to 50% of neonatal malignant tumors and 7 to 14% of childhood malignant neoplasms (2–5). However, neuroblastoma presents with spinal cord compression in only 1 to 4% of cases (4,6,7). The incidence peaks at 2 years of age. The adrenal gland is the most common site of origin, but the tumor may arise from sympathetic nervous system tissue anywhere in the body. Neuroblastoma is located intraabdominally in 60 to 70% of the patients (6–9) and within the chest in 10 to 15%, although in some series, the primary tumor was almost as often mediastinal as retroperitoneal (10). Spreading of the tumor from retroperitoneal and retropleural regions to the spinal canal through the intervertebral foramina and involvement of the spine itself are common. Intraspinal neuroblastoma is uncommon, but is seen preferentially in neonates, in whom it is obviously congenital. Most children with neuroblastoma have distant metastases at the time of diagnosis (8,9,11,12). No difference in sex distribution is observed.

Neural crest tumors arise wherever neural crest cells migrate and proliferate. Malignancy of these tumors depends on the age of the patient, site of origin, the histologic maturity of the cells, and the amount of tumor present.

Clinical Aspects

Primary neuroblastomas can arise in many regions of the body, although most frequently in the adrenal glands, followed by the thoracic, cervical, and abdominal sympathetic ganglia. Neurologic symptoms and signs appear when the disease spreads to the extradural space and compresses the cord. Two-thirds of the children have metastases when first seen; in such cases, the symptomatology is predominantly that of the diseased metastasized organs and that of a systemic illness (13). Neuroblastomas with intraspinal (dumbbell) extension usually present less acutely with irritability, constipation, pain on moving the limbs, or a visible flank mass. Children over 2 years old present with motor signs, pain in the back, legs, buttocks or other sites, urinary symptoms, or constipation.

Spinal cord compression produces limb weakness or paralysis, clonus, sometimes a Babinski sign, and sphincter dysfunction. Horner's syndrome may be present when the tumor is located in the cervical and upper thoracic regions.

Infantile myoclonic encephalopathy (opsoclonus-myoclonus, opsoclonus, "dancing-eyes/dancing-feet syndrome," infantile polymyoclonia, acute cerebellar encephalopathy) (15) is caused by a neuroblastoma in 50% of cases (16,17). Since the first two patients described by Solomon and Chutorian (16), this association has been reported frequently (17–22). The most common location of the neuroblastoma associated with infantile myoclonic encephalopathy is the posterior mediastinum, followed by the abdomen, pelvis, and neck (23). There is a female predominance, as opposed to patients with neuroblastoma without myoclonic encephalopathy, who show a male predominance (23). The mean delay between onset of symptoms and diagnosis is 2.5 months, and the mean age of patients is 17 months (23). Catecholamine excretion is normal in many patients with this disease (23–25). The exact pathophysiology of the myoclonic encephalopathy in patients with neuroblastoma is not known, although many hypotheses have been suggested (24–25).

One patient with a tumor in the pelvic region presented signs of sciatic nerve involvement. Another rare case described by Ljung et al. (26), who had an exclusively intraspinal ganglioneuroma, presented with foot deformities.

Patients with metastasis from neuroblastoma frequently present fever, proptosis, and orbital ecchymosis (Fig. 1), enlarged nodes, weight loss, vomiting, and pallor (13). The peculiar facies of children with cranial metastases of neuroblastoma is well known (27). The interval between the onset of symptoms and diagnosis averaged 4 to 6.5 weeks in some series (10,28). However, delays of several years before diagnosis are common (14). Neuroblastoma should be considered as a possible diagnosis for any unexplained neurologic condition in a child (29).

A particular form of the disease is congenital intraspinal neuroblastoma, which is a rare neoplasm. In a relatively recent review of the English literature, only 21 cases were found (30). However, there are several more cases reported in other languages (19), and, in some series of intraspinal neuroblastomas, 19 to 20% had neurologic disease at birth (10,31). The patients present with paresis of the lower limbs, a patulous anus, urinary incontinence, and may have an abdominal or flank mass at birth. The tumor, which is commonly large, is located in the lower thoracic or upper lumbar region and is extradural in location. Males are affected slightly more often than females. Examination of the primary tumor suggests that the lesion may arise from cell rests or have extended in a dumbbell fashion from a paraspinal mass through the intervertebral foramina (32). Occasionally, the tumor may arise entirely within the spinal canal (33). These tumors can simulate myelodysplasia in some cases. Osseous metastases are uncommon in congenital intraspinal neuroblastoma, but metastases to other structures such as the liver and brain have been observed (34). With appropriate treatment, the tumor can be controlled

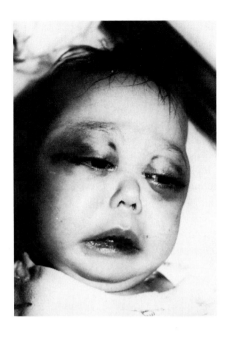

FIG. 1. A 1-year-old child with generalized metastases of neuroblastoma. He shows the typical facies of this disorder, with bilateral orbital ecchymoses, dry lips, and a suffering expression.

in most patients, and the survival rate is high. However, paresis of the legs and urinary and sexual problems persist (32). The current recommendation is for local resection. Radiotherapy and chemotherapy are adjuvant treatments which are considered detrimental to newborns (30,31).

Laboratory Tests

Urine catecholamine levels are elevated up to threefold in 75% of the patients (13,28). Most likely, the catecholamines produced by the tumor are rapidly converted to the inactive vanillylmandelic acid (VMA) and homovanillic acid (HVA) that are eliminated in the urine. The small variations that exist in the excretion of HVA and VMA during different periods of the day result from variations in renal excretion rather than variations in production (35), which indicates that a random urine sample should be as good as a 24-hr collection for diagnosis and follow-up of neural crest tumors. Patients with ganglioneuroma may present only marginally elevated levels of catecholamines.

A significant number of patients with neuroblastomas secrete norepinephrine and epinephrine, but this does not produce hypertension.

An abnormal circulating ganglioside was found in patients with neuroblastoma (36). This ganglioside appears as a single band by resorcinol-HCl staining of thin-layer chromatograms of purified total gangliosides. Measurement of this circulating tumor-associated ganglioside should be useful clinically in neuroblastoma, offering a new approach to the detection of tumor and the evaluation of therapy.

Blood changes, especially anemia, have been observed in patients with neuro-blastomas and bony metastases (37). Bone marrow aspiration or biopsy is required to visualize the tumor cells.

The sympathetic nervous system influences the growth of neuroblastoma both *in vivo* and *in vitro* (38). The sympathetic nervous system exerts a trophic-mitogenic influence on C-1300 mouse neuroblastoma. Sympathetic axotomy suppresses the growth of some clonal lines of neuroblastoma but does not influence the growth *in vivo* of other clonal lines. Sympathetic ganglia-conditioned medium significantly increases the proliferation of some clonal cell lines *in vitro*, while not influencing other clonal cell lines. Chelmicka-Schorr et al. (38) postulate that the sympathetic nervous system secretes a trophic-mitogenic factor that favors growth of C-1300 neuroblastomas *in vivo*, the sensitivity to this factor differing among neuroblas-toma clonal lines.

Genetics

A family history of malignancy or a premalignant condition is elicited in some cases. Carachi et al. (28) stated that 13% of the children of their series had a family with this type of problem. Familial neuroblastoma has sometimes been reported (39–50). Wong et al. (39) described two brothers with neuroblastoma whose father presented with elevated urinary HVA, suggesting the possibility of an autosomal dominant trait. Neuroblastoma and neurofibromatosis are sometimes associated (28). The risk of neuroblastoma in siblings or offspring of most people with neuroblastoma appears to be less than 6% (50). Chromosomal aberrations and oncogenes have been detected recently in embryonal malignancies (51).

Histology

Histologically, tumors originating from the neural crest may be classified as (a) ganglioneuroma, (b) ganglioneuroblastoma, and (c) neuroblastoma. This last type can be subdivided into differentiated and undifferentiated types (28).

The histologic features that define each type are:

(a) *Ganglioneuroma*: Fibroblasts, collagen, and Schwann cells with clumps of ganglion cells; no neuroblasts.

(b) *Ganglioneuroblastoma*: Neuroblastoma cells, usually well differentiated, in-termixed with recognizable ganglion cells. (Ganglioneuromatous areas predomi-nate in regions where the tumor is composed of neuroblasts.)

(c) *Differentiated neuroblastoma*: Neuroblastoma cells with recognizable differ-entiation, with prominent neurofibrillary material between the tumor cells. No differentiated ganglion cells are visible.

(d) *Undifferentiated neuroblastoma*: Diffuse sheets of neuroblasts without sig-nificant neurofibrillary differentiation, although electron microscopy reveals char-acteristic neurosecretory granules.

The term neuroblastoma is commonly used to include categories (a) through (d) above. A majority of authors accept the staging classification for neuroblastoma given by Evans et al. (52) that is shown in Table 1.

Subclassification of Stage II patients into lymph-node-positive and lymph-node-negative groups may help define those patients who might benefit from improved adjuvant postsurgical treatment, because lymph node involvement has adverse prognostic significance (53).

The dura appears to be relatively resistant to infiltration by neuroblastoma in primary paraspinal tumors as well as in intracranial metastasis (27).

Fine-needle aspiration biopsy smears permit one to determine the tumor's cytomorphologic features by light and electron microscopy and is an effective way to diagnose neuroblastomas (54).

Radiology

Radiographs of the spine may show increased interpedicular distances, enlarged intervertebral foramina, thinning or overgrowth of the pedicles, scalloping of the posterior vertebral body, or widening of the spinal canal when a part of the tumor is intraspinal, and rib thinning with an increased distance between ribs which are sometimes subluxated when the tumor is intrathoracic. Paraspinal masses can be seen on chest or abdominal X-rays. Ultrasound can differentiate among abdominal masses with considerable accuracy, especially if they are cystic. Ultrasonically, neuroblastomas have a variable appearance but are usually solid. A retroperitoneal neuroblastoma was discovered in a fetus by ultrasonography during a routine pregnancy check in the 29th week of amenorrhea (55) and was confirmed after birth. About 60% of abdominal neuroblastomas occur in the adrenal glands and, on urography, show caudal and lateral displacement of the kidney (Fig. 2). About 50% of these cases show calcification on conventional radiographs. Brasch et al. (56) found no difference in sensitivity (87%) and specificity (100%) between ultrasound and computerized tomography (CT) studies, although CT yielded a more accurate differential diagnosis. Myelogram with the use of metrizamide, com-

TABLE 1. *Staging for neuroblastoma*

Stage I	Tumors confined to the organ or structure of origin.
Stage II	Tumors extending in continuity beyond the organ or structure of origin but not crossing the midline. Homolateral lymph nodes may be involved.
Stage III	Tumors extending in continuity beyond the midline. Bilateral regional lymph nodes may be involved.
Stage IV	Dissemination with metastases in skeleton, organs, soft tissue, distant lymph nodes, etc.
Stage IV-S *(special category)*	Patients who would be in Group I or II were it not for the fact that they show dissemination in liver, spleen, or bone marrow, but without radiographic evidence of bone metastases after complete skeletal survey.

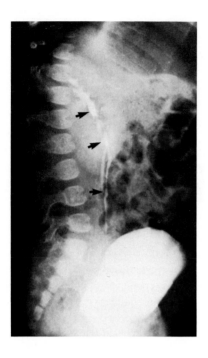

FIG. 2. Neuroblastoma affecting several intervertebral foramina, which are enlarged. Urography shows severe forward displacement of the kidneys and ureters (*arrows*) by the tumor.

bined, if possible, with CT scan, demonstrates a total or partial block, with the typical picture of an extradural mass with paraspinal extension. Comprehensive workup includes intravenous urogram, skeletal survey, and bone and liver scan. Today, ultrasonography, CT scan, and/or magnetic resonance (MR) are the procedures of choice. Comparative studies performed before the availability of MR have shown that CT gave essential information for 47% of management decisions, while non-CT studies provided information for only 28% (57).

Some authors have recommended the routine performance of myelography in all patients with paraspinal tumors, even in those without clinical and radiographic evidence of intraspinal extension (58,59). The retroperitoneal space is an area poorly visualized by conventional radiographic techniques, and, in this respect, CT has a great advantage over conventional studies such as plain X-rays, ultrasound, and scintigraphy. CT also permits the evaluation of the location, extension, calcification, and composition of tumors, particularly in extensive neoplasms (Fig. 3), which may be bilateral and may involve either bone or the spinal canal. CT also enables the assessment of pelvic lesions that may have deep extensions or sacral involvement (60).

CT reveals calcifications in about 40 to 80% of abdominal neuroblastomas. These are likely to have a streaky or curvilinear appearance (58,59). During chemotherapy, the most common change in tumor morphology is a decrease in the size of the mass and an increase in calcification, although a few tumors remain unchanged and become less calcified (59).

MR, with its ability to image sections in the sagittal and coronal as well as the

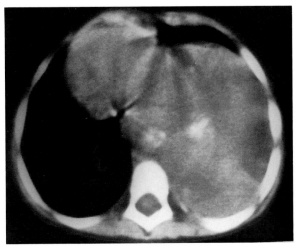

FIG. 3. Intrathoracic giant neuroblastoma. The CT shows a voluminous mass spreading into the right hemithoracic cavity. Note intratumoral calcifications.

axial planes, provides accurate tumor localization and enables management planning. MR may obviate the need for myelography, since it can show the intraspinal extension of the neuroblastoma (61). This tumor is best demonstrated using proton spin lattice relaxation time (T1) and weighted images such as inversion recovery or calculated T1, rather than proton density (62). MR clearly demonstrates the extent of the primary tumor and the presence of bony metastases (62).

Congenital intraspinal neuroblastomas produce more or less the same radiologic findings as postnatal ones. However, punctate and amorphous intraspinal calcification, associated with interpediculate widening in plain films, is probably pathognomonic for congenital intraspinal neuroblastoma (30). CT assists in therapeutic planning such as calculating dose levels and portals of entry for radiotherapy, staging the disease, and evaluating the results of treatment (60), as well as in planning secondary surgery.

In addition to producing moth-eaten lacunae of the vault, cranial metastases of neuroblastomas can produce very wide splitting of the cranial sutures (Fig. 4) (including those of the orbit), irregular thickening of the bones with "hairbrush" images (Fig. 5), displacement of the basal cisterns, obstruction of the carotid siphon, thrombosis of the cavernous sinus, and excessive vascularization of the metastases (11).

Differential Diagnosis

Many benign and malignant tumors occur in children at the same early age as neuroblastomas. Differential diagnosis is usually not difficult, provided attention is paid to the patient's history, physical examination, excretion of catecholamines,

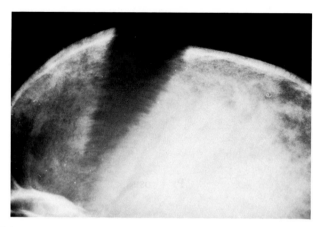

FIG. 4. Cranial metastases of neuroblastoma. The X-ray film shows very wide diastasis of the coronal suture.

and provided appropriate radiologic methods are used. New imaging techniques available today provide an almost definitive diagnosis.

The presence of a paraspinal mass with either a radiographically normal spine or widened spinal canal in a neonate with paralyzed legs should suggest congenital intraspinal neuroblastoma. Multiple lytic bone lesions anywhere on the body, with wide splitting of the skull sutures and a characteristic facies with proptosis and orbital ecchymosis suggest the diagnosis of generalized metastatic neuroblastoma. Intracerebral metastases from neuroblastoma are exceptionally rare. We observed them only once. There is a reported case of cerebellar metastases from an abdominal tumor (27). Many other tumors may present signs or symptoms in a location or with clinical and radiological findings that make it necessary to consider neuroblastoma in the differential diagnosis. Masses in the abdomen must be differenti-

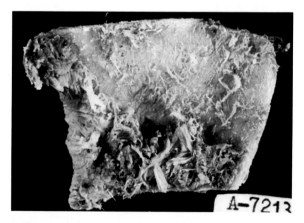

FIG. 5. A small part of the cranial vault in a case of neuroblastoma with generalized metastases showing irregular infiltration of the external table of the skull.

ated from Wilms tumor, pheochromocytoma, multicystic kidney, or other benign or malignant tumors. In the neck, one needs to consider enlarged lymph nodes, cysts, and thyroid enlargement; in the thorax, neurinoma, teratoma, and duplication of the esophagus; and in the head and face, osteoma (very rare), dermoid cyst (quite frequent, but isolated and associated with quite specific lytic lesion in the skull), bumps related to trauma, multiple lytic metastases from a lymphangioma (very easy to distinguish because of an external hemangiolymphangioma or lymphangioma) (27), histiocytosis X, and several other benign and malignant conditions.

Prognosis

Several prognostic factors may be assessed at diagnosis. The main prognostic factors are (a) histopathology, (b) age, (c) tumor site and extent, (d) quantity of neuron-specific enolase in serum, (e) serum ferritin levels, (f) N-myc oncogene, and (g) amount of DNA.

Histopathology

The prognosis for patients with neuroblastoma varies with the stage of the disease and the age at diagnosis. According to the classification by Evans et al. (52) of the different types of neuroblastomas, Stage I, corresponding to localized disease, has the best prognosis, and Stage IV, correlating with widespread disease, has the worst outcome. None of the children with Stage IV at diagnosis could be saved (63). Stage IV-S, a special form of widespread neuroblastoma, is an exception, because it frequently undergoes spontaneous regression and has an excellent prognosis (52,64,65). In all cases, spontaneous regression from the more malignant to the more benign forms may occur (8,66). It has been estimated that at least 1% of all cases of neuroblastoma regress, particularly in children under one year of age. In a compiled series of 126 cases of malignant tumors that regressed unexpectedly, 29 were neuroblastomas (67). The prognosis for patients with neuroblastoma associated with myoclonic encephalopathy is excellent; this may be partially explained by an earlier diagnosis and by a higher percentage (71%) of cases observed with Stage I, II, and IV-S disease (68). However, the prognosis for the myoclonic encephalopathy itself is variable, because there are many patients in whom opsoclonus and myoclonus persist despite complete tumor removal (26). These patients show some improvement following treatment with ACTH or steroids (22,23).

Age

Another variable correlated with prognosis is age at diagnosis. Stage for stage, younger patients have a better outcome (69,70). It is widely known that patients under 1 year of age at the time of presentation (4,6,8–10,63,71–74) have a much better prognosis than children over 1 year of age.

Tumor Site and Extent

Patients with thoracic neuroblastomas have a better prognosis than those with tumors located in any other site of the body (10,28,52,71,73–76). Carachi et al. (28) reported a mortality of 16.5% among patients with thoracic neuroblastomas, which is in striking contrast with the 86.0% mortality in abdominal cases.

The extent of the disease at the time of diagnosis is more important than the site of the primary tumor as a prognostic factor (13). When patients present spinal cord compression, disseminated disease is quite infrequent. This is reflected by the relatively good long-term survival rate reported in some series (10,33,63, 72,74). Tumor growth is believed to be related to prognosis (77). A diameter greater than 5 cm is regarded as less favorable. However, size alone has not been considered decisive by some authors (28). Benign ganglioneuroma and ganglioneuroblastoma have a more favorable prognosis than the more malignant neuroblastomas.

Quantity of Neuron-Specific Enolase in Serum

A good or poor prognosis for children with Stage IV tumors may be predicted through the quantitation of neuron-specific enolase (NSE) in the serum. Zeltzer et al. (78) found that 96% of their patients had levels more than three standard deviations above the mean for age-related normal children. Serum levels greater than 100 ng/ml were associated with a poor outcome, since 7 of 8 children died within 12 months of diagnosis, whereas all 7 of those with serum NSE below 100 ng/ml were alive 36 months and more after diagnosis.

Serum Ferritin Levels

Another test to help assess prognosis of neuroblastoma is the serum ferritin level which differs in patients with Stages IV and IV-S. Ferritin levels are elevated in those with Stage IV disease, whereas patients with Stage IV-S usually show low or normal levels (79). Hann et al. (80) measured serum ferritin levels in a series of 241 patients with neuroblastoma and observed that they were infrequently elevated in patients with Stage I and II disease but were elevated in 37% and 54% of those with Stage III and IV disease, respectively. Moreover, tumors of Stages III and IV with elevated ferritin had a significantly poorer prognosis than those with normal levels. The determination of the level of ferritin in the serum at diagnosis may be helpful for selecting appropriate therapy, especially for patients with Stage III neuroblastoma.

N-myc Oncogene

Aberrant expression of proto-oncogenes is implicated in the causation of various malignant neoplasms. Aberration may occur when regulation of a single gene is faulty, when multiple copies of a gene are formed, or when mutation results in an oncogenic product. Human neuroblastoma cell lines have multiple copies of a DNA sequence that is related to the v-myc and c-myc oncogenes, and is designated N-myc (81,82). Genomic amplification results in production of high levels of RNA specific for N-myc (82). N-myc itself may function as an oncogene when cotransfected with the mutant c-HA-ras 1 (EJ) oncogene in cultured mammalian cells (83). There is a correlation between the amplification of N-myc oncogene in untreated primary neuroblastomas, particularly those that already are disseminated at diagnosis, and early tumor progression (84). Stages II, III, and IV neuroblastomas show a higher number of copies of N-myc than State IV-S, indicating that genomic amplification of N-myc contributes to the aggressiveness of neuroblastoma cells and thus to their malignant phenotype (85). The absence of amplification in all Stage IV-S tumors may indicate that the tumor regresses spontaneously at many sites (86). Genomic amplification and synthesis of large amounts of N-myc mRNA are characteristic of continuously proliferating neuroblastoma cell lines (81,82). The association of a single copy of N-myc with Stage IV-S tumors, and of multiple copies with Stage IV tumors, provides evidence for biological differences between these two types of metastatic neuroblastoma (85). The number of N-myc copies in primary untreated neuroblastoma is a new and clinically important prognostic factor that is independent of the stage of the tumor. Seeger et al. (85) concluded from their study that patients with Stage I, II, III, and IV-S tumors and children with Stage IV disease whose tumors show a single copy of N-myc usually have a good prognosis with conventional therapy, rendering a more aggressive therapy unnecessary. Those with Stage IV disease, diagnosed after 1 year of age, whose tumors have one copy of N-myc, have an intermediate prognosis, but almost all eventually suffer progression of their disease. Why this group has a bad outcome is not known. Patients with Stage II, III, or IV tumors containing multiple copies of N-myc have the worst prognosis, because progressive disease develops soon after diagnosis. Improving survival in the latter two groups requires more aggressive therapy from the moment diagnosis and prognosis have been established.

Amount of DNA

Abnormal DNA content of neuroblastoma cells is an unequivocal marker for malignant disease and has been linked to rate of cell proliferation, stage of cell differentiation, and prognosis in some of the tumor types (87,88). In unresectable neuroblastoma of infants, hyperdiploid DNA content of the malignant cells is a favorable prognostic feature when the tumor is treated with cyclophosphamide and doxorubicin (89). All infants with Stage IV-S disease showed clonal hyperdiploid abnormalities, which were indicative of malignant disease and not of benign hyperplasia (89).

Treatment

Current recommendations for the management of intraspinal neuroblastoma in all age groups include the three modalities of surgery, radiotherapy, and chemotherapy in varying combinations.

Regarding surgery, decompressive laminectomy may be urgently required in cases with signs of spinal cord compression, as well as in cases with intraspinal dumbbell tumors. Some patients need a second laminectomy for recurrence. Total removal of the tumor is feasible only in Stages I and II patients; it is rarely possible in patients with extradural Stage III tumors. Residual tumor is commonly left around nerve roots, ventral to the spinal cord, and in the foramina (14). Thoracotomy or laparotomy may be necessary to remove the tumor when intrathoracic, intra-abdominal, or pelvic structures are compressed. Laminectomy not only avoids neurologic deterioration and growth of tumor but also provides material for histologic diagnosis. It has also been recommended to perform bone marrow aspiration and needle biopsy under the same general anesthetic in order to provide accurate staging, preferably at two sites (10,13). Complete surgical removal of the tumor is the therapy of choice in neuroblastoma associated with myoclonic encephalopathy.

If radiologic studies do not disclose metastases and if the paraspinal mass is well-circumscribed, resection by thoracotomy or laparotomy is recommended (10). Laparotomy might be considered unjustified in cases in which the intraspinal component shows ganglioneuroblastoma, because the extraspinal component tends to be more mature than the intraspinal component (10). Prolonged paralytic ileus may occur after removal of large retroperitoneal tumors, and, in some cases, parenteral nutrition may be necessary (10). Second operations may be necessary in order to eradicate the primary focus of the tumor or selective areas of metastatic disease. Secondary operation should follow the onset of radiotherapy by 4 to 6 weeks, or of chemotherapy by 12 to 24 weeks (90). This delay allows maximum control of primary and generalized disease, as well as maturation, differentiation, encapsulation, and shrinkage of an extensive, initially unresectable primary tumor (90). Postoperative radiotherapy is recommended. Doses depend on the patient's age and particular circumstances. Low doses (between 1,000 and 1,500 rad) are recommended for children under 1 year of age (10,14). The usual dose is 2,500 to 4,000 rad, directed to the tumor site (10,28). Some authors report that patients receiving lower dose radiation (< 2,000 rad) do as well as those receiving higher doses (14).

Chemotherapy is indicated (a) in nonmetastatic cases with immature histology where the abdominal component is unresectable (Stage III), (b) when metastases are present (Stage IV), and (c) when no paraspinal tumor is found, that is, when cord compressing is due to intraspinal metastasis. Several agents are used, including vincristine, cyclophosphamide, vitamin B_{12}, vinblastine, melphalan, Adriamycin, DTIC, and some others, either singly or in combination. Punt et al. (10) recommend induction with vincristine, cyclophosphamide, and Adriamycin, followed by consolidation with high-dose melphalan.

Spinal deformity is one of the sequelae of intraspinal neuroblastoma. In a series of 419 children with malignant neuroblastoma (91), 18% survived more than 5 years, and of the survivors, 20% had spinal deformity severe enough to warrant treatment. The factors associated with the development of spinal deformity were (a) orthovoltage radiation exceeding 3,000 rad, (b) asymmetrical radiation of the spine, (c) thoracolumbar kyphosis, and (d) epidural spread of the tumor.

The systemic and nutritional sequelae of neuroblastoma are related to tumor burden, tumor host-influenced metabolic effects, and surgical, pharmacologic, and radiation therapy (92).

PARAGANGLIOMA OF THE CAUDA EQUINA

Paragangliomas are rare tumors of neural crest origin. The term paraganglioma comes from the histologic pattern resembling the structure of normal paraganglia (carotid body, glomus jugularis).

These tumors are commonly located in the head and neck, although they can be found anywhere in the body. Their spinal location has occasionally been described. The author knows of only eight cases of paraganglioma in the spinal canal reported in the literature, always in the region of the cauda equina-filum terminale (93,94). All but one of the patients were middle-aged adults. The nonadult case was a 13-year-old boy (94) whose symptoms began with low back pain radiating to the left leg and buttock. The pain worsened, increasing with head or body movement, and caused him to limp. Although the duration of the symptoms prior to diagnosis was only 2 months in this child, it is usually longer in adult cases, lasting between 6 months (95) and 15 years (96) before surgical treatment. A characteristic feature of spinal paraganglioma is a marked increase of the cerebrospinal fluid (CSF) protein concentration, which suggests the diagnosis of spinal paraganglioma. X-rays of the spine are usually normal in cases with a short evolution (94,95,97), whereas vertebral erosion or destruction occurs in patients whose symptoms go back several years (93,96,98–100). Myelography shows complete block with the features of an intradural extramedullary mass.

Paraganglioma is characterized by a relatively bland, organoid growth of cells which contain argyrophilic and, ultrastructurally, dense-core granules or vesicles. The presence of mild nuclear pleomorphism with relatively frequent mitotic figures has been reported in only one case of spinal paraganglioma (94), although these features are occasionally seen in paragangliomas located elsewhere. Metastatic spread of paraganglioma has not been reported in spinal cases and is rare in paragangliomas in other locations (101). Complete surgical resection with close follow-up is indicated.

REFERENCES

1. Sawada T. Outcome of 25 neuroblastomas revealed by mass screening in Japan. *Lancet* 1986;i:377.
2. Schneider KM, Becker JM, Krasma IH. Neonatal neuroblastoma. *Pediatrics* 1965;36:350–366.
3. Giuffre R, DiLorenzo N. Primary spinal cord tumors in infancy and childhood. In: Modern problems in pediatrics. *Neurosurgery* Basel: Karger, 1977;18:231–235.
4. Le Pintre J, Schweisguth O, Labrune M, Lemerle J. Les neuroblastomes en sablier. Etude de 22 cas. *Arch Fr Pediatr* 1969;26:829–847.
5. Till K. *Pediatric neurosurgery.* Oxford: Blackwell, 1975;200.
6. Koop CE, Hernandez JR. Neuroblastomas: experience with 190 cases in children. *Surgery* 1964;56:726–733.
7. Jones PG, Campbell PE. *Tumours of infancy and childhood.* Oxford: Blackwell, 1976;543.
8. Gross RE, Farber S, Martin LW. Neuroblastoma sympatheticum. A study and report of 217 cases. *Pediatrics* 1959;23:1179–1191.
9. De Lorimer AA, Braggs KU, Linden G. Neuroblastoma in childhood. *Am J Dis Child* 1969; 118:441–450.
10. Punt J, Pritchard J, Pincott JR, Till K. Neuroblastoma: a review of 21 cases presenting with spinal cord compression. *Cancer* 1980;45:3095–3101.
11. Pascual-Castroviejo I, López-Martín V, Rodriguez-Costa T, Pascual-Pascual JI. Radiological and anatomical aspects of the cranial metastases of neuroblastoma. *Neuroradiology* 1975;9:33–38.
12. Hartmann O, Scopinare M, Tourinade MF, et al. Neuroblastomes traités à l'Institut Gustave-Roussy. Cent soixante-treize cas. *Arch Fr Pediatr* 1983;40:15–21.
13. Evans AE, D'Angio CJ, Koop CE. Diagnosis and treatment of neuroblastoma. *Pediatr Clin N Am* 1976;23:161–170.
14. Holgersen LD, Santulli TV, Schullinger JN, Berdon WE. Neuroblastoma with intraspinal (dumb-bell) extension. *J Pediatr Surg* 1983;18:406–411.
15. Kinsbourne M. Myoclonic encephalopathy of infants. *J Neurol Neurosurg Psychiatry* 1962; 25:271–279.
16. Solomon G, Chutorian AM. Opsoclonus with occult neuroblastoma. *N Engl J Med* 1968; 279:475–477.
17. Bray PF, Ziter FA, Lahey ME, Myers CG. The coincidence of neuroblastoma and acute cerebellar encephalopathy. *J Pediatr* 1969;75:983–990.
18. Dyken P, Kolar O. Dancing eyes, dancing feet. Infantile polymyoclonia. *Brain* 1968;91:305–320.
19. Navarro Gonzalez J, Martinez Caro A, Claro Fernandez F, et al. Encefalopatiá mioclonica infantil y ganglioneuroblastoma. Presentacíon de un caso y ravisión de la literatura. *An Esp Pediatr* 1973;6:398–410.
20. Keating JW, Cromwell LD. Remote effects of neuroblastoma. *Am J Roentgenol* 1978;131:299–303.
21. Boltshauser E, Deonna T, Hirt WR. Myoclonic encephalopathy of infants or "dancing eyes syndrome." *Helv Paediatr Acta* 1979;34:119–133.
22. Nickerson BG, Nutter J Jr. Opsomyoclonus and neuroblastoma: response to ACTH. *Clin Pediatr* 1979;18:446–448.
23. Baker ME, Kirks DR, Korobkin M, et al. The association of neuroblastoma and myoclonic encephalopathy: an imaging approach. *Pediatr Radiol* 1985;15:185–188.
24. Senelick RC, Bray PF, Lahey ME, et al. Neuroblastoma and myoclonic encephalopathy: two cases and a review of the literature. *J Pediatr Surg* 1973;8:623–632.
25. Kinast M, Levin HS, Rothner AD, et al. Cerebellar ataxia, opsoclonus and occult neural crest tumor: abdominal computerized tomography in diagnosis. *Am J Dis Child* 1980;134:1057–1059.
26. Ljung R, Halin I, Stromblad LG. Ganglioneuroma with an uncommon location in a six-year-old girl. *Acta Paediatr Scand* 1984;73:411–413.
27. Pascual-Castroviejo I. *Neurología infantil.* Barcelona: Ed Cientifico-Médica, 1983;1226–1230.

28. Carachi R, Cambell PE, Kent M. Thoracic neural crest tumors. A clinical review. *Cancer* 1983; 51:949–954.
29. Latchaw RE, L'Heureux PR, Young G, Priest JR. Neuroblastoma presenting as central nervous system disease. *Am J Neuroradiol* 1982;3:623–630.
30. Haden MA, Koats TE. Congenital intraspinal neuroblastoma with intraspinal calcification in the neonatal period: report of a case with a 32-year follow-up. *Pediatr Radiol* 1983;13:335–338.
31. Sainte-Rose C, Roux FX, Pierre-Kahn A, et al. Les neuroblastomes intrarachidiens congénitaux. A propos de 7 cas opérés. *Neurochirurgie* 1982;28:409–415.
32. Moschos A, Anagnostakis D. Congenital neuroblastomas with paraplegia. Case report. *Helv Paediatr Acta* 1975;30:521–523.
33. Fagan CJ, Swischuk LE. Dumb-bell neuroblastoma or ganglioneuroma of the spinal canal. *Am J Roentgenol* 1964;120:453–460.
34. Kenney PG, Siegal MJ, McAlister WH. Congenital intraspinal neuroblastoma: a treatable simulant of myelodysplasia. *Am J Roentgenol* 1982;138:166–167.
35. Tuchman M, Robinson LL, Maynard RC, et al. Assessment of the diurnal variations in urinary homovanillic and vanillylmandelic acid excretion for the diagnosis and follow-up of patients with neuroblastoma. *Clin Biochem* 1985;18:176–179.
36. Ladisch S, Wu Z. Detection of a tumor-associated ganglioside in plasma of patients with neuroblastoma. *Lancet* 1985;i:136–138.
37. Mancini AF, Rosito P, Vecchi V, et al. Il neuroblastoma. Aspetti ematologici e considerazioni prognostiche. *Minerva Pediatr* 1978;30:301–312.
38. Chelmicka-Schorr E, Jones KH, Chevinski ME, et al. Influence of the sympathetic nervous system on the growth of neuroblastoma in vivo and in vitro. *Cancer Res* 1985;45:6213–6215.
39. Wong KY, Hanenson IB, Lampkin BC. Familial neuroblastoma. *Am J Dis Child* 1971;121:415–416.
40. Feingold M, Gheradi CJ, Simos C. Familial neuroblastoma. *Am J Dis Child* 1971;121:451.
41. Hardy PC, Nesbit ME Jr. Familial neuroblastoma: report of a kindred with a high incidence of infantile tumors. *J Pediatr* 1972;80:74–77.
42. Knudson AG Jr, Strong LC. Mutation and cancer. Neuroblastoma and pheochromocytoma. *Am J Hum Genet* 1972;24:514–532.
43. Wagget J, Aherne G, Aherne W. Familial neuroblastoma: report of two sib pairs. *Arch Dis Child* 1973;48:63–66.
44. Roberts FF, Lee KR. Familial neuroblastoma presenting as multiple tumors. *Radiology* 1975;116:133–136.
45. Pogelow CH, Ebbin AJ, Powars D, Towner JW. Familial neuroblastoma. *J Pediatr* 1975;87:763–765.
46. Arenson EB, Hutter JJ, Restuccia RD, Holton CP. Neuroblastoma in father and son. *JAMA* 1976;235:727–729.
47. Bond JV. Familial neuroblastoma and ganglioneuroblastoma (letter). *JAMA* 1976;236:561–562.
48. Hecht F, Hecht BK, Northup JC, et al. Genetics of familial neuroblastoma: long-range studies. *Cancer Genet Cytogenet* 1982;7:227–230.
49. Mancine AF, Rosito P, Fadella G, et al. Neuroblastoma in a pair of identical twins. *Med Pediatr Oncol* 1982;10:45–51.
50. Kushner BH, Gilbert F, Helson L. Familial neuroblastoma. Case reports, literature review, and etiologic considerations. *Cancer* 1986;57:1887–1893.
51. Yunis JJ. The chromosomal basis of human neoplasia. *Science* 1983;221:227–236.
52. Evans AE, D'Angio CJ, Randolf J. A proposed staging for children with neuroblastoma. *Cancer* 1971;27:374–380.
53. Ninane J, Pritchard J, Morris Jones PH, et al. Stage II neuroblastoma. Adverse prognostic significance of lymph node involvement. *Arch Dis Child* 1982;57:438–442.
54. Akhtar M, Ali MA, Sabbah RS, et al. Aspiration cytology of neuroblastomas. Light and electron microscopic correlations. *Cancer* 1986;57:797–803.
55. Fénart D, Deville A, Donceau M, Bruneton JN. Neuroblastome rétroperitoneal diagnostiqué in utero. A propos de 1 cas. *J Radiol* 1983;64:359–361.
56. Brasch RC, Abolis IB, Gooding CA, Filly RA. Abdominal disease in children. A comparison of computed tomography and ultrasound. *Am J Roentgenol* 1980;134:153–158.
57. Arger PH, Mulhern CB Jr, Littman PS, et al. Management of solid tumors in children: contribution of computed tomography. *Am J Roentgenol* 1981;137:251–255.

58. Armstrong EA, Harwood-Nash DCF, Fitz CR, et al. CT of neuroblastomas and ganglioneuromas in children. *Am J Roentgenol* 1982;139:571–576.
59. Goldin SJ, McElwain TJ, Husband JE. The role of computed tomography in the management of children with advanced neuroblastoma. *Br J Radiol* 1984;57:661–66.
60. Cremin BJ, Mervis B. Paediatric abdominal computed tomography: the technique and use in neuroblastomas and pelvic mass. *Br J Radiol* 1983;56:291–298.
61. Siegel MJ, Jamroz GA, Glazer HS, Abramson CL. MR imaging of intraspinal extension of neuroblastoma. *J Comput Assist Tomogr* 1986;15:593–595.
62. Smith FW, Cherryman GR, Redpath TW, Grosher G. The nuclear magnetic resonance appearances of neuroblastoma. *Pediatr Radiol* 1985;15:329–332.
63. Traggis DG, Filler RM, Druckman H, et al. Prognosis for children with neuroblastoma presenting with paralysis. *J Pediatr Surg* 1977;12:419–425.
64. D'Angio CG, Evans AE, Koop CE. Special pattern of widespread neuroblastoma with a favorable prognosis. *Lancet* 1971;i:1046–1049.
65. Eklöf O, Sanstedt B, Thönel S, Anström L. Spontaneous regression of stage IV neuroblastoma. *Acta Paediatr Scand* 1983;72:473–476.
66. Bolande RP. Benignity of neonatal tumours and the concept of cancer regression in early life. *Am J Dis Child* 1971;122:12–14.
67. Everson TC, Cole WH. *Spontaneous regression of cancer*. Philadelphia: W.B. Saunders, 1966.
68. Altman AJ, Baehner RL. Favourable prognosis for survival in children with coincident opsomyoclonus and neuroblastoma. *Cancer* 1976;37:846–852.
69. Breslow N, McCann B. Statistical estimation of prognosis for children with neuroblastoma. *Cancer Res* 1971;31:2098–2103.
70. Finklestein JZ, Klemperer MR, Evans A, et al. Multiagent chemotherapy for children with metastatic neuroblastoma: a report from Children's Cancer Study Group. *Med Pediatr Oncol* 1979;6:179–188.
71. Kinier-Wilson KM, Draper CJ. Neuroblastoma: its natural history and prognosis: the study of 487 cases. *Br Med J* 1974;3:301–307.
72. King D, Goodman J, Hawk T, et al. Dumbbell neuroblastomas in children. *Arch Surg* 1975;110:888–891.
73. Filler RM, Traggis DG, Jaffe N, Vawter GF. Favorable outlook for children with mediastinal neuroblastoma. *J Pediatr Surg* 1972;7:136–143.
74. Balakrishnan V, Rice MS, Simpson DA. Spinal neuroblastomas: diagnosis, treatment and prognosis. *J Neurosurg* 1974;40:631–638.
75. Bar-Ziv J, Nogrady MB. Mediastinal neuroblastoma and ganglioneuroma: the differentiation between primary and secondary involvement on the chest roentgenogram. *Am J Roentgenol* 1975;125:380–390.
76. Davidson KG, Walbaum PR, McCormack RJM. Intrathoracic neural tumors. *Thorax* 1978;33:359–367.
77. Adam A, Hochholzer L. Ganglioneuroblastoma of the posterior mediastinum. *Cancer* 1981;47:373–381.
78. Zeltzer PM, Marangos PJ, Parma AM, et al. Raised neuron-specific enolase in serum of children with metastatic neuroblastoma. *Lancet* 1983;2:361–363.
79. Hann HL, Evans AE, Cohen IJ, Leitmeyer JE. Biologic differences between neuroblastoma stages IV-S and IV. Measurement of serum ferritin and E-rosette inhibition in 30 children. *N Engl J Med* 1981;305:425–429.
80. Hann HL, Evans AE, Siegel SE, et al. Prognostic importance of serum ferritin in patients with stages III and IV neuroblastoma: The Children's Cancer Group experience. *Cancer Res* 1985;45:2843–2848.
81. Schwad M, Alitalo K, Klempnauer K-H, et al. Amplified DNA with limited homology to myc cellular oncogene is shared by human neuroblastoma cell lines and a neuroblastoma tumor. *Nature* 1983;305:245–248.
82. Kohl NE, Gee CE, Alt FW. Activated expression of the N-myc gene in human neuroblastoma and related tumors. *Science* 1984;226:1335–1337.
83. Schwab M, Varmus HE, Bishop JM. Human gene N-myc contributes to neoplastic transformation of mammalian cells in culture. *Nature* 1985;316:160–162.
84. Brodeur GM, Seeger RC, Schwab M, et al. Amplification of N-myc in untreated human neuroblastomas correlates with advanced disease stage. *Science* 1984;224:1121–1124.

85. Seeger RC, Brodeur GM, Sather H, et al. Association of multiple copies of the N-myc oncogene with rapid progression of neuroblastomas. *N Engl J Med* 1985;313:1111–1116.

86. Evans AE, Baum E, Chard D. Do infants with stage IV-S neuroblastoma need treatment? *Arch Dis Child* 1981;56:271–274.

87. Barlogie B, Hittelman W, Spitzer G, et al. Correlation of DNA distribution abnormalities with cytogenic findings in human adult leukemia and lymphoma. *Cancer* 1977;37:4400–4407.

88. Barlogie B, Raber MN, Schumann J, et al. Flow cytometry in clinical cancer research. *Cancer Res* 1983;43:3982–3997.

89. Look AT, Hayes FA, Nitscken R, et al. Cellular DNA content as a predictor of response to chemotherapy in infants with unresectable neuroblastoma. *N Engl J Med* 1984;311:231–235.

90. Smith EI, Krous HF, Tunell WP, Hittch DC. The impact of chemotherapy and radiation therapy on secondary operations for neuroblastoma. *Ann Surg* 1980;191:561–569.

91. Mayfield JK, Riseborough EJ, Jaffe N, Nehme ME. Spinal deformity in children treated for neuroblastoma. *J Bone Joint Surg* 1981;63A:183–193.

92. Ziegler MM, Kirby J, McGarrick JW III, et al. Neuroblastoma and nutritional support. Influence on the host-tumor relationship. *J Pediatr Surg* 1986;21:236–239.

93. Taxy JB. Paraganglioma of the cauda equina. Report of a rare tumor. *Cancer* 1983;51:1904–1906.

94. Soffer D, Pittaluga S, Caine Y, Feinsod M. Paraganglioma of cauda equina. A report of a case and review of the literature. *Cancer* 1983;51:1907–1910.

95. Van Alphen HAM, Bellot SM, Stam FC. Paraganglioma of cauda equina. *Clin Neurol Neurosurg* 1977;79:316–322.

96. Miller CA, Torack R. Secretory ependymoma of the filum terminale. *Acta Neuropathol (Berl)* 1970;15:240–250.

97. Horoupian DS, Kerson LA, Saiontz H, Valsamis M. Paraganglioma of cauda equina: clinicopathologic and ultrastructural studies of an unusual case. *Cancer* 1974;33:1337–1348.

98. Legace R, Delange C, Gangne F. Paraganglioma of the filum terminale. *Can J Neurol Sci* 1978;5:257–260.

99. Lerman RI, Kaplan ES, Daman L. Ganglioneuroma-paraganglioma of the intradural filum terminale. Case report. *J Neurosurg* 1972;36:652–658.

100. Llena JF, Hirano A, Rubin RC. Paraganglioma in the cauda equina region. *Acta Neuropathol (Berl)* 1979;46:235–237.

101. Robertson DI, Cooney TP. Malignant carotid body paraganglioma: light and electron microscopic study of the tumor and its metastasis. *Cancer* 1980;46:2623–2633.

9

Tumors of Cartilage and Bone

Ignacio Pascual-Castroviejo

OSTEOCHONDROMA

Osteochondroma is the most common of the benign bone tumors. It is called by many other names, such as multiple cartilaginous exostosis, diaphyseal aclasis, familial osteochondromatosis, hereditary multiple exostosis, and hereditary osteochondromatosis.

Hereditary multiple exostosis was described by Stanley in 1849 (1). Malignant neoplastic transformation to osteochondrosarcoma may occur in 5 to 10% of cases (2,3), although a higher percentage, more than 20% (4), has been reported. Involvement of the spine occurs in approximately 7% of patients (5), commonly affecting the spinous process or neural arch. Spinal osteochondromas account for some 3% of all spinal osseous tumors both in children and adults (6).

Encroachment on the spinal canal with neurologic complications is rare, although almost all series include one or two cases (7–9). Cord involvement may occur at any level below the foramen magnum and produce unilateral or bilateral neurologic signs. The majority of cases involve the cord in the thoracic or lumbar region, few the cervical region. A fatal outcome is particularly likely with high cervical lesions (10,11). The spinal cord is less frequently involved, but these tumors regularly affect the nerve roots. Tumors arising from the heads of the ribs have been reported to invade the spinal canal through the intervertebral foramina (12). Large paraspinal lesions may remain asymptomatic until extensive bony deformity occurs and several foramina are invaded, resulting in a significant compromise of the spinal canal (13). Smaller tumors may cause local pain or focal neurologic findings (14). Occasionally, palpable exostoses are found arising from the vertebrae, mainly near the tips of the spinous processes.

The age in reported cases ranged from 8 (13) to 50 (15) years at diagnosis. Most patients are young adults in their third decade. There is a marked male preponderance, with a male to female ratio of 3:1 (4). An unaffected male does not transmit the disease, but an unaffected female may (16).

Osteochondromas may originate in the periosteum during early childhood. They grow progressively by endochondral ossification of their cartilaginous caps. Compression of the tissues surrounding these growths may cause local discomfort. Many pathologists regard osteochondromas as developmental anomalies rather than true tumors. Their cause is unknown, and they may arise from any part of the skeletal system except membranous bone.

Osteochondroma has the appearance of a firm, sometimes lobulated mass attached to its parent bone by a pedicle. A clear zone of hyaline cartilage covered by a thin layer of fibrous tissue surrounds the tumor. The periosteum around the tumor is continuous with that of the parent bone.

A strong familial inheritance pattern of multiple osteochondromatosis occurs in up to 75% of cases (17). Gardner's syndrome, a familial disease that consists of papillary adenomas of the colon, multiple hamartomas of soft tissues, and multiple osteomas and osteochondromas, may be associated with osteochondromatosis. Since papillary adenomas of the colon may become adenocarcinomas, it is advisable to study all patients with multiple osteochondromas to rule out papillary colonic lesions.

X-ray films show quite characteristic, although not diagnostic, lesions. The tumor develops within the juxtacortical connective tissue, causing erosion with secondary sclerosis of the underlying cortical bone. The cartilaginous matrix is commonly focally calcified. If a soft tissue mass is present, it is small; it occurs in one-third of cases. Plain spine X-rays usually show the size of the tumor. Myelography may be needed to define the extent of the spinal canal invaded by the tumor and deviation or compression of the spinal cord. Computerized tomography (CT) scan and perhaps also magnetic resonance (MR) imaging are now not only convenient, but required for diagnosis. Several authors have reported their experiences with CT scan in the study of osteochondromas (3,6,9,13–15,18–20). Spallone et al. (20) suggested that the following CT scan findings may be considered typical of osteochondroma: (a) a roundish, sharply outlined mass; (b) bonelike density, with scattered calcifications; (c) paraspinal, dumbbell, or eccentric intraspinal location; (d) osteosclerotic changes in neighboring bone; and (e) lack of contrast enhancement.

In cases of spinal cord compression, excision is mandatory and may be critical (3,21–23). These tumors may require extensive bony resection with spinal fusion following removal (12). Radiation is of no benefit in reducing the size of the mass, and the amount needed for such a radioresistant tumor might cause radiation myelitis.

CHONDROMYXOID FIBROMA

Chondromyxoid fibroma is a rare benign tumor of probable cartilaginous origin. It represents less than 1% of primary bone tumors (24). The first case of chondromyxoid fibroma of the spine was described by Benson and Bass (25). A review of the literature showed no more than 12 cases involving the vertebrae (26). About one-third of the patients were children. The tumor occurs predominantly in young adults in the 20- to 30-year range (24). It is rare below age 5 and above age 60 (27). It appears preferentially in the metaphyseal zone of the long bones. Both sexes are affected equally, although there may be a slight male preponderance (27). All segments of the spine can be involved, with the thoracic region affected most frequently. The lesions originate in the spinous processes in half the cases and less frequently in the vertebral bodies and pedicles. Symptomatology of this tumor includes pain in the back, legs, and feet; motor and sensory defects of the lower limbs; genitourinary symptoms; and a tender mass. Occasionally, it can present with paraparesis of sudden onset.

Plain radiographs show features of a benign, expanding and lytic mass. Tumor calcification is rarely visible (24,28). Some cases show erosion or destruction of bone with paravertebral calcification (29), sometimes with an associated pathological fracture suggestive of a malignant primary bone tumor or a metastatic process. If myelography is performed, it demonstrates the extradural location of the tumor. CT scan may show breakthrough of the bony cortex and extension into surrounding tissues (30).

Histologically, this tumor consists of a chondroid component and abundant myxoid, alcian-blue-positive, metachromatic intercellular substance. On section, the tumor is usually firm, somewhat fibrous, and semitranslucent (31). It is well demarcated from surrounding tissues.

Recommended treatment is block excision of the tumor, when feasible. Curettage with or without bone graft may be used as an alternative treatment. Incomplete removal results in recurrence in approximately 10 to 25% of the cases (24,27,32). Young patients have an increased tendency to recur (24), but older people (26), or patients of any age with tumors containing enlarged and pleomorphic nuclei (31) have the same tendency. Malignant transformation has been reported, but only occasionally (24,26). Two cases of sarcoma arising in otherwise classical chondromyxoid fibromas were reported by Dahlin (24); one of these patients had been treated with radiotherapy 6 years after the evolution to a sarcoma. There is little information on the effectiveness of radiotherapy. Dahlin thinks that it is not indicated, except for a surgically inaccessible lesion. Complications, such as fibrosarcomatous degeneration, chronic osteomyelitis, radionecrosis, and postradiation myelitis after high dose radiotherapy, contribute to the opinion that radiotherapy is not a first-line treatment modality.

CHONDROSARCOMA (CLASSICAL)

Chondrosarcoma accounts for about 7.6% of all primary malignant bone tumors (33). Classical chondrosarcomas arising from the spinal column are extremely rare: less than 12 cases were reported before 1976 (34). These tumors occur at every level of the spine and in all ages. They have been found as a primary malignant tumor in the younger age groups and as a secondary malignant change in such conditions as osteochondroma and Paget's disease in older ones. Most investigators believe that these tumors arise from preexisting benign cartilaginous lesions such as chondroma, osteochondroma, multiple exostoses, and Ollier's disease. Chondrosarcomas originate from the surface of the exostoses in chondrodysplasia and multiple cartilaginous exostoses. Malignant changes are reported to occur after a lapse ranging from 18 months to 30 years (35). Metastasis tends to occur late and is disseminated by way of large veins over long distances, especially to the lungs.

Plain radiographs show frank destruction of trabecular bone and cortex by an expanding lesion that contains irregular flecks of calcium or mottling of the calcified tissue. Complete removal of these tumors must always be attempted.

Histologically, the tumor has the appearance of an atypical, more cellular enchondroma, with islands of mature hyaline cartilaginous matrix combined with other areas where the cartilage is poorly developed and contains atypical anaplastic cells. Thomson and Turner-Warwick (36) classified chondrosarcomas into three types:

Type 1: Low-grade, well-differentiated tumor containing increased numbers of cartilaginous cells within a well-formed matrix. Approximately 75% of these patients were alive 10 years after treatment.

Type 2: Average-grade tumor with increased cellularity and less matrix. The cells are variable in size and shape and present nuclear irregularities. Five years after treatment, less than 50% of the patients were alive, and only one-third were alive after 10 years.

Type 3: High-grade tumor with a poorly differentiated picture. Anaplastic cells are common, mitoses are frequent, and islands of cartilage occasionally occur. The behavior of this type is similar to that of the osteosarcoma. Only one of ten patients survived 3 years.

MESENCHYMAL CHONDROSARCOMA

Two types of chondrosarcoma may be distinguished: mesenchymal and classical. Mesenchymal chondrosarcoma of bone or soft tissue was first described by Lichtenstein and Bernstein in 1959 (37). It is a malignant tumor that presents a typical histologic aspect characterized by densely cellular sheets and cords of undifferentiated mesenchymal cells interspersed with islands of hyaline cartilage (38). Fewer than 100 cases have been reported in adults and even fewer in children.

Compression of the spinal cord is a rare complication in the pediatric tumor, as compared to the adult malignancy. Since the case described by Lichtenstein and Bernstein (37), six primary and eleven secondary or metastatic intraspinal mesenchymal chondrosarcomas causing spinal cord compression have been reported. Clinical findings are the same as those observed in any other tumor, that is, local or radicular pain, progressive weakness and paresthesia, almost always of the lower limbs, urinary problems, and thoracic scoliosis.

On examination, patients usually have a stumbling gait, motor paresis or paraplegia, a sensory level, local pain mainly in the shoulder, thoracic, or lumbar regions, hyperreflexia, and unilateral or bilateral extensor plantar reflexes.

Primary as well as metastatic intraspinal mesenchymal chondrosarcomas present with a similar frequency in both sexes. Primary tumors occur in the first two decades of life (39). The metastatic type occurs during the second and third decades. Both types of tumors are thoracic or, less frequently, lumbar and present with acute spinal cord compression. Patients with a metastatic tumor frequently have other metastases when the spinal cord compression is diagnosed; this is a poor prognostic sign.

Radiology

Radiographic findings may be nonspecific. Primary paraspinal tumors extending intraspinally (dumbbell tumors) often cause enlargement of the intervertebral foramina, pedicle erosion, collapse of the vertebral body, and the image of a paravertebral mass. Metastatic intraspinal tumors do not usually show these radiological findings. These features are inadequate for differentiating among the various types of primary and metastatic intraspinal tumors such as lymphoma, neuroblastoma, and sarcomas of the soft tissues and bones (39). The ^{99m}TC-polyphosphate bone scan, ^{69}Ga-citrate total body scan, and perhaps other isotopic substances are useful for detecting metastases to bones. CT scan reveals a lobulated contrast-enhancing mass.

Histology

Grossly, the tumors appear to be well-circumscribed, but they are often invasive. The distinction between mesenchymal chondrosarcoma and classical or non-mesenchymal chondrosarcoma poses little difficulty (40). The latter are commonly well-differentiated tumors with few or no highly cellular mesenchymal components; the cartilaginous element predominate, gradually merges with the stroma and shows considerable pleomorphism. Their preferential localization to the axial skeleton, the infrequent involvement of the soft tissues, and the peak incidence in the sixth decade also serve to distinguish between the two tumors.

The diagnosis and grading of chondrosarcoma of bone are best established by cytologic study of smeared preparations, and by histologic study of sections of the tumor that demonstrate its structure and relationship to the host bone (41). Smear preparations demonstrate the cytologic features of chondrosarcoma with greater clarity and detail than histologic sections. Histology is particularly helpful in the diagnosis of low-grade chondrosarcoma through the demonstration of its invasion of the host bone. A knowledge of the grading of chondrosarcomas is important for elucidating their biological behavior and establishing their prognosis.

The confusion between myxoid chondrosarcoma and chondromyxoid fibroma remains a problem for the general histopathologist. Mesenchymal chondrosarcoma may be erroneously diagnosed at first, as in a patient reported by Harsh and Wilson (42) who was operated on for an intraspinal meningeal tumor originally diagnosed as angioblastic meningioma. There was a recurrence 6 years later, and histologic review of the pathology led to a change in diagnosis to that of mesenchymal chondrosarcoma.

Treatment

A combination of surgery, irradiation, and chemotherapy may improve outcome, especially when applied before the development of metastases. Excessive bleeding from these highly vascular tumors suggests the use of preoperative embolization (42). Hirsh et al. (43) described a patient with primary spinal chondrosarcoma who survived with useful function for over 18 years following repeated local tumor excisions. Resection of the tumor must be accompanied by irradiation therapy of about 5,000 rad and chemotherapy consisting of vincristine, actinomycin D, cyclophosphamide, Adriamycin, or other new chemotherapeutic drugs.

OSTEOBLASTOMA

The term benign osteoblastoma was independently proposed by Jaffe (44) and Lichtenstein (45) to define a vascular osteoid and bone-forming tumor containing numerous osteoblasts with a benign appearance, occurring preferentially in the spine.

This tumor constitutes less than 1% of all bone tumors (46). More than 40% of the reported cases are located in the spine. More than half are associated with scoliosis (47), which is observed in 86% of those located in the thoracic and lumbar spine (48). Benign osteoblastomas also occur in the long bones, ribs, the skull, maxilla, mandible, and the small bones of the hands and feet. Osteoblastoma of the spine usually involves the spinous and transverse processes. The vertebral body is rarely involved primarily. It has been reported in all ages, from 3 to 78 years, with an average of 17 years. About two-thirds of the cases are under 30 years of age (49). The male to female ratio is said to be approximately 2:1 in some series (50), although others show a higher frequency in women (51). Osteoblastoma is also referred to as osteoblastic osteoid tissue-forming tumor, spindle-cell variant of giant cell tumor, osteogenic fibroma, and giant osteoid osteoma. Although quite similar to the osteoid osteoma, it differs from it by its different size, site, and degree of sclerosis (52). The main characteristics of the osteoblastoma are its larger size (giant osteoid osteoma), its predilection for the spinous and transverse processes [although 14% are located within the vertebral body (53)], and its lack of reactive perifocal bone formation.

The importance of a usually painful scoliosis as the most common presenting sign of this tumor has often been emphasized (47,51,54–57). Marked spinal stiffness from paravertebral muscle spasm is also common (51). Neurologic symptoms secondary to spinal cord and root compression, usually accompanied by muscle spasm, have been observed in 26 to 60% of cases. Radicular pain occurs in 50% of the patients (58).

X-ray films show a well-circumscribed radiolucent lesion whose size varies between 2 and 10 cm. The lesion contains areas at different stages of new bone formation, which is commonly accompanied by a soft tissue component and by a small amount of cortical new bone formation along its margin (59,60). Small lesions must be differentiated from osteoid osteoma and aneurysmal bone cyst, while larger, more aggressive lesions must be distinguished from sarcomatous tumors (59,61,62) and also from aneurysmal bone cysts. The osteoblastoma may be located in the concavity of the scoliosis at or near its apex (57). Plain radiographs show the tumor in less than half of patients (8), and other investigations (bone scintigraphy, CT scan, and MR) are usually required.

Bone scan can localize osteoblastomas successfully (47,48,57,63), although the findings are not specific and the differential diagnosis includes infection, injury, fracture, and other benign tumors. A normal bone scan virtually excludes the diagnosis of osteoblastoma (64). CT scanning and MR provide information not only about the exact location of the tumor but also the state of surrounding tissues. CT and MR have supplanted vertebral and selective aortic angiography for diagnosis.

The tumor ranges in size from 2 to 10 cm and may progress in an expansive or destructive manner. Its color depends on the degree of vascularization, calcification, and hemorrhage. Occasionally, giant tumors undergo central softening or cystic degeneration. The main components of osteoblastoma (49,50,65) are well-vascularized fibroblastic tissue, finely lamellar or coarse osteoid tissue, and zones of calcification. Groups of giant osteoblastic cells and atypical cells are infrequent. Osteoblasts line newly formed bony trabeculae. Some cases of initially benign osteoblastoma may undergo malignant transformation (65–70). Only three such cases with metastases have been found in the literature (65,68,70), two of these being located in the spine (68,70). Although malignant transformation is commonly assumed to be secondary to radiotherapy, one of the cases had not received it (68). Sarcomatous transformation of osteoblastoma occurred from 2 to 10 years after the initial pathologic diagnosis and recurrence was common in such cases.

Surgical treatment is recommended for small and medium-sized tumors. Local resection is the treatment of choice for tumors located in the spinous processes. If the tumor invades the spinal canal, urgent removal of the tumor is required to relieve spinal cord compression (53) and avoid the risk of a permanent scoliosis when symptoms have been present for more than 15 months (48). Patients undergoing resection of vertebral osteoblastoma may expect to be "cured" when total gross removal has been achieved, without the requirement for adjunctive radiotherapy. Even subtotal excision produces permanent remission, whether or not it is followed by radiotherapy (46,61). Patients with osteoblastoma must be followed for many years because tumor recurrence and even malignant transformation have been reported as late as 11 or 12 years postoperatively (46,67).

OSTEOID OSTEOMA

The term osteoid osteoma was introduced by Jaffe (71). He described a benign bone tumor characterized by a nidus of vascular osteoid tissue surrounded by dense sclerotic bone. It is a well-circumscribed growth, measuring less than 2 cm in diameter, which usually is not accompanied by a soft tissue component. In a review of 860 cases of osteoid osteoma (72), 10% occurred in the spine. Fifty-nine percent of these were located in the lumbar spine, 27% in the cervical region, 12% in the thoracic region, and 2% in the sacral vertebrae. Involvement of the vertebral body is unusual (7%); most osteoid osteomas occur in the vertebral arches (75%), articular facets (19%), pedicles (15%), and, especially, the lamina (33%). In one series, 100% of cases affected the pedicle (51). The exact nature of this tumor remains unclear, but it is interesting that this site corresponds with the primary ossification center for each half of the neural arch. Females are somewhat more likely to be affected than males. These tumors are most frequent in the first two decades of life, with an average age of 13.5 years at onset of symptoms (51).

The two most important signs of the tumor are painful scoliosis (54–56) and marked stiffness of the spine (51,73). The pain increases gradually, worsens at night, but can be relieved promptly by aspirin. Spinal stiffness results from paravertebral muscle spasm. A bizarre gait, restricted joint motion, and other neurologic symptoms have also been observed, the most frequent being gait disturbance, radicular pain, and limb atrophy. As reported in a number of studies (51,54,55), there is usually a delay of about 19 months between the onset of symptoms and definitive diagnosis. The majority of the patients had consulted three or more specialists before the correct diagnosis was made.

The distinction between osteoid osteoma and osteoblastoma has come to be regarded as one of size, site, and degree of sclerosis (52). The osteoblastoma, also known as giant osteoid osteoma (74), is larger (sometimes up to 10 cm in diameter) and is often accompanied by a soft tissue mass, with little or no osseous reaction around it (49,74).

Plain X-ray films clearly show a lucent lesion less than 1.5 cm in diameter with a surrounding well-defined sclerotic area in long bones. In some cases, visualization may require X-ray tomography. In the spine, the complex anatomy of multiple superimposed bony structures can make it very difficult to detect and diagnose osteoid osteoma, not only with conventional radiographs but even with tomography (75). Nearly 100% of osteoid osteomas can be visualized on bone scan with pyrophosphate (76) or other tracers (51,64,73,75–79) (Fig. 1A).

Scintigraphic findings are not specific, and differential diagnosis includes infection, injury, fracture, or other benign tumors. A normal bone scan virtually excludes the diagnosis of osteoid osteoma (64). Intraoperative skeletal scintigraphy as an aid to the localization of the tumor has sometimes been performed (79).

CT scans show the precise location of the lesion and distinguish its center from the surrounding sclerosis (Fig. 1B). The CT appearance of osteoid osteoma has three characteristics (75): (a) a well-defined round or oval low-density area; (b) a high density area in the center of the lesion surrounded by a halo of low density (this high density area represents mineralized osteoid, often misnamed sequestrum). The high density area may be absent or minimal in osteoma without a low density halo; (c) various degrees of surrounding reactive bone changes,

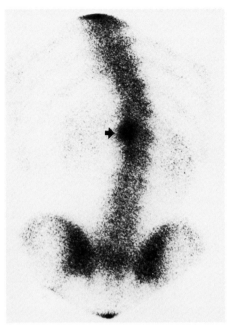
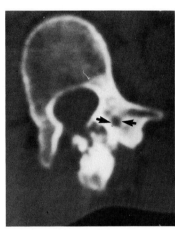

A,B

FIG. 1. A: A 16-year-old boy with osteoid osteoma. The tumor (*arrow*) is very evident in the radioisotopic study. It is located in the apex of the vertebral curve. (Courtesy of Dr. Sanchez-Girón. Scoliosis Unity. Hospital "La Paz," Madrid.) **B:** Same case as A. CT shows the tumor as a well-defined, round, low-density area (*arrows*) in the sclerotic area of the mass.

ranging from mild cancellous sclerosis to an exhuberant periosteal reaction resulting in thickening of the bone harboring the osteoma. Osteomas are located in the concavity of the scoliosis, the tumor usually being situated at the apex of the curve (51). L3 is the vertebra affected most frequently (63). Osteoid osteomas may undergo spontaneous remission (72,80); nevertheless, the tumor should be removed promptly. Surgical intervention brings immediate relief of pain, a rapid return of spinal mobility, and return to daily activities within a few months. Delay in treatment in a growing child results in a progressive scoliosis with significant vertebral rotation, which leads to a permanent structural scoliosis in some patients (51). Symptoms present for more than 15 months before diagnosis make it unlikely that scoliosis will improve postoperatively (48).

GIANT CELL TUMOR

Giant cell tumors are quite rare. They represent 4.2% of all bone tumors (81). Most occur at the ends of the long bones, the majority around the knee. These tumors account for about 4% of all vertebral tumors (82). 1.3% of all giant cell tumors affect the spine above the sacrum (83) and 4% of all giant cell tumors involve the vertebrae (84). Most occur in the second and third decades (range, 2 to 66 years) according to the most extensive series (85), which included 31 cases involving the spine above the sacrum. Most of the patients were female, with a female to male ratio of 3:1. Another name for this tumor is osteoclastoma (86,87).

Their clinical symptomatology depends on the location of the tumor. Neck pain and stiffness are present when the tumor is in the cervical spine. The common symptoms in the case of tumors located lower in the spine include progressive neurologic compromise, usually affecting the legs, local pain or radiculopathy, sphincter disturbance, and sexual impotence.

Plain X-ray films and CT scans usually reveal a destructive lesion, which may be mistaken for a metastasis or other malignant tumor, but also for benign processes such as an aneurysmal bone cyst or eosinophilic granuloma. However, giant cell tumors have features that may help in the differential diagnosis (85). They involve the body of the vertebra with secondary involvement of the pedicle and vertebral arch. In contrast, aneurysmal bone cysts and osteoblastomas almost always arise in the posterior elements and infrequently originate in the vertebral body. Technetium-99 bone scans show a "hot spot" in the area corresponding to the tumor (88). Since total removal is the treatment of choice, it is important to know the precise location and extent of the tumor. CT and MR may help define the extent of the tumor in bone and soft tissue, which is important since infiltration may compromise the spinal canal and neural elements. The characteristic finding in cervical CTs is a soap-bubble pattern that is enhanced after venous injection of contrast medium (88). CT, combined with myelography, is a useful diagnostic tool. Vertebral angiography is required to visualize the tumor and surrounding regions in preparation for embolization of the feeding arteries (88).

The histologic appearance of osteoid osteoma is that of multinucleated cells, together with collagen, and cyst formation. There are sheets of exuberant but nonanaplastic mononuclear cells admixed with osteoclast-like giant cells containing from several to several hundred nuclei. Invasion of striated muscle and mitotic figures are frequent (89).

Radical resection after embolization of the arteries feeding the tumor is the treatment of choice. Cryosurgery is an extremely effective method for curing this tumor if it can be totally frozen (90). In cases in which it is uncertain whether the entire tumor was frozen, especially in the region of the odontoid peg, some authors supplement cryosurgery with irradiation. Mirra et al. (91) followed cryosurgery with a course of radiotherapy (4,600 rad) in a patient with a tumor in the second cervical vertebra who was asymptomatic 30 months later. Irradiation of the cervical spine may produce adverse side effects such as radiation edema and necrosis of the spinal cord (92). Nonetheless, postoperative low-dose irradiation seems advisable (88,91). There are patients who have survived without recurrence for more than 20 years after a nonradical operation (93). Giant cell tumors are believed to be semimalignant tumors because, although they appear benign on pathological examination, they can evolve into malignant tumors which recur after high-dose irradiation. The recurrence rate is high according to most large series and is reported to range between 25 and 50% of cases, usually within 2 years of the initial therapy (85).

EWING'S SARCOMA

Following osteosarcoma, Ewing's sarcoma is the most common malignant bone tumor in children and young adults. Ewing (98,99) collected and described a series of round-cell sarcomas of the bone and considered them to be a single entity. It is a relatively infrequent lesion, comprising approximately 3.5 to 7.0% of all vertebral tumors, including those of adults (94,95). Excluding the sacrum, primary Ewing's sarcoma of the spine is even rarer, accounting for less than 1% of primary vertebral tumors (97). The predominant age is between 5 and 15 years. It is very rare below the age of 5, although Kozlowski et al. (96) described three cases of Ewing's sarcoma in children under 5 in a series of seven patients. Males are affected more often than females.

Patients with involvement of the vertebral body have a short clinical history, more often weeks than months (96). Common signs and symptoms include local pain, an abnormal gait, loss of muscle tone and power, sensory disturbances, paraplegia, and general malaise. Lumbar disc protrusion has been reported (100,101).

The most frequent radiographic findings are variable degrees of osteolysis or osteosclerosis with partial or complete vertebral collapse. The disc space may be narrowed or, rarely, widened. Paravertebral soft tissue masses and spread to adjacent vertebral bodies may also be seen in association with intraspinal involvement. Myelography reveals complete or partial extradural block. Other studies, such as urography, barium enema, or esophagography, may show invasion of soft tissues. CT shows destruction of the vertebral body and, less frequently, of the neural arches or spinous and lateral processes, extending into the spinal canal and paravertebral areas (96,102). CT may be complemented with metrizamide myelography to evaluate spinal cord compression and the size of the tumor (103). Differential diagnosis includes other diseases, notably neuroblastoma (because of paravertebral calcification) and aneurysmal bone cyst (because of expansion of a transverse process) (102).

Ewing's sarcoma is a firm mass, arising from a long bone, which often contains areas of hemorrhage and necrosis that are often extensive, resulting in hemorrhagic cavities and liquefied areas. The tumor is a cellular neoplasm composed of sheets of relatively uniform and closely packed round cells. The cells have an indistinct outline and an indented round to oval nucleus with fine glycogen granules, demonstrable by histologic and ultrastructural study. Rarely, osseous, cartilaginous, and fibroblastic tissue may form within the tumor. The histologic differential diagnosis includes several other neoplasms with morphological similarities such as neuroblastoma, reticulum cell sarcoma (histiocytic lymphoma), alveolar rhabdomyosarcoma, and undifferentiated carcinoma. The development of pulmonary and osseous metastases is characteristic of Ewing's sarcoma. Most patients with Ewing's sarcoma present with the clinical and radiographic features of a primary osseous tumor. However, extraosseous primary Ewing's sarcoma in the paravertebral area spreading by contiguity to the epidural space has been described, more frequently in young adults (100,101,104–108). These lesions arise in soft tissue at various anatomic sites and do not involve adjacent bone.

Treatment of Ewing's sarcoma must be aggressive (16), with initial and maintenance chemotherapy to eradicate completely all metastatic microfoci of disease which are presumed to be present at the time of diagnosis in patients with an isolated primary tumor or with metastases presenting before the primary tumor. The drugs used for chemotherapy are dactinomycin, Adriamycin, vincristine, and cyclophosphamide. Surgery alone or in combination with moderate dose radiotherapy is a reasonable approach for patients who are predicted to have a high probability of local recurrence. Rosen et al. (109) obtained a survival rate of at least 5 disease-free years in 75% of twenty children with only a primary tumor. Children with metastatic disease had complete responses to chemotherapy, but tumor recurrence was high. Treatment failures were attributed to relapse after positive response to chemotherapy. High dose radiotherapy, greater than 6,000 to 7,000 rad, may be dangerous to the spinal cord, especially in children.

PRIMARY AND SECONDARY OSTEOGENIC SARCOMAS

Primary osteogenic sarcoma arising in the spine is a rare tumor, comprising only 0.85 to 2.00% of all osteogenic sarcomas (110). The distribution is fairly equal between the lumbar and thoracic regions, with cervical involvement less common. Of over 1,000 patients with osteogenic sarcoma of bone studied at Memorial Hospital, only 10 cases had their origin within the spine (110). There were 17 cases of osteogenic sarcoma of the spine among 600 cases of osteogenic sarcoma in another series (111), 3 in the cervical, 3 in the thoracic, 2 in the thoracolumbar, and 5 in the lumbar regions, and 4 in the sacrum.

Osteogenic sarcoma of the spine may be primary or secondary. Males are more often affected than females in both types. Some series indicate a moderate predominance of primary tumors (110).

Though most cases of primary osteogenic sarcoma are found in the second and third decades, the highest prevalence is at 12 years in females and 16 years in males (112). Age ranges from 3 to 70 years, with a mean age of 35 years. Only three patients with thoracic and lumbar tumors were younger than 25 years. A cervical location is even rarer than a thoracic or lumbar location. Sarcoma arising in vertebrae affected by Paget's disease occurs in the sixth and seventh decades (110,113,114). Radiation has been implicated as a predisposing factor in vertebral osteosarcoma (115). The case published by Dowdle et al. (116) is very unusual. A 3-year-old girl who had a pilocytic astrocytoma at C2–C4 was operated on and radiated. After a latent period of 11 years, she had a rapidly fatal clinical course; necropsy showed osteosarcoma.

In the series of Barwick et al. (110), all seven patients with a primary osteogenic sarcoma involving the spine were males, whereas the three cases of osteogenic sarcoma secondary to Paget's disease were female, and older than patients with primary tumors. Of the 600 cases of osteogenic sarcoma reported by Dahlin and Coventry (111), which included osteoblastic, fibroblastic, and chondroblastic varieties, 3.3% arose in bones affected by Paget's disease, but none of them affected the spine.

Osteogenic sarcoma of the spine has a predilection for the lumbar and thoracolumbar segments. Neurologic symptoms are due to compression of the spinal cord or roots. They include pain and stiffness, limb weakness, a staggering gait, paraplegia or quadriplegia, hyperreflexia, clonus and Babinski signs when the tumor involves the spinal cord, and hyporeflexia or areflexia with radicular sensory involvement in cases of compression of roots. Generalized sensory disturbances may be observed in cervical tumors. Neurologic deficit is common and often progresses rapidly to cord transsection. A majority of the patients have neurological symptoms at the time of presentation. (110).

The alkaline phosphatase is commonly elevated and tends to increase as the disease progresses (110), although this finding may be lacking in localized Paget's disease (110,117). Patients with Paget's disease present with cortical osteosclerotic thickening of the bodies and pedicles, which take on a typical puffy appearance.

The radiographic findings are usually distinctive, with dense sclerosis and new bone formation involving the vertebral body, and, sometimes, the neural arches. Findings are unilateral. Some cases show radiolucent or densely sclerotic destructive lesions. Occasionally, osteogenic sarcoma may be mistaken for a benign osteoblastoma (110).

Myelography shows partial or complete extradural block of the contrast medium. CT scan reveals an expansive lytic lesion of the body and sometimes of the pedicles, with the tumor spreading to the soft tissues and encroaching on the spinal canal (118).

All cases show the histologic picture of osteoid within a sarcomatous stroma. On the basis of their predominant microscopic features, the tumors are classified into several types. In the series of Dahlin and Coventry (111), 54.7% were osteoblastic sarcomas, 23.5% fibroblastic sarcomas, and 22.0% chondroblastic sarcomas. In the series of ten cases described by Barwick et al. (110), four were osteoblastic, two chondrosarcomatous, two fibrohistiocytic, and one fibrosarcomatous. The remaining case exhibited an unusual pattern with abundant myxoid ground substance containing spindle and stellate tumor cells. The more anaplastic sarcomas are associated with a poorer prognosis (111). Errors in interpretation or malignant transformation of an osteoblastoma to an osteogenic sarcoma occur (119,120). Merryweather et al. (70) described a patient who presented with metastatic sclerosing osteoblastic osteosarcoma 9 years after the diagnosis of osteoblastoma. There are histologic criteria, however, that distinguish osteoblastoma from osteogenic sarcoma (110). Osteogenic sarcoma shows frequent mitoses and cellular pleomorphism, whereas osteoblastic lining of bone spicules is uncommon. Tumor cells are usually crowded by a dense cellular stroma, and there are frequent cartilaginous foci and tumorous giant cells. In osteoblastoma, on the other hand, mitoses are absent or rare, cellular pleomorphism is usually absent, osteoblastic lining of bone spicules is common, the stroma is usually delicate with dilated thin-walled vessels and rare cartilaginous foci, and tumorous giant cells are absent unless the lesion is complicated by a fracture or by a previous biopsy that revealed cartilaginous foci.

One variety of vertebral sarcoma, hardly referred to in the literature, is fibrosarcoma. Some authors believe that fibrosarcoma is a variant of osteosarcoma (121), while others consider it a primary tumor arising from the osseous connective tissue stroma (122). The difference between fibroblastic osteosarcoma and fibrosarcoma rests on the absence of malignant bone or osteoid in the former and the presence of malignant changes in the latter (123). When fibrosarcoma originates in a bone with preexisting pathology, such as Paget's disease (123), it is known as secondary fibrosarcoma.

Surgical treatment is the therapy of choice and should be performed when feasible, although the spine has inaccessible portions and outcome is poor, with short survival (115,116,119,120,123). Radiotherapy is not very effective and should be regarded as palliative (124). However, cases treated with radiotherapy alone are known to have survived for more than 10 years (125) and more than 4 years (126). Barwick et al. (110) described a 3-year-old boy with vertebral osteosarcoma treated by radiotherapy and chemotherapy who survived more than 6 years before he finally died of multiple metastases. Ogihara et al. (127) reported the case of a 15-year-old boy with complete paraplegia resulting from compression by an osteogenic sarcoma of the fourth thoracic vertebra, who was treated solely by arterial infusion of Adriamycin (doxorubicin) and systemic chemotherapy consisting of cyclophosphamide, Oncovin (vincristine), methotrexate, phenylalanine mustard, and Adriamycin (doxorubicin) according to the (COMPADRI)-III regimen. The patient regained normal function and had been disease-free without any neurologic deficit for 6 years at the time of the report.

Patients with osteogenic sarcoma of the spine commonly have a poor prognosis, with a short course prior to demise. In the series of Barwick et al. (110), only 1 patient survived for more than 2 years and most were dead within a year of diagnosis. The prognosis of fibrosarcoma is similar to that of the more common osteosarcoma.

ANEURYSMAL BONE CYST

Generalities

Aneurysmal bone cysts are usually benign expanding lesions which are not true neoplasms. Jaffe and Lichtenstein (128) described two cases of a peculiar cyst which they named aneurysmal bone cyst. This lesion had previously been called such names as atypical giant cell tumor and benign bone aneurysm. These lesions accounted for 1.5% of all primary tumors of bone treated at the Mayo Clinic

(129). They may be located in all parts of the skeleton, including the skull and vertebrae.

Aneurysmal bone cysts are most common in patients under the age of 20, the average age being 16.6 years. Females are somewhat more often affected than males (130). Twenty-two to 47% occur in the cervical spine, 30 to 40% in the thoracic, 17 to 31% in the lumbar, and 6 to 13% in the sacral regions (130,131). Aneurysmal bone cysts have occurred at the craniovertebral junction (132). Forty percent of the lesions occur in the vertebral bodies and 60% in the pedicles, transverse processes, laminae, and spinous processes. Occasionally, vertebrae adjacent to the cyst may be partially involved, but complete destruction of several contiguous vertebrae, simulating a malignant tumor, is uncommon (133).

According to Mirra (134), aneurysmal cysts go through three phases: (a) an incipient phase, (b) a midphase, and (c) a stabilization phase. Lytic lesions in the incipient phase may be overlooked during a routine exam.

Needle biopsy may be carried out, but deep bone penetration is usually necessary; there is a risk of extradural hematoma (130), and the biopsy is likely to be negative.

Histology

Macroscopically, aneurysmal bone cysts appear as large, communicating cavities, usually filled with unclotted blood. Microscopically, the walls of the cavernous spaces are lined by an indistinct epithelium and do not contain elastic laminae or muscle tissue. The walls separating the spaces are fibrous and frequently show osteoid or fibrous tissue with several giant cells. Extravasated blood and hemosiderin-laden phagocytes are also present.

Clinical Findings

Neurologic symptoms depend upon the location of the lesion and include localized back pain, radicular symptoms, signs of spinal cord compression such as paresthesias, weakness or paresis of the limbs and, occasionally, paraplegia and the presence of a tender mass to palpation. At first, pain is mild and intermittent, but it becomes severe and constant with growth of the lesion which may press on the nerve roots and produce radicular pain, including severe sciatica (131). The average duration of symptoms is 8 months, and is less than 3 months in 30% of the patients (130).

Radiology

Plain radiographs of the spine are indicated as soon as symptoms present. A destructive lesion with expansion and trabeculae, and a "blown out" appearance are characteristic. The surrounding bone is often sclerotic. In the spinous or transverse processes, it appears as a cystlike expanding lesion surrounded by an egg-shell-thin border of bone. Advanced disease may result in fracture of the vertebral body with possible compression or destruction. Involvement of several vertebrae is fairly common (129,135) (Fig. 2A). Tomography improves visualization of the lesion. Angiography shows its blood supply along with pathological circulation (129,131,136,137). Myelography defines the extent of the lesion inside the spinal canal, especially if combined with CT scanning (Fig. 2B). Its appearance on cross-sectional CT, although not pathognomonic, gives additional information about bone and soft-tissue components of the lesion, spinal cord and nerve root compression, as well as about the relationship of the lesion with surrounding spinal and intraspinal structures (138). CT shows an osteolytic lesion with a multi-loculated aspect and low-density cavities (131,139–141). It enhances after intravenous contrast (131,139). CT also reveals its extension into the spinal canal (140). MR imaging demonstrates an intact rim of low-intensity signal completely surrounding the lesion (142). Acute hemorrhage is not well defined on MR owing to relatively prolonged T1 (142).

Differential Diagnosis

The radiologic differential diagnosis includes hydatic cyst, giant cell tumor, eosinophilic granuloma, hemangioma of bone, osteoblastoma, fibrous dysplasia, and metastatic disease (malignant lymphoma, leukemia, and neuroblastoma) (130,131).

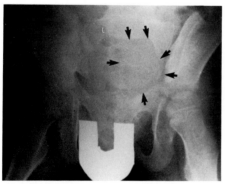
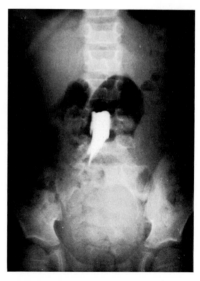

A,B

FIG. 2. A: Aneurysmal cyst in a 6-year-old boy. X-ray film of the sacral region showing a destructive lesion (*arrows*). **B:** Same case as A. Pantopaque myelography presents the image of an extradural mass pushed up and to the right by the aneurysmal cyst.

Pathogenesis

Many theories regarding the pathogenesis of aneurysmal bone cysts have been advanced over the years and include the following (130): a vascular disturbance of the bone, a secondary manifestation of a preexisting condition, a reparative process, trauma and subsequent hemorrhage, a skeletal hemangioma, and a hematoma that may have arisen as the result of leakage from a congenital hemangioma or trauma. Ameli et al. (131) suggest that aneurysmal bone cysts may occur from hemodynamic alterations in a bone that is the site of a congenital vascular anomaly. These changes might be triggered by trauma or by some other process interfering with venous drainage of the area, since the rate of growth of the lesion seems to be inversely related to venous drainage.

Treatment

Total excision of the lesion is the treatment of choice, but it is not always feasible (131). When complete excision is not feasible, some authors advocate simple curettage of the lesion followed by bone grafting and fusion. This situation arises principally when both the anterior and posterior portions of the vertebra are involved or when the body of the vertebra must be removed (141,143). Bone grafting does not appear to influence the prevalence of recurrence, which must be treated by further attempts at partial or total excision, with or without curettage (130). Recurrence may occur even after complete removal followed by radiotherapy. Patients younger than 15 years of age are more predisposed to recurrence than older ones. Most commonly, recurrence develops within a few months of the operation; it is quite unusual after 2 years and rare after 4 years (129). It appears that there will be no recurrence if all the spaces are opened and curetted at the first operation. Prognosis is generally good, and recurrence is exceptional after a second curettage. Disappearance of the disease has been reported to occur following biopsy alone (144) and may even occur spontaneously (145).

Treatment of aneurysmal bone cyst of the spine is controversial. While some authors (130) believe that radiotherapy should be reserved for the few cases where operation is inadvisable, others (136,146) claim it is superior to surgery. The recommended dose must not exceed 2,000 rad because of the possibility of radionecrosis of the spinal cord and the development of malignant changes, although doses of 2,000 to 3,000 rad have been advocated by others as primary method of treatment (146). It is believed that the curative effect of radiotherapy may be damage to small arteries, resulting in a diminished blood supply to the lesion (131).

CHORDOMA

Chordoma is a malignant and relatively rare tumor. It represents approximately 3% of all primary bone tumors (147). Less than 4% of cases are observed below age 20 years (148). The mean annual incidence in Finland between 1953 and 1971 was 0.30 in males and 0.18 in females per one million population (149). Chordomas arise from notocordal rests, with approximately 85% occurring in the skull base and sacrococcygeal region (150,151) and about 50 to 60% having a sacrococcygeal location (152–155). The remaining 15% occur in the lumbar, thoracic, and cervical spine. The distribution in three important series was: 10 cervical, 2 thoracic, 2 lumbar and 40 sacrococcygeal (10); 5 cervical, 2 thoracic, 11 lumbar, and 36 sacrococcygeal (156); 3 cervical, 0 thoracic, 2 lumbar, and 13 sacrococcygeal (157). Aberrant tumors in the scapula, mandible, frontal bone, ethmoid, and maxillary sinuses have been described (147,150,151). Chordomas have little metastatic potential but produce considerable local destruction. They are usually slow growing. Some 10 to 34% of chordomas metastasize (148,150, 153,158–160). Most of these originate in the sacrococcygeal region, although in the series of Sundaresan et al. (148) they originated more frequently in other spinal zones. Most metastatic nodules are located in the lung, liver, lymph nodes, and adjacent soft tissues (148,161). Metastases have been observed in very young children, such as the 4-year-old boy described by Rosenqvist and Saltzman (162) with a sacrococcygeal chordoma who died with extensive metastases. Metastases probably spread via the hematogeneous route.

There is a male preponderance of about 2:1 (148,151). Intracranial chordomas are more common than spinal ones in younger patients (150,152,154,155), whereas sacrococcygeal ones predominate in the older age groups. These tumors can occur at any age. Patients range from 7 to 79 years of age in the series of O'Neill et al. (155). Chordoma of the coccyx has been reported in a 7-month-old fetus (163), in neonates, and in children in the first three years of life (164,165).

In general, the symptomatology of vertebral chordomas is neurologic because they compress the spinal cord and roots. Pressure on the spinal cord may affect sensory pathways, producing numbness and pain. As the neoplasm enlarges, motor paresis or paralysis may occur. Extravertebral extension can produce associated symptoms resulting from pressure on various other structures. Clinical symptoms and signs vary with the site and extent of tumor growth. Paraplegia or quadriplegia occurs late in the course of the disease. Posterolateral extension produces early-onset radicular symptoms. There are no pathognomonic clinical signs that identify chordomas.

Chordoma of the cervical spine can present as a mass in the nasopharynx or hypopharynx (147), although, on most occasions, it is confined to paravertebral soft tissues or the cervical vertebrae. The majority of cervical chordomas presented initially with pain, occasionally with dysphagia, and rarely with respiratory difficulty (148,150,154,166,167). Few cases presented with symptoms of upper airway obstruction.

Intrathoracic chordomas are usually located in the posterosuperior part of the mediastinum. In a review of 1,271 reported cases of chordomas from all sites up to 1954 (156), there were only 20 located in the thoracic spine. Only three cases of persons younger than 20 years of age had been described up to 1983 (168); the mass was asymptomatic for several years in all cases. Symptoms in patients with posterior mediastinal tumors frequently include chest pain and cough, resulting from pressure of the mass on such structures as the esophagus, aorta, or trachea.

Lumbar chordomas represent 20% of the spinal and sacrococcygeal chordomas, (148). They have essentially the same symptoms and signs as the sacrococcygeal ones.

Sacrococcygeal chordoma is the most frequent of the chordomas. In 90% of patients, the primary symptom is pain, commonly centered at the base of the spine. Other symptoms include constipation and bladder dysfunction and pain due to nerve compression. Diagnosis may be delayed for a few weeks to several years. When a patient complains of pain in the lower spine, plain radiographs must be obtained and studied carefully in order to arrive at an early diagnosis of this tumor. A history of prior trauma is elicited in about 20% of the patients, but it probably bears no etiologic relation to the tumor (169).

Histopathology

Chordomas are lobulated, gray, cystic or solid, partially translucent masses of varied consistency. Their extensions into soft tissues appear encapsulated, which is not the case of their bony extensions. Microscopically, chordomas are characterized by a lobular architecture with "physaliphorous" (dewdrop-like) cells with ample vacuolated cytoplasm and "signet-ring" cells (148,154). The size of intracytoplasmic mucus droplets varies greatly; they show a positive staining reaction for both mucin and glycogen. Sometimes, only small numbers of the vacuolated cells are present. Occasionally, anaplastic spindle cells occur (170). The size and chromatin content of the nuclei vary greatly, but mitotic figures are rare. The frequent finding of clusters or columns of chordoma cells invading between muscle planes and along nerve trunks shows the infiltrating capacity of the tumor. Ultrastructural studies reveal two distinct types of tumor cells; some are large and have an epitheleal appearance, while others are elongated and spindly. Transitional forms between these two types may also be seen (171,172).

Radiology

Chordomas of the spine are usually osteolytic and destroy multiple adjacent vertebral bodies. They produce a paravertebral or precervical soft tissue mass, osteosclerosis (seen mainly at the periphery of the destructive lesion), and involvement of the intervening intervertebral disc space (173). Chordomas occurring in the sacrococcygeal region destroy several segments, while those higher in the spine appear to originate in a single vertebral body.

The tumor may surround the vertebral body before destroying the neural arches and encroaching on the spinal canal. Chordomas have a demonstrable intraspinal extension on myelography, usually presenting as an epidural mass. The appearance of an intradural mass indicates dural invasion by the neoplasm (173). Selective angiography may demonstrate abnormal vascularization in the tumor (173). Ultrasound, conventional tomography, intravenous pyelography, and venography have all been used to help define the extravertebral extension of the mass, but these studies have been replaced by more sophisticated methods of evaluation, such as CT and MR.

Chordomas at different levels of the spine have characteristic findings on plain X-ray films. Most cervical chordomas produce destructive changes in the vertebral body which may be lytic, blastic, or both. Adjacent cervical disc spaces may be narrowed, and invasion of contiguous vertebral bodies is frequent (151,160). Enlargement of the intervertebral foramina, mimicking a neurofibroma, has occasionally been observed (174). CT, alone or combined with metrizamide myelography and MR, not only shows the erosion or destruction of the vertebral bodies but also the size and extent of the mass and its relation to the spinal cord and roots. Cervical chordoma is usually anterolaterally situated and has a homogeneous density comparable to that of muscle (175). CT shows the soft tissue component of the tumor, which is disproportionately large compared with the area of bony involvement. CT findings include septated areas of low attenuation within the tumor, amorphous soft tissue calcification, tumor extension into the spinal canal, disc space involvement, and contrast enhancement (176). The presence of solitary or multiple areas of low attenuation within a soft tissue mass usually supports the diagnosis of chordoma and has been observed in more than 50% of cases studied by CT (176). The areas of low attenuation probably represent the myxoid, gelatinous, or semiliquid material described macroscopically in chordomas (148,152).

MR offers several advantages over CT because of its superior resolution of soft tissue lesions and because the images can be orientated in any plane. The signal pattern from chordoma is quite distinct from that of other tumors, suggesting that MR has the potential for making a specific diagnosis (177) (Fig. 3A,B).

Thoracic chordomas presenting as a mediastinal tumor produce a large soft tissue mass, usually located in the posterosuperior mediastinum, occasionally displacing or compressing the esophagus or trachea. They indent the bodies of vertebrae anteriorly (178) and, on occasion, may opacify and impart an ivory aspect to the bodies of the vertebrae. The general aspect, size, and location of the tumor and its relationship to adjacent structures are easily seen on CT (168) and MR studies.

The most frequent radiological finding in sacrococcygeal chordoma is destruction of several segments associated with a soft tissue mass anterior to the sacrum (148). Calcification in the tumor is demonstrable in 15% of the cases (148). Amorphous calcifications in the periphery of the tumor are common in chordomas of the sacrum (89%) (175).

Plain radiographs alone are usually inadequate for detecting many of the abnormalities in this area, especially soft tissue extension. CT is superior and shows the total extent of bone and soft tissue involvement (179). MR has important advantages over CT in the evaluation of sacrococcygeal chordoma (180). The exact

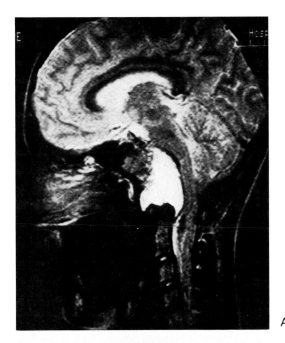

FIG. 3. A: Chordoma of the clivus and foramen magnum in a 15-year-old female. Lateral view of MR in T2 (TE 100, TR 2067) showing a voluminous mass destroying the clivus, protruding into the cavum and posterior fossa. The brainstem appears displaced backward and the odontoid seems unaffected. (Courtesy of Dr. Luis Lopez-Ibor.) **B:** Same case as A. The axial views show destruction of the clivus and narrowing of the occipital foramen by the tumor. (Courtesy of Dr. Luis Lopez-Ibor.)

craniocaudal extent of the lesion is well seen in sagittal images. Invasion of adjacent soft tissue and muscles is easy to detect because of the prolonged T1 and T2 times of the tumor. Either MR or CT can demonstrate tumor involvement of the sacral nerve roots (180).

Differential Diagnosis

Very few processes need to be differentiated from chordomas. The most common ones are giant cell tumors, chondrosarcomas, adenocarcinomas, metastatic carcinomas, and ependymomas.

Treatment and Prognosis

Complete surgical resection is rarely possible with current methods because of the tumor's widespread extension into soft tissues and bone at the time of primary diagnosis. The initial treatment usually involves decompressive laminectomy with removal of as much as possible of the extradural tumor and involved bone. Laparatomy or thoracotomy with intraoperative biopsy, or biopsy in cervical-retropharyngeal chordomas is also recommended, followed by radiotherapy. Several surgical techniques have been described for sacrococcygeal chordomas in an attempt to conserve anorectal and urogenital function (181,182). Occasionally, cordotomy or other techniques for the relief of intractable pain are required several years after the initial surgery. Irradiation, although not curative, offers the possibility of palliation in primary and recurrent chordoma, which is a relatively radioresistant tumor. Large doses may be more effective than lower ones. Tewfik et al. (183) recommend 6,000 to 6,500 rad following surgical removal of chordoma and 7,000 to 7,500 rad if surgical treatment is not feasible. Sundaresan et al. (148) give doses of 6,000 to 7,000 rad over 6 to 10 weeks for radical treatment and 4,000 to 5,000 rad over 4 to 6 weeks for palliation. The dose given in recurrent cases depends on how much radiation the patient has already received and on the condition of the normal tissues. High-dose proton-beam radiation may constitute a significant progress (184,185). This modality allows a higher dose to be administered accurately to the tumor with less radiation of adjacent and surrounding structures than can be achieved with standard radiotherapy. Although primary results are encouraging, more experience is needed. Chemotherapy seems to have no effect on this tumor (148).

In general, the prognosis for chordomas is poor. Several circumstances account for this, such as the difficulty of surgical excision, a relentlessly progressive biologic behavior, and relative radio resistance. The average length of survival is between 5 and 6 years (148,150,154,167). In the series of Sundaresan et al. (148), the 5-year survival rate for the sacrococcygeal group was 66%, and 50% for chordosarcomas in other regions of the spine. Approximately 40% of patients with sacral chordomas lived 10 years whereas very few of those with other vertebral location were alive at 10 years. There are cases with a long survival. For example, Shallat et al. (186) described a 17-year-old woman with a pharyngocervical chordoma which was subtotally resected, with no other therapy given. She showed recurrence 16 years later in the form of an epidural spinal cord compression. Subtotal resection was again accomplished via laminectomy followed by an uneventful recovery. O'Neill et al. (155) reported the case of a 9-year-old girl with a chordoma involving the C5 and C6 vertebrae; she remained well and disease-free 20 years after her initial presentation. Sundaresan et al. (148) referred to two patients in a series of 54 cases who survived 17 and 20 years following surgery only. Isolated instances of survival for 21 years (187) and 26 years (162) have been documented. It seems that high dose radiation may provide a recurrence-free survival (188).

REFERENCES

1. Stanley E. *Illustrations of the effects of disease and injury of the bone.* London: Longman, Brown, etc., 1849;29.
2. Larson NE, Dodge HW Jr, Rushton JG, Dahlin DC. Hereditary multiple exostoses with compression of the spinal cord. *Proc Staff Meet Mayo Clin* 1957;32:728–734.
3. Palmer FJ, Blum PW. Osteochondroma with spinal cord compression. Report of three cases. *J Neurosurg* 1980;52:842–845.
4. Greenfield GB. *Radiology of bone disease*, 3rd ed. Philadelphia: J.B. Lippincott, 1980;577–580.
5. Carmel PW, Cramer FJ. Cervical cord compression due to exostosis in a patient with hereditary multiple exostoses. Case report. *J Neurosurg* 1968;28:500–503.
6. Fortuna A, DiLorenzo N, Noletti A, Nardi P. Chondromes et osteochondromes solitaires du rachis entrainant une compression myéloradiculaire. A propos de 6 cas traités chirurgicalement. *Neurochirurgie* 1983;29:271–278.
7. Vinstein AL, Franken EA. Hereditary multiple exostoses: report of a case with spinal cord compression. *Am J Roentgenol* 1976;112:405–407.
8. Karian JM, De Filipp G, Buchheit WA, et al. Vertebral osteochondroma causing spinal cord compression. Case report. *Neurosurgery* 1984;14:483–484.
9. Linkowski GD, Tsai FY, Recher L, et al. Solitary osteochondroma causing spinal cord compression. *Surg Neurol* 1985;23:388–390.
10. Rose EF, Fekete A. Odontoid osteochondroma causing sudden death. Report of a case and review of the literature. *Am J Clin Pathol* 1964;42:606–609.
11. Chiurco AA. Multiple exostoses of bone with fetal spinal cord compression. Report of a case and a brief review of the literature. *Neurology* 1970;20:275–278.
12. Twersky J, Kassner E, Tenner M, Camera A. Vertebral and costal osteochondroma causing spinal cord compression. *Am J Roentgenol* 1975;124:124–128.
13. Novick GS, Pavlov H, Bullough PG. Osteochondroma of the cervical spine: report of two cases in preadolescent males. *Skeletal Radiol* 1982;8:13–15.
14. Lanzieri CF, Solodnik P, Sacher M, Herman G. Computed tomography of solitary spinal osteochondromas. *J Comput Assist Tomogr* 1985;9:1042–1044.
15. Lord G, Massare C, Guillamon JL, Bard M. Intérêt de la tomodensitométrie axiale transverse dans le diagnostic et le traitement d'algies vertébrales inexpliquées (à propos d'un cas d'ostéochondrome pédiculaire dorsal). *Chirurgie* 1978;104:360–366.
16. Jaffe HL. Hereditary multiple exostosis. *Arch Pathol* 1943;36:335–357.
17. Bell MS. Benign cartilaginous tumors of the spine. A report of one case together with a review of the literature. *Br J Surg* 1971;58:707–711.
18. Bléry M, Chagnon S, Chanzy M, Turmel L. Tumeur cartilagineuses axiales. A propos de 3 cas avec symptomatologie neurologique. *J Radiol* 1981;62:31–36.
19. Loftus CM, Rozario RA, Prager R, Scott RM. Solitary osteochondroma of T4 with thoracic cord compression. *Surg Neurol* 1980;13:355–357.

20. Spallone A, DiLorenzo N, Nardi P, Nolletti A. Spinal osteochondroma diagnosed by computed tomography. Report of two cases and review of the literature. *Acta Neurochir* 1981;58:105–114.
21. Thomas ML, Andress MR. Osteochondroma of the cervical spine causing cord compression. *Br J Radiol* 1971;44:549–550.
22. MacGee EE. Osteochondroma of the cervical spine: a cause of transient quadriplegia. *Neurosurgery* 1979;4:259–260.
23. O'Connor GA, Roberts TS. Spinal cord compression by an osteochondroma in a patient with multiple osteochondromatosis. *J Neurosurg* 1984;60:420–423.
24. Dahlin DC. *Bone tumors. General aspects and data on 6221 cases*, 3rd ed. Springfield, Ill.: Charles C Thomas, 1978;57–70.
25. Benson WR, Bass S. Chondromyxoid fibroma: first report of occurrence of this tumor in vertebral column. *Am J Clin Pathol* 1955;25:1290–1292.
26. Nuñez C, Bennett T, Bohlman HH. Chondromyxoid fibroma of the thoracic spine. Case report and review of the literature. *Spine* 1982;7:436–439.
27. Spejut HJ, Dorfman HD, Fechner RE, Ackerman LV. Tumors of bone and cartilage. In: Armed Forces Institute of Pathology, eds. *Atlas of tumor pathology*, 2nd series, fascicle 5. Washington, DC: Armed Forces Institute of Tumor Pathology. 1971;50–59.
28. Feldman F, Hecht HL, Johnston AD. Chondromyxoid fibroma of bone. *Radiology* 1970;94:249–260.
29. Standefer M, Hardy RW Jr, Marks K, Cosgrove DM. Chondromyxoid fibroma of the cervical spine—a case report with a review of the literature and a description of an operative approach to the lower anterior cervical spine. *Neurosurgery* 1982;11:288–292.
30. Shulman L, Bale P, De Silva M. Sacral chondromyxoid fibroma. *Pediatr Radiol* 1985;15:138–140.
31. Rahimi A, Beabout JW, Ivins JC, Dahlin DC. Chondromyxoid fibroma: a clinicopathologic study of 76 cases. *Cancer* 1972;30:726–736.
32. Schajowicz F, Gallardo H. Chondromyxoid fibroma (fibromyxoid chondroma) of bone. A clinicopathological study of thirty-two cases. *J Bone Joint Surg* 1971;53B:198–216.
33. Dahlin DC, Enderson ED. Chondrosarcoma: a surgical and pathological problem. Review of 212 cases. *J Bone Joint Surg* 1956;38A:1025–1058.
34. Blaylock RL, Kempe LG. Chondrosarcoma of the cervical spine. Case report. *J Neurosurg* 1976;44:500–503.
35. Coley BL. *Neoplasms of bone*, 2nd ed. New York: Paul Hoeber, 1960.
36. Thomson AD, Turner-Warwick RT. Skeletel sarcomata and giant cell tumor. *J Bone Joint Surg* 1955;37B:266–303.
37. Lichtenstein L, Bernstein D. Unusual benign and malignant chondroid tumors of bone: a survey of some mesenchymal cartilage tumors and malignant chondroblastic tumors, including a few multicentric ones, as well as many atypical benign chondroblastomas and chondromyxoid fibromas. *Cancer* 1959;12:1142–1157.
38. Dahlin DC. Mesenchymal chondrosarcoma. In: Dahlin DC, ed. *Bone tumors*, 3rd ed. Springfield, Ill.: Charles C Thomas, 1978;218–225.
39. Chan HSL, Turner-Gomes SO, Chuang SH, et al. A rare cause of spinal cord compression in childhood from intraspinal mesenchymal chondrosarcoma. A report of two cases and review of the literature. *Neuroradiology* 1984;26:323–327.
40. Scheithauer BW, Rubinstein LJ. Meningeal mesenchymal chondrosarcoma: report of 8 cases with review of the literature. *Cancer* 1980;42:2744–2752.
41. Sanerkin NG. The diagnosis and grading of chondrosarcoma of bone. A combined cytologic and histologic approach. *Cancer* 1980;45:582–594.
42. Harsh GR IV, Wilson CB. Central nervous system mesenchymal chondrosarcoma. Case report. *J Neurosurg* 1984;61:375–381.
43. Hirsh LF, Thanki A, Spector HB. Primary spinal chondrosarcoma with eighteen-year follow-up. Case report and literature review. *Neurosurgery* 1984;14:747–749.
44. Jaffe HL. Benign osteoblastoma. *Bull Hosp Joint Dis* 1956;17:141–151.
45. Lichtenstein L. Benign osteoblastoma: category of osteoid- and bone-forming tumours other than classical osteoid osteoma which may be mistaken for giant-cell tumour or osteogenic sarcoma. *Cancer* 1956;9:1044–1052.
46. Lichtenstein L, Sawyer WR. Benign osteoblastoma. Further observations and report of twenty additional cases. *J Bone Joint Surg* 1964;46A:755–765.

47. Marsh BW, Bonfiglio M, Brady LP, Enneking WF. Benign osteoblastoma. Ranging of manifestations. *J Bone Joint Surg* 1975;57A:1–9.
48. Pettine KA, Klassen RA. Osteoid-osteoma and osteoblastoma of the spine. *J Bone Joint Surg* 1986;68A:354–361.
49. Huvos AG. *Bone tumors. Diagnosis, treatment and prognosis*, 1st ed. Philadelphia: W.B. Saunders, 1979;33–46.
50. Alp H, Ceviker N, Baykaner K, et al. Osteoblastoma of the third lumbar vertebra. *Surg Neurol* 1983;19:276–279.
51. Kirwan W O'G, Hutton PAN, Pozo JL, Ransford AO. Osteoid osteoma and benign osteoblastoma of the spine. Clinical presentation and treatment. *J Bone Joint Surg* 1984;66B:21–26.
52. Byers PD. Solitary benign osteoblastic lesions of bone. Osteoid osteoma and benign osteoblastoma. *Cancer* 1968;22:43–57.
53. Epstein N, Benjamin V, Pinto R, Budzilovich G. Benign osteoblastoma of a thoracic vertebra. Case report. *J Neurosurg* 1980;53:710–713.
54. MacLellan DI, Wilson FC. Osteoid osteoma of the spine: a review of the literature and report of six new cases. *J Bone Joint Surg* 1967;49A:111–121.
55. Keim HA, Reina EG. Osteoid osteoma as a cause of scoliosis. *J Bone Joint Surg* 1975;57A:159–163.
56. Metha MH, Murray RO. Scoliosis provoked by painful vertebral lesions. *Skeletal Radiol* 1977;1:223–230.
57. Akbarnia BA, Rocholamini SA. Scoliosis caused by benign osteoblastoma of the thoracic or lumbar spine. *J Bone Joint Surg* 1981;63A:1146–1155.
58. Janin Y, Epstein JA, Carras R, Khan A. Osteoid osteoma and osteoblastoma of the spine. *Neurosurgery* 1981;8:31–38.
59. Pozachesky R, Yen YM, Sherman RS. The roentgen appearance of benign osteoblastoma. *Radiology* 1960;75:429–437.
60. Stutch R. Osteoblastoma—a benign entity? *Orthop Rev* 1975;4:27–33.
61. McLeod RA, Dahlin DC, Beabout JW. The spectrum of osteoblastoma. *Am J Roentgenol* 1976;126:321–335.
62. De Souza Dias L, Frost HM. Osteoblastoma of the spine. A review and report of eight new cases. *Clin Orthop* 1973;91:141–151.
63. Azouz EM, Kozlowski K, Marton D, et al. Osteoid osteoma and osteoblastoma of the spine in children. Report of 22 cases with brief literature review. *Pediatr Radiol* 1986;16:25–31.
64. Papanicolaou N, Treves S. Bone scintigraphy in the preoperative evaluation of osteoid osteoma and osteoblastoma of the spine. *Ann Radiol* 1984;27:104–110.
65. Lichtenstein L. *Bone tumors*, 4th ed. St. Louis: C.V. Mosby, 1972;103–120.
66. Schajowicz F, Lemos C. Malignant osteoblastoma. *J Bone Joint Surg* 1976;58B:202–211.
67. Scranton PE Jr, De Cicco FA, Totten RS, Yunis EJ. Prognostic factors in osteosarcoma. A review of 20 years experience at the University of Pittsburgh Health Center Hospitals. *Cancer* 1975;36:2179–2191.
68. Seki T, Fukuda H, Ishii Y, et al. Malignant transformation of benign osteoblastoma. *J Bone Joint Surg* 1975;57A:424–426.
69. Jackson JR, Bell MEA. Spurious "benign osteoblastoma." *J Bone Joint Surg* 1977;59A:397–401.
70. Merryweather R, Middlemiss JH, Sanerkin NG. Malignant transformation of osteoblastoma. *J Bone Joint Surg* 1980;62B:381–384.
71. Jaffe HL. "Osteoid osteoma." Benign osteoblastic tumor composed of osteoid and atypical bone. *Arch Surg* 1935;31:709–728.
72. Jackson RP, Reckling FW, Mautz FA. Osteoid osteoma and osteoblastoma: similar histologic lesions with different natural histories. *Clin Orthop* 1977;128:303–313.
73. Wedge JH, Tchang S, MacFadyen DJ. Computed tomography in localization of spinal osteoid osteoma. *Spine* 1981;6:423–427.
74. Dahlin DC, Johnson EW. Giant osteoid osteoma. *J Bone Joint Surg* 1954;36A:559–572.
75. Gamba JL, Martinez S, Apple J, et al. Computed tomography of axial skeletal osteoid osteoma. *Am J Roentgenol* 1984;142:769–772.
76. Lisbona R, Rosenthall L. Role of radionuclide imaging in osteoid osteoma. *Am J Roentgenol* 1979;132:77–80.
77. Nelson OA, Greer RB. Localization of osteoid-osteoma of the spine using computerized tomography. *J Bone Joint Surg* 1983;65A:263–265.

78. Smith FW, Gilday DL. Scintigraphic appearances of osteoid osteoma. *Radiology* 1980;137:191–195.
79. Rinsky LA, Goris M, Bleck EE, et al. Intraoperative skeletal scintigraphy for localization of osteoid osteoma in the spine. *J Bone Joint Surg* 1980;62A:143–144.
80. Sabanas AO, Bickel WH, Moe JH. Natural history of osteoid osteoma of the spine. Review of the literature and report of three cases. *Am J Surg* 1956;91:880–889.
81. Dahlin DC. *Bone tumors*, 2nd ed. Springfield, Ill.: Charles C Thomas, 1970.
82. Cohen DM, Dahlin DC, MacCarty CS. Vertebral giant cell tumor and variants. *Cancer* 1964; 17:461–472.
83. Johnson KA, Riley LH. Giant cell tumor of bone. *Clin Orthop* 1969;62:187–191.
84. Goldenberg R, Cambell CS, Bonfiglio M. Giant cell tumor of bone. *J Bone Joint Surg* 1970; 52A:619–664.
85. Dahlin DC. Giant cell tumor of vertebrae above the sacrum. *Cancer* 1977;39:1350–1356.
86. Windeyer BW, Woodyatt PB. Osteoclastoma. A study of thirty-eight cases. *J Bone Joint Surg* 1949;31B:252–267.
87. Gonem MN. Osteoclastoma of the thoracic spine. Case report. *J Neurosurg* 1976;44:748–752.
88. Shirakuni T, Tamaki N, Matsumoto S, Fujiwara M. Giant cell tumor in cervical spine. *Surg Neurol* 1985;23:148–152.
89. Swimer SR, Bassett LW, Mancuso AA, et al. Giant cell tumor of the cervicothoracic spine. *Am J Roentgenol* 1981;136:63–67.
90. Marcove RC, Weiss LD, Vaghaiwalla MR, et al. Cryosurgery in the treatment of giant cell tumors of bone. A report of 52 consecutive cases. *Cancer* 1978;41:957–969.
91. Mirra JM, Rand F, Rand R, et al. Giant-cell tumor of the second cervical vertebra treated by cryosurgery and irradiation. *Clin Orthop* 1981;154:228–233.
92. DiLorenzo N, Spallone N, Nolletti A, Nardi P. Giant cell tumor of the spine: a clinical study of six cases, with emphasis on the radiological features, treatment, and follow-up. *Neurosurgery* 1980;6:29–34.
93. Fabiani A, Brignolio F, Favero M, et al. Benign and malignant craniospinal giant cell tumours: report of four cases. *Acta Neurochir (Wien)* 1982;64:133–150.
94. Dahlin DC. Ewing's tumor. In: Dahlin DC, ed. *Bone tumors*, 3rd ed. Springfield, Ill.: Charles C Thomas, 1978;274.
95. Schajowicz F. *Tumours and tumorlike lesions of bone and joints.* New York, Heidelberg, Berlin: Springer Verlag, 1981.
96. Kozlowski K, Beluffi G, Masel J, et al. Primary vertebral tumours in children. Report of 20 cases with brief literature review. *Pediatr Radiol* 1984;14:129–139.
97. Whitenhouse GH, Griffiths GJ. Roentgenologic aspects of spinal involvement by primary and metastatic Ewing's tumor. *J Can Assoc Radiol* 1976;27:290–297.
98. Ewing J. Diffuse endothelioma of bone. *Proc NY Pathol Soc* 1921;27:17–24.
99. Ewing J. Further report on endothelial myeloma of bone. *Proc NY Pathol Soc* 1924;24:92–101.
100. Fink LH, Meriwether MW. Primary epidural Ewing's sarcoma presenting as a lumbar disc protrusion. Case report. *J Neurosurg* 1979;51:120–123.
101. Bollar Zabala A, Gelabert Gonzalez M, García Allut A, et al. Sarcoma de Ewing de localización epidural lumbar. *Rev Neurol (Barcelona)* 1986;14:75–79.
102. Weinstein JB, Siegel MJ, Griffith RC. Spinal Ewing sarcoma: misleading appearances. *Skeletal Radiol* 1984;11:262–265.
103. Vacher H, Vacher-Lavenu MC, Sauvegrain J. Etude anatomo-radioclinique des sarcomes d'Ewing du rachis lombaire. Sarcomes à cellules rondes. A propos de trois cas. *J Radiol* 1981; 62:425–428.
104. Tefft M, Vawter GF, Mitus A. Paravertebral "round cell" tumors in children. *Radiology* 1969;92:1501–1509.
105. Angervall L, Enzinger FN. Extraskeletal neoplasm resembling Ewing's sarcoma. *Cancer* 1975; 36:240–251.
106. Scheithauer BW, Egbert BM. Ewing's sarcoma of the spinal epidural space: report of two cases. *J Neurol Neurosurg Psychiatry* 1978;41:1031–1035.
107. Soule EH, Newton W Jr, Moon TE, Tefft M. Extraskeletal Ewing's sarcoma. A preliminary review of 26 cases encountered in the Intergroup Rhabdomyosarcoma Study. *Cancer* 1978; 42:259–264.

108. Spaziante R, De Divitiis E, Giamundo A, et al. Ewing's sarcoma arising primarily in the spinal epidural space: fifth case report. *Neurosurgery* 1983;12:337–341.
109. Rosen G, Caparros B, Mosende C, et al. Curability of Ewing's sarcoma and considerations for future therapeutic trials. *Cancer* 1978;41:888–899.
110. Barwick KW, Huvos AG, Smith J. Primary osteogenic sarcoma of the vertebral column. A clinicopathologic correlation of ten patients. *Cancer* 1980;46:595–604.
111. Dahlin DC, Coventry MB. Osteogenic sarcoma. A study of six hundred cases. *J Bone Joint Surg* 1967;49A:101–110.
112. Larsson S-E, Lorentzon R. The incidence of malignant primary bone tumors in relation to age, sex, and site. A study of osteogenic sarcoma, chondrosarcoma and Ewing's sarcoma diagnosed in Sweden from 1958 to 1968. *J Bone Joint Surg* 1974;56B:534–540.
113. Greditzer HG, McLeod RA, Unni KK, Beabout JW. Bone sarcomas in Paget disease. *Radiology* 1983;146:327–333.
114. McKenna RJ, Schwinn CP, Soong KY, Higinbotham NL. Sarcomata of the osteogenic series (osteosarcoma, fibrosarcoma, chondrosarcoma, parosteal osteogenic sarcoma and sarcomata arising in abnormal bone). An analysis of 552 cases. *J Bone Joint Surg* 1972;54A:1479–1489.
115. Sim FH, Cupps RE, Dahlin DC, Ivins JC. Postradiation sarcoma of bone. *J Bone Joint Surg* 1972;54A:1479–1489.
116. Dowdle JA, Winter RB, Dehner LP. Postradiation osteosarcoma of the cervical spine in childhood. A case report. *J Bone Joint Surg* 1977;59A:969–971.
117. Woodard HQ. Long-term studies of blood chemistry in Paget's disease of bone. *Cancer* 1959;12:1226–1237.
118. Patel DV, Hammer RA, Levin B, Fisher MA. Primary osteogenic sarcoma of the spine. *Skeletal Radiol* 1984;12:276–279.
119. Marsh HO, Choi C. Primary osteogenic sarcoma of the cervical spine originally mistaken for benign osteoblastoma. A case report. *J Bone Joint Surg* 1970;52A:1467–1471.
120. Fielding JW, Fietti VG, Hughes JEO, Gabrielian JCZ. Primary osteogenic sarcoma of the cervical spine. A case report. *J Bone Joint Surg* 1976;58A:892–894.
121. Spejut HJ, Dorfman HD, Fechner RE, Ackerman LV. Tumors of bone and cartilage. In: Armed Forces Institute of Pathology, eds. *Atlas of tumor pathology*, 2nd series, fascicle 5. Washington, DC: Armed Forces Institute of Pathology, 1970;174–177.
122. Dahlin DC. Fibrosarcoma. In: Dahlin DC, ed. *Bone tumors*, 2nd ed. Springfield, Ill.: Charles C Thomas, 1967;212–221.
123. Gandolfi A, Brizzi R, Tedeschi F, et al. Fibrosarcoma arising in Paget's disease of the vertebra: review of the literature. *Surg Neurol* 1983;19:72–76.
124. Gandolfi A, Bordi C. Primary osteosarcoma of the cervical spine causing neurological symptoms. *Surg Neurol* 1984;21:441–444.
125. Poppe E, Liverud K, Efskind J. Osteosarcoma. *Acta Chir Scand* 1968;134:549–556.
126. Beck JC, Wara WM, Bovill EG Jr, Phillips TL. The role of radiation therapy in the treatment of osteosarcoma. *Radiology* 1976;120:163–165.
127. Ogihara Y. Sekiguchi K, Tsuruta Y. Osteogenic sarcoma of the fourth thoracic vertebra. Long-term survival by chemotherapy only. *Cancer* 1984;53:2615–2618.
128. Jaffe HL, Lichtenstein L. Solitary unicameral bone cyst with emphasis on the roentgen picture, the pathologic appearance and the pathogenesis. *Arch Surg* 1942;44:1004–1025.
129. Tillman BP, Dahlin DC, Lipscomb PR, Stewart JR. Aneurysmal bone cyst: an analysis of ninety-five cases. *Mayo Clin Proc* 1968;43:478–495.
130. Hay MC, Paterson D, Taylor TKF. Aneurysmal bone cysts of the spine. *J Bone Joint Surg* 1978;60B:406–411.
131. Ameli NO, Abbassioun K, Saleh H, Eslamdoost A. Aneurysmal bone cysts of the spine. Report of 17 cases. *J Neurosurg* 1985;63:685–690.
132. Verbiest H. Tumors involving the cervical spine. In: Cervical Spine Research Society, eds. *The cervical spine*. Philadelphia: J.B. Lippincott, 1983;430–477.
133. Stillwell WT, Fielding JW. Aneurysmal bone cyst of the cervicodorsal spine. *Clin Orthop* 1984; 187:144–146.
134. Mirra JM. *Bone tumors. Diagnosis and treatment*. Philadelphia: J.B. Lippincott, 1980.
135. Karparov M, Kitov D. Aneurysmal bone cyst of the spine. *Acta Neurochir (Wien)* 1977;39:101–113.
136. Cambelles G, Delcambre B, Madelain M, et al. Le kyst anévrismal rachidien. Considérations thérapeutiques à propos de 6 observations. *Neurochirurgie* 1983;29:1–11.

137. Billings KJ, Werner LG. Aneurysmal bone cyst of the first lumbar vertebra. *Radiology* 1972;104:19–20.

138. Wang A-M, Lipson SJ, Haykal HA, et al. Computed tomography of aneurysmal bone cyst of the L_1 vertebral body. *J Comput Assist Tomogr* 1984;8:1186–1189.

139. Calliaw L, Roels H, Caemaert J. Aneurysmal bone cysts in the cranial vault and base of the skull. *Surg Neurol* 1985;23:193–198.

140. Volikas Z, Stingounas E, Saridakes G, Tsioulias A. Aneurysmal bone cyst of the spine. *Acta Radiol [Diagn] (Stockh)* 1982;23:643–646.

141. Bret P, Confavreux C, Thouard H, et al. Aneurysmal bone cyst of the cervical spine: report of a case investigated by computed tomographic scanning and treated by a two-stage surgical procedure. *Neurosurgery* 1982;10:111–115.

142. Beltran J, Simon DC, Levy M, et al. Aneurysmal bone cysts: MR imaging at 1.5 T1 *Radiology* 1986;158:689–690.

143. Nicastro JF, Leatherman KD. Two-stage resection and spinal stabilization for aneurysmal bone cyst. A report of two cases. *Clin Orthop* 1983;180:173–178.

144. Murray RO, Jacobson JG. Aneurysmal bone cyst. In: *The radiology of skeletal disorders*. London, Edinburgh: Churchill Livingstone, 1971;382–386,946–949.

145. Sherman RS, Soong KY. Aneurysmal bone cyst: its roentgen diagnosis. *Radiology* 1957;68:54–64.

146. Nobler MP, Higinbotham NL, Phillips RF. The cure of aneurysmal bone cysts. Irradiation superior to surgery in an analysis of 33 cases. *Radiology* 1968;90:1185–1192.

147. Wright D. Nasopharyngeal and cervical chordoma—some aspects of their development and treatment. *J Laryngol Otol* 1967;81:1335–1337.

148. Sundaresan H, Galicich JH, Chu FCH, Huvos AG. Spinal chordomas. *J Neurosurg* 1979; 50:312–319.

149. Paavolainen P, Teppo L. Chordoma in Finland. *Acta Orthop Scand* 1976;47:46–51.

150. Kamrin RP, Potanos JN, Pool JL. An evaluation of the diagnosis and treatment of chordoma. *J Neurol Neurosurg Psychiatry* 1964;27:157–165.

151. Higinbotham NL, Phillips RF, Farr HW, Hustu HO. Chordoma: thirty-five year study at Memorial Hospital. *Cancer* 1967;20:1841–1850.

152. Dahlin DC. *Bone tumors. General aspects and data on 6221 cases*. Springfield, Ill.: Charles C Thomas, 1978;329–343.

153. Huvos AG. *Bone tumors*. Philadelphia: W.B. Saunders, 1979;373–391.

154. Mindell ER. Chordoma. *J Bone Joint Surg* 1981;63A:501–505.

155. O'Neill P, Bell BA, Miller JD, et al. Fifty years of experience with chordomas in Southeast Scotland. *Neurosurgery* 1985;16:166–170.

156. Utne JR, Pugh DG. The roentgenologic aspects of chordoma. *Am J Roentgenol* 1955;74:593–608.

157. Volpe R, Mazabraud A. A clinicopathologic review of 25 cases of chordoma (a pleomorphic and metastasizing neoplasm). *Am J Surg Pathol* 1983;7:161–170.

158. Want CC, James AE. Chordoma with a brief review of the literature and a report of a case and widespread metastases. *Cancer* 1968;22:162–167.

159. Fox JE, Batsakis JG, Owano LR. Unusual manifestations of chordomas. A report of two cases. *J Bone Joint Surg* 1968;50A:1618–1628.

160. Firooznia H, Pinto RS, Lin JP, et al. Chordoma: radiologic evaluation of 20 cases. *Am J Roentgenol* 1976;127:797–805.

161. Chambers J, Head BE. A metastasizing chordoma. *J Bone Joint Surg* 1972;54B:526–529.

162. Rosenqvist H, Saltzman GF. Sacroccygeal and vertebral chordomas and their treatment. *Acta Radiol (Stockh)* 1959;52:177–192.

163. Henning L. Ueber congenitale echte Sacraltumoren. *Beitr Pathol Anat* 1900;28:593–619.

164. Nix VL, Steuber CP, Hawkins EP, et al. Sacrococcygeal chordoma in a neonate with multiple anomalies. *J Pediatr* 1978;93:995–998.

165. Richards AT, Stricke L, Spitz L. Sacrococcygeal chordomas in children. *J Pediatr Surg* 1973;8:911–914.

166. Murali R, Rovit RL, Benjamin MW. Chordoma of the cervical spine. *Neurosurgery* 1981;9:253–256.

167. Erikson B, Gunterberg B, Kindblom LG. Chordoma. A clinicopathologic and prognostic study of a Swedish national series. *Acta Orthop Scand* 1981;52:49–58.

168. Cotler HB, Cotler JM, Cohn HE, et al. Intrathoracic chordoma presenting as a posterior superior mediastinal tumor. *Spine* 1983;8:781–786.
169. Gray SW, Sughabhandu B, Smith RA, Skandalakis JE. Sacrococcygeal chordoma: report of a case and review of the literature. *Surgery* 1975;78:573–582.
170. Knechtges TC. Sacrococcygeal chordoma with sarcomatous features (spindle cell metaplasia). *Am J Clin Pathol* 1970;53:612–616.
171. Murad TM, Murthy MSN. Ultrastructure of a chordoma. *Cancer* 1970;25:1204–1215.
172. Pena CE, Horvat BL, Fisher ER. The ultrastructure of chordoma. *Am J Clin Pathol* 1970; 53:544–551.
173. Pinto RS, Lin JP, Firooznia H, Lefleur RS. The osseous and angiographic features of vertebral chordoma. *Neuroradiology* 1975;9:231–241.
174. Wang A-M, Joachim CL, Shillito J Jr, et al. Cervical chordoma presenting with intervertebral foramen enlargement mimicking neurofibroma: CT findings. *J Comput Assist Tomogr* 1984; 8:529–532.
175. Krol GH, Sundaresan N, Deck M. Computed tomography of axial chordoma. *J Comput Assist Tomogr* 1983;7:286–289.
176. Meyer JE, Lepke RA, Lindfors KK, et al. Chordomas: their CT appearance in the cervical, thoracic, and lumbar spine. *Radiology* 1984;153:693–696.
177. Patterson H, Hudson T, Hamlin D, et al. Magnetic resonance imaging of sacrococcygeal tumors. *Acta Radiol [Diagn] (Stockh)* 1985;26:161–165.
178. Schwarz SS, Fisher WS III, Pulliam MW, Weistein ZR. Thoracic chordoma in a patient with paraparesis and ivory vertebral body. *Neurosurgery* 1985;16:100–102.
179. Hudson TM, Galceran M. Radiology of sacrococcygeal chordoma: difficulties in detecting the soft tissue extension. *Clin Orthop* 1983;175:237–242.
180. Rosenthal DI, Scott JA, Mankin HJ, et al. Sacrococcygeal chordoma: magnetic resonance imaging and computed tomography. *Am J Roentgenol* 1985;145:143–147.
181. Gunterberg B, Romanus B, Stener B. Pelvic strength after major amputation of the sacrum. An experimental study. *Acta Orthop Scand* 1976;47:635–642.
182. Stener B, Gunterberg B. High amputation of the sacrum for extirpation of tumors. Principles and techniques. *Spine* 1978;3:351–366.
183. Tewfik HH, McGinnis WL, Nordstrom DG, Latourette HB. Chordoma. Evaluation of clinical behavior and treatment modalities. *Int J Radiol Oncol Biol Physiol* 1977;2:959–962.
184. Suit HD, Goitein M, Munzenrider J, et al. Definitive radiation therapy for chordoma and chondrosarcoma of base of skull and cervical spine. *J Neurosurg* 1982;56:377–385.
185. Saunders WM, Castro JR, Chen GTY, et al. Early results of ion beam radiation therapy for sacral chordoma. A Northern California Oncology Group study. *J Neurosurg* 1986;64:243–247.
186. Shallat RF, Taekman MS, Nagle RC. Unusual presentation of cervical chordoma with long-term survival. Case report. *J Neurosurg* 1982;64:243–247.
187. Pearlman AW, Friedman M. Radical radiation therapy of chordoma. *Am J Roentgenol Rad Nucl Med* 1970;108:333–341.
188. Lybeert MLM, Meerwaldt JH. Chordoma. Report on treatment results in eighteen cases. *Acta Radiol Oncol* 1986;25:41–43.

10

Tumors of the Soft Tissues

Ignacio Pascual-Castroviejo

SARCOMAS OF SOFT TISSUES

Sarcomas of soft tissues affecting the spinal cord or roots are rare tumors arising from tissues formed from mesenchyme. Some originate in the connective tissue elements in the meninges and their derivatives. Distinguishing between meningeal sarcomas and malignant meningiomas may be difficult.

Many types of soft tissue sarcomas occasionally spread to the spinal cord or roots. The following are specific designations of the tumors (1):

1. Alveolar soft tissue sarcoma
2. Angiosarcoma
3. Extraskeletal chondrosarcoma
4. Extraskeletal osteosarcoma
5. Fibrosarcoma
6. Leiomyosarcoma
7. Liposarcoma
8. Malignant fibrohistiocytoma
9. Malignant mesenchymoma
10. Malignant schwannoma
11. Rhabdomyosarcoma
12. Sarcoma, undefined type
13. Synovial sarcoma

Some of these tumors can be subclassified (2). There is insufficient information to categorize the following types (1): (a) malignant embryonal mesenchymal tumor, (b) epithelioid sarcoma, (c) fibrosarcoma with areas of chondrosarcoma, (d) malignant hemangiopericytoma, and (e) mesothelioma. A system for determining the clinical status of patients with soft tissue sarcomas is based on the characteristics of the primary tumor (size, extension), the involvement of lymph nodes, the presence of metastases, and the histologic grade of the tumor (1). Perhaps the most common and malignant soft tissue sarcoma is the rhabdomyosarcoma.

Sarcomas affect the meninges more frequently in children than in adults; the most malignant and undifferentiated forms occur in young infants (3–5). These tumors may be located anywhere along the spine. Symptoms include postural disturbances; weakness; back, neck, or limb pain; torticollis; and a sickly aspect. Associated signs are commonly flaccid or spastic paralysis, sensory deficits, abnormal reflexes, scoliosis, and a painful stiff back. Tumors located in the cervical region may cause neck stiffness or tenderness. When the tumor is in the dorsolumbar region, flaccid paraparesis may result. The cerebrospinal fluid (CSF) is usually xanthochromic with an elevated protein and moderate pleocytosis.

Plain X-rays of the spine are abnormal in at least 50% of cases, with such features as postural scoliosis, loss of lumbar lordosis, a paraspinal mass, and widening of the spinal canal at one or several segments. Myelography shows complete or incomplete block at the level of the tumor. Computerized tomography (CT) scan may not reveal any definite abnormality (5). Many of these tumors respond well to radiotherapy and surgical removal. Some types of tumors, such as reticulum cell sarcomas, respond favorably to steroid therapy (6).

The age of the patient may be an important factor in determining the aggressiveness of sarcomas. For example, a child with fibrosarcoma has a better prognosis than an adult (1).

Childhood malignant soft tissue fibrous histiocytoma appears to be similar to childhood rhabdomyosarcoma in its modes of spread and response to therapy (7). It rarely affects the spine. Successful therapy must include removal of the tumor. Combined treatment with radiotherapy, at doses similar to those used for other soft tissue sarcomas in childhood, and with chemotherapy, seems beneficial. The role of multiple-agent chemotherapy is unclear. Adriamycin is the most promising single agent.

Fibrosarcoma very rarely spreads to the spine or paraspinal region. Among 110 cases of fibrosarcoma, 40 appeared in children (8). Fibrosarcoma was located in the lumbosacral area in only one patient. The tumor was discovered and operated on at birth, but the patient died at 5.5 years of age with metastases to the central nervous system (CNS) and lungs.

Extraskeletal masses resembling Ewing's sarcoma are usually found in children and in adolescents (average age, 20 years) (9). They are quite commonly located in paraspinal muscles or in the epidural region anywhere along the spine (9–11). The presence of a mass, local pain or tenderness, sciatic pain, progressive weakness, numbness of the legs, cramps, paresis or paralysis of the legs are the most common symptoms and signs. The average duration of symptoms prior to surgery is usually a few months. Microscopically, these tumors show solidly packed small round or ovoid cells of great uniformity, arranged in sheets or lobules separated by strands of fibrous connective tissue. The nuclei of the tumor cells contain finely divided chromatin, a distinct nuclear membrane, and, frequently, a minute nucleolus. Metastatic lesions may develop within a few months after the primary tumor is excised (9).

Malignant fibrous histiocytomas arising from soft tissue are rare (12). The neoplasm is not visible on plain X-ray films, whereas myelography shows an extradural mass extending from T2 to T5. They may occasionally originate from a congenital malformation, such as a myelomeningocele (13).

Neurofibrosarcomas are rare neoplasms that may arise independently or in association with neurofibromatosis. They constitute only 5% of all soft tissue sarcomas

(1). These tumors rarely affect the spine (14). They are commonly located in the extremities. Three stages—I, II, and III—are distinguished in neurofibrosarcomas. Eighty percent of Stage I tumors have a 5-year survival rate, whereas less than 20% of Stages II and III survive (15). Prognosis is equally dismal in clinical Stages II and III patients. Both moderate and high-grade primary neurofibrosarcomas are highly malignant neoplasms that should be treated by radical resection. Adriamycin and radiotherapy may be beneficial.

Malignant mesenchymomas are rare. Diagnosis of this tumor requires the coexistence of two or more different malignant tissue types, other than fibrosarcoma, in the same mass. Malignant mesenchymomas are not associated with spinal disease. Ectomesenchymomas are a subtype of mesenchymoma restricted to infants and children. They are neoplasms with rhabdomyoblastic elements which contain foci of ganglioneuromatous tissue and characteristically occur in the head and neck. These tumors behave similarly to rhabdomyosarcomas. Few cases have been reported, with none causing spinal disease.

Liposarcomas are the most common malignant soft tissue tumors of adults, but they rarely occur in children (16,17). They do not affect the spinal region directly. Histologic classification into well-differentiated myxoid, round cell, and pleomorphic types is applicable to tumors in children. Response to radiotherapy and chemotherapy may allow complete surgical excision (17).

Soft tissue mesenchymal chondrosarcomas are malignant tumors that may cause acute or subacute spinal cord compression. They can arise in paraspinal muscles (18), in the thoracic region (19), or in the meninges (19–21). Primary and metastatic tumors can affect the spinal canal. Patients with primary intraspinal tumors usually present early and often respond well to a combination of surgery, irradiation, and chemotherapy. The presence of metastases carries a poor prognosis, since surgical removal is the main treatment of this tumor, and the role of radiotherapy and chemotherapy is still undefined. These tumors tend to recur locally, not necessarily immediately.

Rhabdomyosarcoma

Rhabdomyosarcomas are malignant tumors that usually occur in childhood, but may be seen at any age. These tumors represent 10 to 15% of solid tumors in childhood. Primary head and neck rhabdomyosarcomas account for more than one-third of all childhood cases. Among 554 reported patients with rhabdomyosarcoma, the head and neck were the most frequent primary sites (38%); parameningeal sites were involved in 46% (22). Of the head and neck tumors, about 80% presented in children below 12 years of age and 55% in children less than 5 years of age. The term parameningeal is used to include those sites anatomically adjacent to the meninges (23). Mastoid, ear canal, middle ear, nasal cavity, paranasal sinus, nasopharynx, and infratemporal fossa are the regions included under this term. Males are affected more than females (24). The spine and structures within the spinal cord may be invaded by paraspinal tumors, which are very rare, accounting for less than 1% of all spinal tumors in our series. Head and neck tumors tend to invade the meninges; that involvement was as high as 35% in some series (23).

The symptoms and signs of root and cord compression depend on the size and site of the mass. If the tumor is located in the lower cervical region, Horner's syndrome may appear on one or both sides.

Plain films and conventional tomography show bony destruction surrounded by a soft tissue mass. Angiography may be helpful for visualizing soft tissue masses and ascertaining the vascular supply of the tumor in order to facilitate operation. CT and MR have made the study of rhabdomyosarcomas simple and at the same time sophisticated, by defining the extent of the tumor (Fig. 1), recurrence in both soft tissue and bone metastases, and response to treatment.

Rhabdomyosarcomas may arise wherever striated muscle is found. The Intergroup Rhabdomyosarcoma Study proposed a clinical classification (22) that is important for prognosis. The classification includes the following groups:

  I.   Localized disease, completely resected
 II.   Grossly resected tumor with microscopic residual disease
III.   Incomplete resection or biopsy with gross residual disease
 IV.   Distant metastatic disease present at onset

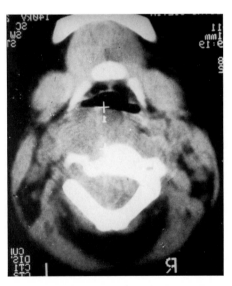

FIG. 1. Cervical rhabdomyosarcoma. CT shows destruction of the left anterior aspect of the atlas and a voluminous soft tissue mass which causes narrowing of the nasopharynx.

Most cases of head and neck rhabdomyosarcoma are in Group III with extensive local disease at diagnosis (25).

Horn and Enterline (26) subclassified rhabdomyosarcomas into three types: embryonal–botryoid, alveolar, and pleomorphic. The pleomorphic rhabdomyosarcomas are seen almost exclusively in adults. Histologically, the embryonal form is the most common among the rhabdomyosarcomas of the head and neck. Sutow et al. (25) found 78% were embryonal–botryoid, 9% alveolar, 10% undifferentiated, and 3% extraosseous Ewing types. The embryonal type presents long, spindle-shaped cells with a single nucleus and eosinophilic cytoplasm. Some cells are larger and oval-shaped, with bright abundant eosinophilic cytoplasm. Occasionally, the cells may appear undifferentiated with round nuclei and little cytoplasm.

The botryoid type is distinguishable from the embryonal variant only by its location and size. It is covered by a normal mucous membrane, with a multi-layered band of cells situated under the epithelium. These cells are oval to spindle-shaped, having little cytoplasm and a high frequency of mitosis.

The alveolar type is characterized by the presence of alveoli that are separated by connective tissue trabeculae. One or several layers of cells are closely attached to the trabeculae. Some of these cells are multinucleated striated giant cells.

The pleomorphic form is a spindle-cell tumor of adults, which presents bizarre, pleomorphic, giant cells containing abundant eosinophilic cytoplasm. Striations are frequent. Local recurrence and distant metastases are both common. These metastases can be found anywhere in the body, although they occur most frequently in the lungs, bones, and lymph nodes. The head and neck region has a very low incidence of lymphatic metastases (27).

In children with a localized mass with histologically clear margins, complete surgical resection should be attempted. Children with paraspinal rhabdomyosarcoma can rarely be treated surgically. Radiotherapy is the most suitable treatment for parameningeal tumors. The dose is 4,500 to 5,000 rad, although a primary tumor dose of at least 5,000 rad resulted in a significantly greater survival rate compared with lesser doses (28). Radiotherapy may result in serious problems. After radiotherapy for head and neck tumors, facial growth may be asymmetrical and normal dentition disturbed (29). The main risk of radiotherapy is spinal cord atrophy. Because of this, it is believed that, if the parameningeal tumor can be resected with adequate margins, prophylactic radiation of the craniospinal axis brings little or no benefit (28). Moderate doses of radiotherapy with intensive combination chemotherapy have been recommended (30). Only 30% of children with rhabdomyosarcoma survived prior to the use of maintenance systemic chemotherapy (31).

Chemotherapy is administered to all patients of rhabdomyosarcoma. A combination of vincristine, cyclophosphamide, and actinomycin D, with the possible addition of Adriamycin, is used for improved focal control and prevention of metastatic disease. Secondary acute side effects as well as immunosuppression are common risks in children.

The survival rate for parameningeal primary rhabdomyosarcomas is lower than in other tumor locations. Forty-five percent have a 3-year relapse-free survival rate, in comparison with 91% for tumors of the eye and orbit and 75% for other sites in the head and neck (25). Most relapses are seen within the first 2 years of diagnosis (32).

MALIGNANT MELANOMA

The spinal axis is an uncommon site for malignant melanoma. Two types of melanoma involve the spine: primary malignant melanoma of the meninges (34), and metastatic malignant melanoma. There are also melanotic variants of certain types of tumor (meningioma, medulloblastoma, medulloepithelioma, schwannoma, neurofibroma). Savitz and Anderson (35) collected 69 cases of spinal cord primary malignant melanoma from the literature in patients of all ages. Rokitansky (33) described a 14-year-old girl who had a giant hairy nevus and had diffuse melanoma of the brain and cord. In a review of 40 cases presenting neurocutaneous melanosis, diffuse spinal cord pigmentation was found in 20% (36). The disease affects both sexes similarly, usually occurs in Caucasians, and is rare in non-Caucasian patients (37). In children and adolescents, spinal melanoma is usually associated with neurocutaneous melanosis and congenital hairy nevi. Autopsy reveals spinal cord melanosis and infiltration of the spinal cord leptomeninges and nerve roots (37–43).

Although the cutaneous nevi are histologically benign, the pial melanin-bearing cells have a potential for malignant transformation. This has been observed not only in giant hairy nevi but also in blue nevi (44). Spinal metastatic malignant melanoma may be secondary to malignant melanoma of the skin (45). The capacity of this tumor to spread appears to be greater than that of the majority of other tumors. Pregnancy increases its activity and it has the potential for transplacental spread (46,47). Prognosis is commonly poor. Neurologic disturbances develop early. These include back pain, paresis and paresthesias of the legs as well as the arms, occasionally, and urinary and fecal retention or incontinence. Symptoms progress until the patients are unable to walk.

Roentgenograms are rarely diagnostic. Myelography commonly reveals incomplete or complete block at the level of the tumor. Diffuse spinal leptomeningeal melanomatosis may produce the myelographic picture of chronic arachnoiditis (48). Cytologic examination of the CSF may show malignant epithelioid cells that contain melanin pigment and are diagnostic of malignant melanoma (37,39).

Melanin-containing cells are the origin of leptomeningeal melanomatosis and of melanotic tumors of CNS. Melanoma is the tumor with the highest prevalence of metastasis to the CNS. Three types of CNS melanopathies need to be clearly differentiated, in the order of their frequency: metastatic melanoma, primary malignant melanoma, and leptomeningeal melanomatosis. The primary malignant melanoma of the leptomeninges may occur in isolation and spread diffusely, or it may be localized and associated with a giant hairy nevus of the skin or with Ota's nevus.

When the tumor is localized, the primary treatment is excision. If the tumor is disseminated, surgery must be supplemented by other forms of treatment such as radiotherapy, starting the day after surgery, and by chemotherapy. Although prognosis is generally poor in patients with this disease, new forms and combinations of therapies have been shown to be increasingly effective (49).

ELASTOFIBROMA

Elastofibromas are benign connective tissue tumors containing pathognomonic elastinophilic fibers. They usually occur at the inferomedial angle of the scapula and, rarely, have an intraspinal location. Since the original description of this tumor in 1961 (50), over 60 cases have been reported in the medical literature. Only one was located intraspinally, in the epidural space of the cervical region (51). This occurred in an adult who experienced neck pain radiating into the upper extremity and radiculopathy; there was no evidence of spinal cord compression. Radiographs showed narrowing of the disc spaces with rheumatoid changes. Myelography provided evidence of extradural root sleeve defects. The patient recovered following removal of the tumor.

Elastofibromas are not true neoplasms, but degenerative pseudotumors that may develop as a consequence of local mechanical stress resulting in vascular injury, ischemia, and massive regeneration and hypertrophy of elastin fibers (52). These tumors can be confused with neoplasms such as sarcomas, because both entities infiltrate surrounding tissues and lack a capsule. The histologic appearance of elastofibromas is characteristic on hematoxylin and eosin preparations (51). Distinctive curly eosinophilic fibers are scattered among collagen fibrils and lobules of fat. These eosinophilic fibers take up all known elastin stains.

MYXOMA

Myxomas are rare neoplasms of mesenchymal origin that were defined by Stout (53) as tumors composed of spindle-shaped or stellate cells in a loose mucoid stroma crossed by fine fibrils going in various directions, with no admixture of other differentiated cells, such as lipoblasts, chondroblasts, or rhabdomyoblasts.

Myxomas arising from within the spinal canal have only occasionally been reported. We know only of one adult patient with an epidural myxoma causing compression of the cauda equina (54), and another with a myxoma of the paraspinal musculature eroding the spine and causing spinal cord compression (55).

Clinical symptoms are consistent with a slowly growing lesion involving the spinal cord or roots. A diagnosis of fibrous dysplasia may have been made several years prior to that of myxoma (56).

Myelography demonstrates a partial or complete block of the spinal canal with the image of an extradural mass. Cure requires complete removal of the tumor.

REFERENCES

1. Russell WO, Cohen J, Enzinger F, et al. A clinical and pathological staging system for soft tissue sarcomas. *Cancer* 1977;40:1562–1570.
2. Favara BE, Galliani CA, Wakely PE Jr. Advances in the care of the child with cancer. The importance of histologic subclassification of tumors. *Cancer* 1986;58:426–441.
3. Mosberg WH. Spinal tumors diagnosed during the first year of life with report of a case. *J Neurosurg* 1951;8:220–224.
4. Tarlov IM, Keener EB. Subarachnoid hemorrhage and tumor implants from spinal sarcoma in an infant. *Neurology* 1953;3:384–390.
5. Zwartverwer FL, Kaplan AM, Hart MC, et al. Meningeal sarcoma of the spinal cord in a newborn. *Arch Neurol* 1978;35:844–846.
6. Clarke PRR, Saunders M. Steroid-induced remission in spinal canal reticulum cell sarcoma. Report of two cases. *J Neurosurg* 1975;42:346–348.
7. Raney RB Jr, Allen A, O'Neill J, et al. Malignant fibrous histiocytoma of soft tissue in childhood. *Cancer* 1986;57:2198–2201.
8. Soule EH, Pritchard DJ. Fibrosarcoma in infants and children. A review of 110 cases. *Cancer* 1977;40:1711–1721.
9. Angervall L, Enzinger FM. Extraskeletal neoplasm resembling Ewing's sarcoma. *Cancer* 1975;36:240–251.
10. Scheithauer BW, Egbert BM. Ewing's sarcoma of the spinal epidural space: report of two cases. *J Neurol Neurosurg Psychiatry* 1978;41:1031–1035.
11. Spaziante R, de Divitiis E, Giamundo A, et al. Ewing's sarcoma arising primarily in the spinal epidural space: fifth case report. *Neurosurgery* 1983;12:337–341.
12. Guarnaschelli JJ, Wehry SM, Serratoni FL, Ozenitis AJ. Atypical fibrous histiocytoma of the thoracic spine. Case report. *J Neurosurg* 1979;51:415–1416.
13. Helle TL, Hanbery JW, Becker DH. Meningeal malignant fibrous histiocytoma arising from a thoracolumbar myelomeningocele. Case report. *J Neurosurg* 1983;58:593–597.
14. Thomeer RTWM, Bots GTAM, Van Dulken H, et al. Neurofibrosarcoma of the cauda equina. Case report. *J Neurosurg* 1981;54:409–411.
15. Storm FK, Eilber FR, Mirra J, Morton DL. Neurofibrosarcoma. *Cancer* 1980;45:126–129.
16. Shmookler BM, Enzinger FM. Liposarcoma occurring in children: an analysis of 17 cases and review of the literature. *Cancer* 1983;52:567–574.
17. Castleberry RP, Kelly DR, Wilson ER, et al. Childhood liposarcoma: report of a case and review of the literature. *Cancer* 1984;54:579–584.
18. Salvador AH, Beabout JW, Dahlin DC. Mesenchymal chondrosarcoma—observations on 30 new cases. *Cancer* 1971;28:605–615.
19. Scheithauer BW, Rubinstein LJ. Meningeal mesenchymal chondrosarcoma: report of 8 cases with review of the literature. *Cancer* 1978;42:2744–2752.
20. Chan HSL, Turner-Gomes SO, Chuang SH, et al. A rare cause of spinal cord compression in childhood from intraspinal mesenchymal chondrosarcoma. A report of two cases and review of the literature. *Neuroradiology* 1984;26:323–327.
21. Harsh GR IV, Wilson CB. Central nervous system mesenchymal chondrosarcoma. Case report. *J Neurosurg* 1984;61:375–381.
22. Maurer HM. The Intergroup Rhabdomyosarcoma Study: update, November 1978. *Natl Cancer Inst Monog* 1981;56:61–68.
23. Tefft M, Fernandez C, Donaldson M, et al. Incidence of meningeal involvement by rhabdomyosarcoma of the head and neck in children. A report of the Intergroup Rhabdomyosarcoma Study (IRS). *Cancer* 1978;42:253–258.
24. Humphreys RP, McGreal D, Fitz CR, et al. Rhabdomyosarcoma of the head and neck in children. *Can J Neurol Sci* 1983;10:119–125.

25. Sutow MW, Lindberg RD, Gehan EA, et al. Three-year relapse-free survival rates in childhood rhabdomyosarcoma of the head and neck. Report from the Intergroup Rhabdomyosarcoma Study. *Cancer* 1982;49:2217–2221.
26. Horn RC, Enterline HT. Rhabdomyosarcoma: a clinico-pathological study and classification of 39 cases. *Cancer* 1958;11:181–199.
27. Lawrence W Jr, Hays DM, Moon TE. Lymphatic metastasis with childhood rhabdomyosarcoma. *Cancer* 1977;39:556–559.
28. Berry MP, Jenkin RDT. Parameningeal rhabdomyosarcoma in the young. *Cancer* 1981;48:281–288.
29. Nwoka AL, Koch H. Effects of radiation injury on the growing face. *J Maxillofac Surg* 1975; 3:28–34.
30. Jereb B, Ghavimi F, Exelby P, Zang E. Local control of embryonal rhabdomyosarcoma in children by radiation therapy when combined with chemotherapy. *Int J Radiat Oncol Biol Phys* 1980; 6:827–833.
31. Donalson S, Castro JR, Wilbur JR, Jesse RH. Rhabdomyosarcoma of the head and neck in children. *Cancer* 1973;31:26–35.
32. Pratt CB, Hustu HO, Kumar APM, et al. Treatment of childhood rhabdomyosarcoma at St. Jude Children's Research Hospital, 1962–78. *Natl Cancer Inst Monog* 1981;56:93–101.
33. Rokitansky C. Ein ausgezeichneter Fall von Pigment—mal mit ausgebreiteter pigmentierung der inner Hirn—und Rückenmarkshäute. *Allg Wien Med Ztg* 1861;6:113–116.
34. Russell DS, Rubinstein LJ. *Pathology of tumours of the nervous system*, 3rd ed. London: Arnold, 1971;40:317.
35. Savitz MH, Anderson PJ. Primary melanoma of the leptomeninges: a review. *Mt Sinai J Med (NY)* 1974;41:774–791.
36. Fox H. Neurocutaneous melanosis. In: Vinken PJ, Bruyn GW, eds. *The phakomatoses. Handbook of clinical neurology*, vol. 14. Amsterdam: Elsevier, 1972;414–428.
37. Kaplan AM, Itabashi HH, Hanelin LG, Lu AT. Neurocutaneous melanosis with malignant leptomeningeal melanoma. A case report with metastases outside the nervous system. *Arch Neurol* 1975;32:669–671.
38. Tveten I. Primary meningeal melanosis. A clinicopathological report of two cases. *Acta Pathol Microbiol Scand* 1965;63:1–10.
39. Hoffman HJ, Freman A. Primary malignant leptomeningeal melanoma in association with hairy nevi. Report of two cases. *J Neurosurg* 1967;26:62–71.
40. Slaughter JC, Hardman JM, Kempe LG, Earle KM. Neurocutaneous melanosis and leptomeningeal melanomatosis in children. *Arch Pathol* 1969;88:298–304.
41. Battin J, Vital C, Alberty J, et al. La mélanose neurocutanée. *Arch Fr Pediatr* 1968;25:277–289.
42. Faillace WJ, Okawara S-H, McDonald JV. Neurocutaneous melanosis with extensive intracerebral and spinal cord involvement. Report of two cases. *J Neurosurg* 1984;61:782–785.
43. Humes RA, Roskamp J, Einsenbrey AB. Melanosis and hydrocephalus. Report of four cases. *J Neurosurg* 1984;61:365–368.
44. Graham DI, Paterson A, McQueen A, et al. Melanotic tumours (blue nevi) of spinal nerve roots. *J Pathol* 1976;118:83–89.
45. Corkill G, Duncan CC. Absence of dural pulsation as an indication for dural opening in malignant melanoma metastatic to the spine. *Surg Neurol* 1983;19:35–37.
46. Conybeare R. Malignant melanoma and pregnancy. Report of three cases. *Obstet Gynecol* 1964; 24:451–454.
47. Demaille A, Cappelaere P. Placental metastasis. *Bull Cancer (Paris)* 1979;66:139–145.
48. Jacobsen HH, Lester J. A myelographic manifestation of diffuse spinal leptomeningeal melanomatosis. *Neuroradiology* 1970;1:30–31.
49. Spitler L, Levin A, Wybrand J. Combined immunotherapy in malignant melanoma: regression of metastatic lesions in two patients concordant in timing with systemic administration of transfer factor and bacillus calmette-guerin. *Cell Immol* 1976;21:1–19.
50. Jarvi OH, Saxon AE. Elastofibroma dorsi. *Acta Pathol Microbiol Scand* 1961;52(Suppl. 144):83–144.
51. Prete PE, Henbest M, Michalski JP, Porter RW. Intraspinal elastofibroma. A case report. *Spine* 1983;8:800–802.
52. Barr JR. Elastofibroma. *Am J Clin Pathol* 1966;45:679–683.

53. Stout AP. Myxoma, the tumor of primitive mesenchyme. *Ann Surg* 1948;127:706–719.
54. Bell WO, Gill A, Babiak T, Patterson RH. Epidural myxoma causing compression of the cauda equina: a case report. *Neurosurgery* 1983;12:325–326.
55. Tahmouresie A, Farmer PM, Stokes N. Paraspinal myxoma with spinal cord compression. *J Neurosurg* 1981;54:542–544.
56. Ireland DCR, Soule EH, Ivins JC. Myxoma of somatic soft tissues. A report of 58 patients, 3 with multiple tumors and fibrous dysplasia of bone. *Mayo Clin Proc* 1973;48:401–410.

11

Spinal Metastases

Ignacio Pascual-Castroviejo

Metastases affecting the vertebrae, spinal meninges, spinal cord, and roots are quite common in children and adolescents. Approximately 13 to 25% of the tumors located along the spinal canal are metastases (1,2). Half the cases of leptomeningeal dissemination of primary central nervous system (CNS) tumors of children occur before diagnosis of the primary tumor (3). Extracranial metastases from intracranial tumors are three times more frequent in adults than in children (4). Primitive neuroectodermal tumors, anaplastic gliomas, and ependymomas are the neoplasms with the greatest propensity for seeding (4). Both myelography and cerebrospinal fluid (CSF) cytological examination are required for the diagnosis of metastases (3).

Tumors producing skeletal metastases in children are mainly neuroblastoma, rhabdomyosarcoma, teratoma-teratocarcinoma, Wilms tumor, lymphoma, hemangioblastoma, embryonal carcinoma of the testis, and carcinoma of the kidney (5). Eighty percent of cases involve the spine (5). Metastatic skeletal involvement is more frequent in younger children (5,6). Pathologic fractures and paraplegia with spinal cord compression occur in many patients. The radiographic appearance of spinal metastases is usually bony destruction. Pathologic fracture is a particularly bad prognostic sign (5). Carcinomas are responsible for 12% of the spinal metastases of children (1). In some series, sarcomatous tumors were the origin of nearly two-thirds of all spinal metastatic lesions (2). Metastatic deposits can occur either from distant tumors or from tumors located in adjacent structures. A large majority of metastatic tumors within the spinal canal are epidural. Intradural metastases account for no more than 5% of all spinal metastases (7,8). Intradural metastases can be intradural intramedullary, intradural extramedullary, or present as meningeal carcinomatosis (9). Three main types of intradural extramedullary metastases have been described: subarachnoid, intradural extra-arachnoid, and epidural with secondary invasion of the meningeal layers.

Almost every type of malignant tumor of the body has been responsible for spinal metastases on some occasion, although they are rare in some neoplasms. In the series of Baten and Vannucci (1), tumor types giving spinal metastases included neuroblastoma, osteogenic sarcoma, embryonal rhabdomyosarcoma, lymphoma, Ewing sarcoma, chondrosarcoma, synovial sarcoma, ovarian carcinoma, vaginal embryonal adenocarcinoma, presacral teratoma (adenosarcoma), and retinoblastoma. Diffuse spinal cord pigmentation has been found in 20% of patients presenting neurocutaneous melanosis (10), although clinical disturbances were not observed in every case. Patients with spinal metastases exhibit symptoms of back pain, leg or arm pain, difficulty in walking, frequent falls, weakness progressing to paralysis, paraparesis, atrophy and sensory loss below the neck, stiff neck, and sore neck.

Medulloblastomas are brain tumors that most often give rise to intraspinal implants in infants and adolescents (11–13) followed by, in approximate order of frequency, ependymomas, pineal neoplasms, astrocytomas, choroid plexus papillomas, and retinoblastomas. The brain tumor that metastasizes to bone most frequently is glioblastoma multiforme (14). Although intraspinal spread from intracranial tumors by seeding along CSF pathways is a common finding at autopsy, it is rarely diagnosed during life (15). This is true in both children and adults. Although seeding occurs most often after removal of primary tumors (17), it can also occur in cases without previous surgery due to fragmentation of tumors bathed with CSF (16). Subarachnoid seeding has been seen at the time of the original craniotomy (18,19), and it has also been observed by myelography within 3 weeks of the craniotomy (13). This may indicate that spread was present before removal of the primary tumor. Very late presentation of extradural metastases has also been reported. Stolzenberg et al. (20) described a patient with cerebellar medulloblastoma who was operated on and underwent irradiation of the head and the spine, who, 10 years later, presented with lumbar metastasis.

Skeletal metastases from medulloblastoma are uncommon (21), and only 43 cases were reported in a relatively recent review of the English literature (22). Eighteen cases below the age of 20, only 14 of whom were verified histologically, were vertebral (14,20–30). Additional cases have been reported more recently (31–33). Metastases commonly occur early, sometimes within weeks or months (32), and usually within 2 years of the original diagnosis. They are rare after 4 years. However, an extradural spinal tumor was observed in a patient who presented with an intracerebral metastasis 3 years after treatment of a spinal metastasis (20). A recent review of the literature (33) indicated that medulloblastoma seeded to the spinal canal in 62% of cases. Patients ranged in age from 6 months to 48 years, with a mean of 13 years; two-thirds of the patients were male. Shunting was a factor causing metastases to appear earlier. Metastases occurred an average of 2 years after diagnosis of the primary tumor in patients without a shunt and 1.3 years in patients with a shunt. Approximately 5% of shunted patients with medulloblastoma develop systemic metastases which are associated with increased morbidity and a shortened life expectancy. Hoffman et al. (34) incorporated a millipore filter in their shunts in an effort to prevent metastatic spread through the shunt.

Spinal intramedullary metastases, in the absence of surface leptomeningeal seeding, are the rarest of the metastases from medulloblastoma. They are well recognized at autopsy but may not always be diagnosed during life (15). Only a few cases of metastatic medulloblastoma presented as an intramedullary spinal cord tumor (12,13,35,36).

The presence of malignant cells in the CSF, either preoperatively or postoperatively, has some value for the detection of spinal involvement, but is too unreliable to be truly helpful for diagnosis or prognosis (12). Myelography shows the presence of spinal metastases in many patients (12,13) [e.g., 43% in the series of Deutch and Reigel (12)] who are clinically asymptomatic. The lumbosacral region is affected most often, with nerve root thickening, nodularity, and irregularity of the dural sac; in the cervical and thoracic areas, cord thickening, nodularity, and meningeal disease are common (13). Computerized tomography (CT) scan may show nodularity on the cord surface, with obliteration of the subarachnoid space (13). Magnetic resonance (MR) imaging has been used to localize intramedullary lesions and has provided much better diagnostic information than either CT or myelography (36).

Treatment depends on the clinical and radiologic characteristics of the disease. A solitary extramedullary metastasis that compresses the spinal cord must be removed as soon as possible. Local radiotherapy, chemotherapy, and analgesics are the main therapeutic approaches. In the series of Kleinman et al. (33), average survival was 7 months after the appearance of systemic metastases for patients both with and without shunts. Longer survivals, such as 7.5 years (11), 6.9 years (14), and 13 years (in an adult) (26), have been reported.

Although less frequent than in medulloblastoma, spinal metastases (seeding) from other intracranial tumors, such as pineal germinoma (32,37) and ependymoma (32), can occur. When we systematically used MR for detecting spinal metastases, we found them in a high proportion of cases, although they had rarely caused clinical symptoms.

Intracranial gliomas (astrocytomas, glioblastomas, and oligodendrogliomas) may metastasize along the spinal canal, as well as to other regions outside the CNS. In a recent review of the literature (38), only four patients below 21 years of age were reported (26,39–41), although some other cases have been described (32,42–44). In the series of Eade and Urich (40), malignant gliomas with widespread dissemination through CSF pathways occurred in five patients under 25 years of age; the primary tumor was in the spinal cord in four cases, and both ependymal and subependymal metastases were found. Spinal spread of brainstem glioma (astrocytoma) has been documented in children as well as in adults (45). Spinal subarachnoid metastases from primary intracranial glioblastoma multiforme seem to be more prevalent in both adults and children according to the findings in autopsy series (44). The spinal cord was commonly invaded from adjacent leptomeningeal metastases. Symptoms and signs of spinal disease were not discovered during the illness; perhaps they were overshadowed by the severe problems caused by the primary intracranial tumor. Salazar and Rubin (46), in an autopsy study of 43 cases of intracranial glioblastoma, claimed that 6% of their supratentorial and 50% of their infratentorial glioblastomas had seeded to the spinal cord. McLaughlin (47) reported five cases of juvenile astrocytoma with subarachnoid spread, three of which were spinal. The thoracic region was the main site of metastasis (44). Duration of symptoms ranged from a few weeks to 3 years (44). The CSF very seldom contained malignant cells. Myelography showed multiple filling defects in the spinal subarachnoid space (48). CT scan and MR provided conclusive diagnostic images. CT scans show spinal lesions very well (49). Most patients with spinal metastases had been operated previously for their primary tumor, although there are reports of cases without previous surgery (17,50,51). The majority also had intracranial metastases. Both lymphatic and bloodstream routes of spread to extracranial sites have been observed (49,52).

Spinal metastases from oligodendrogliomas are very rare in adults and exceptional in children. Only 2 of 170 cases operated for cerebral oligodendrogliomas had spinal involvement in the series of Arseni et al. (53). Clinical manifestations of spinal disease occurred 1 to 2 years after removal of the intracranial tumor. Spinal seeding commonly affects the leptomeninges, but involvement of the underlying spinal cord and vertebrae may also be seen (53,54). Clinical manifestations are those of spinal cord compression. Dissemination occurs through the CSF pathways after removal of cerebral oligodendroglioma. Occurrence following several operations, was reported in some of the children (54). Multiple deposits at several levels of the spinal leptomeninges are commonly found (54). Myelography, metrizamide-CT scan myelography, and MR imaging show the metastases.

Radiotherapy and chemotherapy are the usual treatments for the spinal metastases of malignant gliomas. Surgery is appropriate only for cases with an isolated extramedullary metastasis compressing the spinal cord or for reestablishing the circulation of the CSF. Prognosis is poor, and the survival time ranges from a few months to 3 years (44).

Neuroblastoma is the most common malignant tumor producing vertebral metastases (Fig. 1A,B). Half of the patients show skeletal involvement at the time of diagnosis. The skull and the vertebrae are sites of predilection (Fig. 2). They are involved in 80% of cases (5). Radiologic study shows lytic or punctate lesions, or a moth-eaten appearance of the vertebrae, with cortical destruction, occasional periosteal reaction (Fig. 3), and, commonly, fracture.

Spinal metastases always present a more severe radiologic appearance than predicted from their clinical symptomatology. These radiologic alterations are not specific to neuroblastoma. Therefore, when these radiologic findings are observed in patients who are not known to harbor a neuroblastoma, differential diagnosis includes other diseases, such as leukemia, histiocytosis X, osteomyelitis, lymphoma, osteosarcoma, and Ewing's sarcoma. Treatment of these patients is that described for neuroblastomas (see Chapter 8, Tumors of the Neural Crest).

Metastatic intramedullary spinal cord neuroblastomas seem to be quite rare. Only 70 cases, encompassing all ages, had been reported by 1972 (55). They accounted for less than 1% to 3.4% of all metastatic tumors involving the spinal cord (55). Most of the tumors causing intramedullary lesions are limited to adults, encompassing carcinoma of the lung, malignant melanoma, and lymphoma (55). Medulloblastomas are the most frequent cause of intramedullary metastases in children (12,13,35). As in the case of extramedullary metastases, their main location is the upper thoracic region (55). Signs and symptoms are not different from those of extramedullary metastases: local or radicular pain, paresthesias, bladder or bowel disturbances, a sensory level to pinprick, dissociated sensory loss, spas-

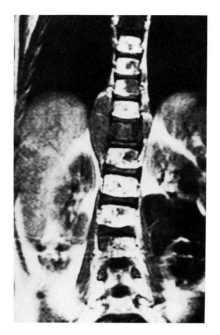 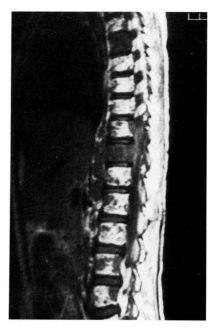

A,B

FIG. 1. A: A 6-year-old boy with neuroblastoma. MR in T1 (TE 30, TR 350). The frontal projection shows metastases to almost all the vertebral bodies (zones of signal attenuation) and to the contiguous paravertebral structures. (Courtesy of Dr. Luis Lopez-Ibor.) **B:** Same case as A. MR in T1 (TE 30, TR 450). The lateral projection shows metastases affecting almost all the vertebral bodies more or less severely, as well as the intra- and extraspinal structures. (Courtesy of Dr. Luis Lopez-Ibor.)

ticity, and paraplegia. The course is very rapid from initial symptoms to the fully developed neurologic deficit. Seventy percent of patients are paraplegic within 2 months and 100% of them within 6 months (55). The pathogenesis of intramedullary metastasis from medulloblastoma remains a matter of speculation. Three hypotheses have been suggested: (a) direct arterial seeding, (b) spread via the vertebral venous system, and (c) direct extension from nerve roots to the CSF. Involvement of the vertebrae is very unusual. Plain X-ray films are most frequently normal. Myelography may or may not be abnormal, which is characteristic of an intramedullary lesion. CT scan and MR images are the definitive tests to ascertain the presence of intramedullary metastases, their number, size, and exact location. Radiotherapy and chemotherapy are the treatments of choice. However, survival is short, usually less than 1 year, and the majority of cases die within 6 months.

There are nonneural tumors that are rarely seen in children, but that may occasionally cause spinal metastases in adolescents and young adults. A prolonged survival of at least 5 years after the onset of paraplegia is expected in patients with these tumors (Hodgkin's disease, multiple myeloma, prostatic and testicular tu-

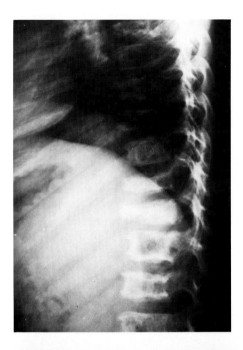

FIG. 2. A 10-year-old boy with generalized metastases of neuroblastoma. X-ray film of the spine in lateral projection shows metastatic alteration of almost all vertebral bodies.

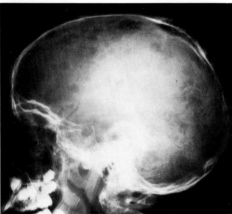

FIG. 3. Cranial metastases of neuroblastoma in a 10-year-old boy. The X-ray film of the skull shows many lytic lacunae, cortical destruction, and periosteal reaction, as well as eroded posterior clinoids.

mors), provided they are appropriately treated by prompt spinal decompression (56), or high dose steroids and radiotherapy in appropriate cases.

Successful treatment of spinal metastases has been achieved recently (59) with combination chemotherapy consisting of cis-platinum, vinblastine, doxorubicin HC1 (Adriamycin), and bleomycin (cis-VAB). A child who received this therapy was well with no sign of tumor 3.5 years after the appearance of the metastatic lesion and 2.5 years after all therapy was discontinued.

Other tumors such as the extragonadal endodermal sinus (yolk sac) tumor (Fig. 4), can metastasize to the lumbosacrococcygeal region (57,58), and, in the past, have had an unfavorable prognosis. This tumor presents in children and adolescents of either sex.

There are exceptional reports of spinal metastases from other tumors. Wilms tumor rarely metastasizes to the vertebrae (60–62). Its roentgenologic features are of a destructive character, with progressive involvement of the body of the vertebrae, occasional periosteal reaction, and a soft tissue mass (5,63). Affected vertebral bodies tend to collapse, causing severe deformity of the vertebral column (63). There are few radiographic differences between metastatic Wilms tumor and neuroblastoma. In contrast to neuroblastoma, bone lesions in Wilms tumor are rarely found during the patients' first admission (63). Skeletal metastases in Wilms tumor are only a part of widespread dissemination of tumor emboli, invari-

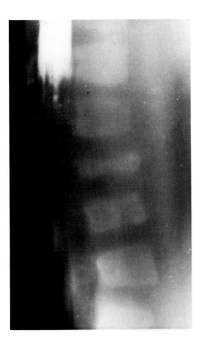

FIG. 4. A 6-year-old boy with extragonadal endo-dermal (yolk sac) tumor. X-ray tomography with myelography shows destruction of the vertebral body of several lumbar vertebrae and the picture of complete extradural block of the contrast medium.

ably resulting in a fatal outcome. Periosteal new bone formation is sparse. Response to radiotherapy and administration of cytostatics is poor.

Renal cell carcinoma may cause spinal metastases at any age, but is quite rare in children (5,64). X-ray films show destruction of the bony cortex, little periosteal response, and, often, an expansile lesion; fracture is common. Mesenchymal chondrosarcoma has sometimes caused intraspinal metastases in children and young people, mostly in the thoracic region (65–68). It carries a poor prognosis, since surgical excision of this tumor is the main modality of treatment (68).

Occasionally, other types of tumors have been reported to metastasize to the spine, usually only in adults. Although they rarely metastasize, leiomyomas (69) and leiomyosarcomas (70) have some tendency to involve the spine (70).

REFERENCES

1. Baten M, Vannucci RC. Intraspinal metastatic disease in childhood cancer. *J Pediatr* 1977; 90:207–212.
2. Haft H, Ransohoff J, Carter S. Spinal cord tumours in children. *Pediatrics* 1959;23:1152–1159.
3. Packer RJ, Siegel KR, Sutton LN, et al. Leptomeningeal dissemination of primary central nervous system tumors of childhood. *Ann Neurol* 1985;18:217–221.
4. Glasauer FE, Yuan RHP. Intracranial tumors with extracranial metastases. *J Neurosurg* 1963; 20:474–493.
5. Leeson MC, Makley JT, Carter JR. Metastatic skeletal disease in the pediatric population. *J Pediatr Orthop* 1985;5:261–267.
6. Young JL Jr, Miller RW. Incidence of malignant tumors in U.S. children. *J Pediatr* 1975;86:254–258.
7. Barron KD, Hirano A, Araki S, Terry RD. Experience with metastatic neoplasms involving the spinal cord. *Neurology (Minneap)* 1959;9:91–106.
8. Black P. Spinal metastasis: current status and recommended guidelines for management. *Neurosurgery* 1979;5:726–746.
9. Barolat-Romana G, Benzel EC. Spinal intradural extraarachnoid metastasis. *Surg Neurol* 1983; 19:137–143.
10. Fox H. Neurocutaneous melanosis. In: Vinkin PJ, Bruyn GW, eds. *The phakomatoses. Handbook of clinical neurology*, vol. 14. Amsterdam: Elsevier, 1972;414–428.
11. McFarland DR, Horowitz H, Saenger EL, Bahr GK. Medulloblastoma—a review of prognosis and survival. *Br J Radiol* 1969;42:198–214.
12. Deutch M, Reigel DH. The value of myelography in the management of childhood medulloblastoma. *Cancer* 1980;45:2194–2197.
13. Stanley P, Senac MO Jr, Segall HD. Intraspinal seeding from intracranial tumors of the central nervous system. *Am J Roentgenol* 1985;144:157–161.
14. Smith DR, Hardman JM, Earle KM. Metastasizing neuroectodermal tumors of the central nervous system. *J Neurosurg* 1969;31:50–58.
15. Bryan P. CSF seeding of intracranial tumours: a study of 96 cases. *Clin Radiol* 1974;25:355–360.
16. Svien HJ, Mabon RF, Kernohan JW, Craig WM. Ependymoma of the brain: pathological aspects. *Neurology* 1953;3:1–15.
17. Cairns H, Russell DS. Intracranial and spinal metastases in gliomas of the brain. *Brain* 1931; 54:377–420.
18. Tarlow IM, Davidoff LM. Subarachnoid and ventricular implants in ependymal and other gliomas. *J Neuropathol Exp Neurol* 1946;5:213–224.
19. Ingrahan FD, Bailey OT, Barker WF. Medulloblastoma cerebelli. *N Engl J Med* 1948;238:171–174.
20. Stolzenberg J, Fischer JJ, Kligerman MM. Extradural metastasis in medulloblastoma 10 years after treatment. Report of a case. *Am J Roentgenol* 1970;108:71–74.

21. Debnam JW, Staple TW. Osseous metastases from cerebellar medulloblastoma. *Radiology* 1973; 107:363–365.
22. Booher KR, Schmidtknecht TM. Cerebellar medulloblastoma with skeletal metastases. *J Bone Joint Surg* 1977;59A:684–686.
23. Paterson E. Distant metastases from medulloblastoma of the cerebellum. *Brain* 1961;84:301–309.
24. Drachman DA, Winter TS III, Karon M. Medulloblastoma with extracranial metastases. *Arch Neurol* 1963;9:518–530.
25. Black SPW, Keats TE. Generalized osteosclerosis secondary to metastatic medulloblastoma of the cerebellum. *Radiology* 1964;82:395–400.
26. Rubinstein LJ, Northfield DWC. The medulloblastoma and the so-called "arachnoidal cerebellar sarcoma." A critical reexamination of a nosological problem. *Brain* 1964;87:379–412.
27. Corrin B, Meadows JC. Skeletal metastases from cerebellar medulloblastoma. *Br Med J* 1967; 2:485–486.
28. Lassman LP, Pearce GW, Banna M, Jones RD. Vincristine sulphate in the treatment of skeletal metastases from cerebellar medulloblastoma. *J Neurosurg* 1969;30:42–49.
29. Banna M, Lassman LP, Pearce GW. Radiological study of skeletal metastases from cerebellar medulloblastoma. *Br J Radiol* 1970;43:173–179.
30. Brutschin P, Culver GJ. Extracranial metastases from medulloblastoma. *Radiology* 1973;107:359–362.
31. Damuth HD, Staple TW. Case report 212. *Skeletal Radiol* 1982;9:64–67.
32. Pezeshkpour GH, Henry JM, Armbrustmacher VW. Spinal metastases. A rare mode of presentation of brain tumors. *Cancer* 1984;54:353–356.
33. Kleinman GM, Hochberg FH, Richardson EP Jr. Systemic metastases from medulloblastoma: report of two cases and review of the literature. *Cancer* 1981;48:2296–2309.
34. Hoffman HJ, Hendrick EB, Humphreys RP. Metastasis via ventriculoperitoneal shunt in patients with medulloblastoma. *J Neurosurg* 1976;44:562–566.
35. Zumpano JB. Spinal intramedullary medulloblastoma. *J Neurosurg* 1978;48:632–635.
36. Barnwell SL, Edwards MSB. Spinal intramedullary spread of medulloblastoma. Case report. *J Neurosurg* 1986;65:253–255.
37. Rubery ED, Wheeler TK. Metastases outside the central nervous system from a presumed pineal germinoma. Case report. *J Neurosurg* 1980;53:562–565.
38. Pasquier B, Pasquier D, N'Golet A, et al. Extraneural metastases of astrocytomas and glioblastomas. Clinicopathological study of two cases and review of literature. *Cancer* 1980; 45:112–125.
39. Wolf A, Cowen D, Stewart WB. Glioblastoma with extracranial metastasis by way of a ventriculopleural anastomosis. *Trans Am Neurol Assoc* 1954;79:140–142.
40. Eade DE, Urich H. Metastasizing gliomas in young subjects. *Pathol* 1971;103:245–256.
41. Russell DS, Rubinstein LJ. *Pathology of tumors and the nervous system*, 4th ed. London: Edward Arnold, 1977;238–239,244.
42. Thierry A, Tommasi M, Fischer G, et al. Glioblastomas multiformes intracraniens du jeune sujet, se manifestant primitivement par une compression radiculomédullaire basse. *Neurochirurgie* 1969; 15:545–555.
43. Steimle R, Charlin A, Jacquet G, et al. Metastase médullaire d'un gliome cérébral. *Neurochirurgie* 1974;20:267–274.
44. Erlich SS, Davis RL. Spinal subarachnoid metastasis from primary intracranial glioblastoma multiforme. *Cancer* 1978;42:2854–2864.
45. Kepes JJ, Striebinger CM, Brackett CE, Kishore P. Gliomas (astrocytomas) of the brainstem with spinal intra- and extradural metastases: report of three cases. *J Neurol Neurosurg Psychiatry* 1976; 39:66–76.
46. Salazar OM, Rubin P. The spread of glioblastoma multiforme as a determining factor in the radiation treated volume. *Int J Radiat Oncol Biol Phys* 1976;1:627–637.
47. McLaughlin JE. Juvenile astrocytomas with subarachnoid spread. *J Pathol* 1976;118:101–107.
48. Wood EH, Taveras JM, Pool JL. Myelographic demonstration of spinal cord metastases from primary brain tumors. *Am J Roentgenol* 1953;69:221–230.
49. Sadik AS, Port R, Garfinkel B, Bravo J. Extracranial metastasis of cerebral glioblastoma multiforme. Case report. *Neurosurgery* 1984;15:549–551.
50. Anzil AP. Glioblastoma multiforme with extracranial metastasis in the absence of previous craniotomy. Case report. *J Neurosurg* 1970;33:88–94.

51. Rubinstein LJ. Development of extracranial metastasis from a malignant astrocytoma in the absence of previous craniotomy. Case report. *J Neurosurg* 1967;26:542–547.
52. Dietz R, Burger L, Merkel K, Schimrigk K. Malignant gliomas—glioblastoma multiforme and astrocytoma III-IV with extracranial metastases. Report of two cases. *Acta Neurochir (Wien)* 1981;57:99–105.
53. Arseni C, Horvath L, Carp N, et al. Spinal dissemination following operation on cerebral oligodendroglioma. *Acta Neurochir (Wien)* 1977;37:125–137.
54. Spataro J, Sacks O. Oligodendroglioma with remote metastases. *J Neurosurg* 1968;28: 373–379.
55. Edelson RN, Deck MDF, Posner JB. Intramedullary spinal cord metastases. Clinical and radiographic findings in nine cases. *Neurology* 1972;22:1222–1231.
56. Jameson RM. Prolonged survival in paraplegia due to metastatic spinal tumours. *Lancet* 1974; i:1209–1211.
57. Huntington RW Jr, Bullock WK. Yolk sac tumours of extragonadal origin. *Cancer* 1970;25:1368–1376.
58. Roth LM, Panganiban WG. Gonadal and extragonadal yolk sac carcinoma. A clinicopathologic study of 14 cases. *Cancer* 1976;37:812–820.
59. Thomas WJ, Kelleher JF, Duval-Arnould B. Successful treatment of metastatic extragonadal sinus (yolk sac) tumor in childhood. *Cancer* 1981;48:2371–2374.
60. Bever CT, Koenigsberger MR, Antunes JL, Wolff JA. Epidural metastasis by Wilms tumor. *Am J Dis Child* 1981;135:644–646.
61. Beckwith JB, Palmer NF. Histopathology and prognosis of Wilms tumor. *Cancer* 1978;41:1937–1948.
62. Merandian MH, Rakchan M, Kouchanfar A, Chafei M. Paraplégie flasque par compression médullaire révélatrice de tumeur de Wilms à l'âge de douze ans. *Arch Fr Pediatr* 1985;42:695–697.
63. Rudhe U. Skeletal metastases in Wilms' tumor. *Ann Radiol (Paris)* 1969;12:337–342.
64. Marsden HB, Lennox E, Lawler W, Kinnier-Wilson LM. Bone metastases in childhood renal tumours. *Br J Cancer* 1980;41:875–879.
65. Rengachary SS, Kepes JJ. Spinal epidural metastatic "mesenchymal" chondrosarcoma. A case report. *J Neurosurg* 1969;30:71–73.
66. Sears WP, Tefft M, Cohen J. Postirradiation mesenchymal chondrosarcoma. A case report. *Pediatrics* 1967;40:254–258.
67. Salvador AH, Beabout JW, Dahlin DC. Mesenchymal chondrosarcoma—observations on 30 new cases. *Cancer* 1971;28:605–615.
68. Chan HSL, Turner-Gomes SO, Chuang, et al. A rare cause of spinal cord compression in childhood from intraspinal mesenchymal chondrosarcoma. A report of two cases and review of the literature. *Neuroradiology* 1984;26:323–327.
69. Gatti JM, Morvan G, Henin D, et al. Leiomyomatosis metastasizing to the spine. *J Bone Joint Surg* 1983;65A:1163–1165.
70. Paley D, Fornaiser VL. Leiomyosarcoma in bone: primary or secondary? A case report and review of the literature. *Skeletal Radiol* 1983;10:147–153.

12

Tumors of Systemic Disease Origin

Ignacio Pascual-Castroviejo

HISTIOCYTOSIS X

Generalities

The name histiocytosis X originates from the abundant proliferation of histiocytes in the lesion. Included under the term histiocytosis X are the eosinophilic granuloma, the Hand-Schüller-Christian syndrome, and the Letterer-Siwe syndrome (1). These syndromes are different clinical and radiologic expressions of the same disease. The basis for classification of histiocytosis X is the extent of the lesion (2,3): (a) disease affecting only one bone (eosinophilic granuloma), (b) disease affecting more than a bone (Hand-Schüller-Christian syndrome), and (c) disease affecting bones and soft tissues, or only soft tissues (Letterer-Siwe syndrome).

On the basis of the presence of immature and mature macrophages, and its histologic and histochemical characteristics, histiocytosis X can be further classified into (4): (a) benign histiocytosis X, which may appear either as solitary or multiple bone lesions, or as benign disseminated histiocytosis X; and (b) malignant histiocytosis X.

The spine is rarely affected, but lesions in vertebrae cause severe neurologic involvement.

Clinical Findings and Pathology

Lesions may be located anywhere in the body, causing a symptomatology that varies depending on the organ affected and the spread of the disease. Spinal lesions can be found at any level from the atlas to the coccyx. Neurologic symptoms reflect the level of the affected segment. Although vertebral lesions are commonly isolated, several vertebrae may be involved (5).

Root compression is common in cervical and cervicodorsal cases, whereas lumbar lesions produce a cauda equina syndrome. We have observed torticollis, retrocollis, radicular pain, muscular atrophy in a shoulder, Horner's syndrome, and paresis of an upper limb in a child who had a lesion of the fifth cervical vertebra, and radicular pain, paraparesis, and moderate sphincter disturbances in a case with a lumbar lesion. Spinal involvement usually occurs in patients with previously diagnosed histiocytosis X (6), although there are descriptions (7) of neurologic involvement as the first symptom of the disease. Neither of the two cases we studied had previously shown any sign or symptom of histiocytosis X outside the vertebrae, and both presented with only neurologic symptomatology and isolated radiologic findings in the spine. It is difficult to think in terms of a diagnosis of histiocytosis X, yet it enters in the differential diagnosis in a child showing spinal or spinal cord symptomatology. All patients with a spinal lesion should undergo a skeletal survey.

In spite of the rarity of nonneurologic symptomatology in children with vertebral lesions, one needs to consider the more common clinical symptoms of histiocytosis X (8): hepatosplenomegaly, lymphadenopathy, pallor, fever, bone lesions, otitis, mastoiditis, lung infections, retarded growth, various skin lesions, exophthalmos, diabetes insipidus, and visceral as well as bone lesions.

Lesions are most common in the lymph glands, skin, liver, bones, and lung. Assessment of those organs is necessary in every case. Histiocytic infiltration is the hallmark of the disease. The lesions in benign forms of histiocytosis X show a combination of eosinophils and histiocytes, whereas histiocytic infiltration characterizes the malignant forms (9,10). Differentiation is not always easy. The cause of histiocytosis X is still unknown.

Chronic histiocytosis X may be located anywhere along the spine. It produces lesions, known as xanthogranulomatous reactions, that involve several roots and

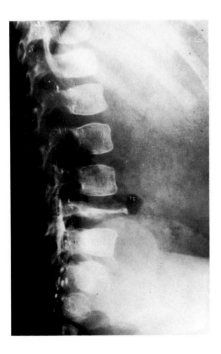

FIG. 1. Histiocytosis X. Flattening with anterior and posterior protrusion of the affected vertebral body 3 years after radiotherapy.

appear as yellow, well-circumscribed nodules that are usually located extradurally (6,7). Microscopically, these nodules contain large numbers of lipid-laden macrophages and giant cells against a background of granulomatous inflammation, with destruction of axons and myelin sheaths.

Radiology

Bone lesions occur as frequently as skin lesions (11) but do not alter the prognosis. Osteolytic lesions are common. Most of the lesions appear gradually as the disease progresses (11), but they are often discovered accidentally before clinical symptoms appear. Bone lesions are located anywhere in the skeleton but more often in the skull, femur, ribs, and vertebrae. They have the appearance of eosinophilic granulomas. X-ray films and computerized tomography (CT) show destruction of the vertebral body and/or pedicles. Affected vertebral bodies appear flattened and protrude in any direction. Protrusion into the spinal canal or into the intervertebral foramina causes spinal cord compression or radicular symptoms. The intervertebral space is always respected (Fig. 1). Myelography usually shows an incomplete block of the contrast medium which, rarely, may be complete. CT and magnetic resonance (MR) may show partial or total destruction of the vertebral body (Fig. 2).

Treatment and Prognosis

Spontaneous regression of bone lesions occurs in some cases (12). Although several types of treatment exist for systemic histiocytosis X (surgery, irradiation,

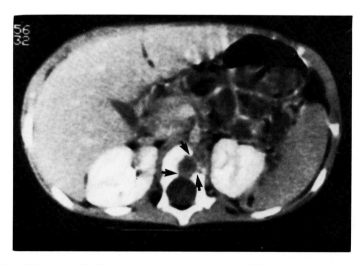

FIG. 2. Histiocytosis X. CT showing destruction of a part of the vertebral body (*arrows*).

chemotherapy with a variety of drugs), spinal involvement is often isolated. Local treatment alone (surgical curettage and/or irradiation) may be indicated for such patients. Most authors recommend local irradiation with 600 to 1,000 rad with fractionated doses of 200 rad in the case of a solitary lesion (13). Higher doses do not seem to be more effective. Flattening of vertebrae is not altered by radio-therapy. In spite of this, the patient is usually asymptomatic.

Recommended doses of corticosteroids and cytostatic agents are (4): Pred-nisone: 40 mg/m^2/day for 6 weeks; vincristine: 2.0 mg/m^2/week for 6 weeks; mer-captopurine: 50 mg/m^2/day for 5 weeks; methotrexate: 30 mg/m^2/week for 5 weeks; cyclophosphamide: 200 mg/m^2/week for 6 weeks.

In the case of multiple bone lesions, the same treatment recommended for soli-tary lesions may be administered. Benign disseminated histiocytosis X can be treated with chemotherapy: prednisone and vincristine for the induction phase, mercaptopurine and methotrexate for the maintenance phase, vincristine and pred-nisone for the consolidation phase. Duration of therapy is 12 months after induc-tion of remission. Malignant disseminated histiocytosis X can be treated with che-motherapy: vincristine, methotrexate, cyclophosphamide, and prednisone as drugs of induction; mercaptopurine, methotrexate, and cyclophosphamide as mainte-nance drugs. Medication has to be continued for 12 months after remission.

The prognosis of histiocytosis X has improved considerably since the introduc-tion of therapy with corticosteroids and cytostatic agents. Nonetheless, patients with solitary or multiple bone lesions should be watched closely for a long time in order to detect any further involvement. Occurrence of extraskeletal lesions is common within 6 months of the first symptoms of the initial bone lesions (8,14). Follow-up of patients with histiocytosis X should continue for many years because relapse remains possible for many years. The term "complete cure" must be used with reservation.

MYELOMA (PLASMACYTOMA)

Localized solitary plasmacytoma (SP) is regarded by some as a disorder related to, but distinct from, multiple myeloma (MM), whereas others see SP as an un-usual presentation of MM.

MM (plasma cell myeloma) is the most common plasma cell neoplasm. Its prevalence increases progressively with age. It is very rare in children. Well-documented cases of myeloma rarely occur in people under 30 years old (15,16). Less than 1% to 2% of patients are younger than 40 years of age at diagnosis (15). Spinal plasmacytoma is extremely rare below that age. Yet Jacoby (17) described an 8-year-old girl with collapsed vertebrae that were found to contain plasma cells at postmortem; however, the diagnosis of myeloma cannot be unequivocally ac-cepted according to current concepts. Large series of spinal plasmacytomas de-scribe only isolated cases below 30 years of age, all above 20 years (18,19).

The central nervous system (CNS) is affected in a large number of adult patients with myeloma. The incidence of spinal cord compression varies from 6% to 16%

(20,21). It may result from intradural and extradural myeloma. Intradural myeloma is extremely rare. Spinal cord compression by an extradural mass may result from vertebral collapse, extradural compression without local bone disease, or extradural extension of plasmacytoma from an adjacent vertebra. The latter possibility is the most common. Some series report that 20% of their MM patients with epidural lesions had no radiologic evidence of bone disease (22). Tumors occurring in the epidural space seem to have a predilection for the thoracic region (22,23). This may be due to the relative paucity of the blood supply and to a greater susceptibility to cord compression in this area. Epidural plasmacytoma often reflects systemic myelomatous involvement and usually has a poor prognosis. The isolated spinal plasmacytoma, however, is a lesion with the potential for long-term remission or even cure in some cases (24).

The primary abnormality is a slow, uncontrolled proliferation of immature and mature plasma cells in the bone marrow. This population of cells is believed to be monoclonal with homogeneous production of immunoglobulin composed of a single class of heavy chains and one type of light chain, often referred to as the M protein (16). The diagnosis is commonly based on the presence of plasmacytoma in tissues, plasmacytosis of the bone marrow, and IgA-$\varkappa$ monoclonal immunoglobulin in the cytoplasm of the tumor cells and in the serum. Lytic bone lesions are another important finding.

The tumor is soft, grayish, and usually is moderately vascularized. It commonly involves the diploë, and respects the bony cortex. The paraspinal muscles may be involved, but this is rare (24). The tumor usually invades the body of the vertebra and, in at least 20% of cases, also compromises the pedicles (21,24).

The neurologic manifestations of the disease are related to compression of the neural structures because of spinal collapse and compression by an epidural tumor. The most consistent symptom is back pain. Motor, sensory, bladder, or sexual deficits may also be observed. When the pedicles are involved, radicular pain is likely. Neurologic involvement is usually minimal (24).

Skeletal roentgenographic abnormalities were seen in 79% of a large series of multiple myelomas (25). The body of the involved vertebra may present a mottled appearance, undergo partial destruction, show multiple lucent lytic defects, sclerosis, and partial or total collapse, with involvement of the pedicles in some cases. The disc spaces are usually narrowed, but may be preserved. Myelography commonly shows an extradural defect. Currently, CT scan and MR are the studies of choice. Both show destruction of the vertebral body and, occasionally, the pedicles as well as tumor extension into paravertebral structures. MR has revealed abnormalities in every myeloma patient. Metastatic lesions show decreased signal intensity on T1-weighted spin-echo images (26).

Medical and surgical treatment must be aggressive (24). Surgical decompression with stabilization of the spine followed by radiotherapy, and chemotherapy when indicated, has afforded excellent symptomatic relief and the potential for long-term remission or even cure (27). The median survival for spinal myeloma is 30 months. Long-term survivors have a younger median age and a lower incidence of renal insufficiency and hypercalcemia, and they also present a better response to therapy, especially chemotherapy (28). The prognosis of patients with single myelomatous lesions of the spine is more favorable than that of patients with metastatic disease of the spine (29–31). Doses of radiotherapy should be at least 4,000 rad (32). Doses of 5,000 to 6,500 rad have been recommended for solitary plasmacytoma (19,33).

Chemotherapy is indicated in all patients with a positive bone marrow biopsy, obviously after surgical decompression. Some authors do not advise chemotherapy in patients with solitary plasmacytoma of bone unless the paraproteinemia or proteinuria persists after treatment of the primary lesion (18,24). The majority of chemotherapeutic drugs, such as melphalan (L-phenylalanine mustard), predisone, cyclophosphamide doxorubicin, carmustine (BCNU), lomustine (CCNU), Adriamycin, vincristine, and galactitol, have been used with more or less success. The agents of choice, however, may be melphalan and prednisone (28,34,35).

SARCOIDOSIS

Sarcoidosis can involve practically every organ system of the body. The spine is affected only occasionally, although intraspinal and vertebral sarcoidosis has been observed in children and adolescents.

Intraspinal sarcoidosis is a rare disease. Since the first pathologic description (36), only about 30 cases of histologically proven spinal sarcoidosis have been reported (37), and most of these patients had disseminated disease. Spinal cord involvement is a serious complication of pulmonary sarcoidosis. Spinal compression does not occur in children. Most patients described were between 20 and 40 years of age. The majority of them had a mass in the cervical spine, and very few cases had symptoms limited to the spinal cord. These tumors may be diagnosed initially as an intramedullary malignant mass such as an ependymoma (38) until histology discloses the true nature of the disease (39). The diagnosis can be suspected, however, from a history of pulmonary sarcoidosis.

The many similarities in the clinical course and radiographic evidence make preoperative distinction from other intraspinal masses very difficult. Difficulties in walking, with hemiparesis or tetraparesis, amyotrophy in one or both hands, fasciculations, decreased sensation, brisk tendon reflexes, and uni- or bilateral extensor plantar responses can occur (37). The cerebrospinal fluid (CSF) usually shows moderate pleocytosis (37,39).

Electromyography may show denervation in muscles of the upper limbs. Radiographs are often normal. Myelography shows widening of the spinal cord, most often in the cervical region, suggesting an intramedullary lesion.

Sarcoidosis must be considered in the differential diagnosis of tumors, syringomyelia, and progressive spinal muscular atrophy.

Vertebral sarcoidosis is surprisingly rare. Very few cases have been reported in children and adolescents. Bloch et al. (40) described a 15-year-old Bantu boy.

Stump et al. (41) observed two black patients, 14 and 13 years of age. One of them complained of fatigue and persistent neck pain, and the other one complained of abdominal pain, chest pain, and fatigue. X-ray showed lytic destruction of a portion of a vertebral body with a sclerotic rim and narrowed disc space. Paraspinal masses, as well as flattening of the affected vertebrae and narrowing of the disc space, are better seen by tomography (41). The differential diagnosis includes fungal infections, tuberculosis, pyogenic osteomyelitis, Hodgkin's disease, and metastatic disease (41).

Histology shows noncaseating granulomas containing lymphocytes and giant and epithelioid cells, surrounded by interstitial fibrosis.

Conservative treatment with high doses of steroids is currently the recommended way to stabilize or even improve the neurologic involvement (42–46). Patients' response is variable, and some undergo spontaneous resolution. Surgery should be limited to extramedullary masses, which appear to improve after excision (47). On the contrary, surgery performed on intramedullary lesions can result in further neurologic deterioration (48,49).

LEUKEMIA

Spinal cord compression occasionally occurs as a complication of childhood leukemia. This has been observed in lymphoid leukemia (50,51) as well as in myeloid leukemia (52), although it is three times more frequent in myeloid leukemia than in lymphoid leukemia (52) and higher in the acute form than in the chronic form (52). Males are affected considerably more often than females. Compression most often occurs at the thoracic level, although diffuse compression is also observed. Weakness, pain, bladder and bowel dysfunction, numbness, and paresthesias are the most frequent symptoms and signs. Paraplegia or quadriplegia with sphincter incontinence may develop if the spinal compression is not treated. Spinal involvement can produce a conus medullaris syndrome (52). Spinal cord compression often occurs after multiple CNS relapses. Lymphoblasts or myeloblasts are commonly encountered in the CSF when lumbar puncture is performed.

X-ray films are usually normal. Myelography reveals a partial or complete block, with the appearance of either an intra- or an extramedullary tumor. CT, especially when combined with metrizamide myelography, shows the exact location of the mass and its relation to the spinal cord (50). MR may also show the lesion.

Spinal leukemic infiltrates are highly radiosensitive. A total of approximately 3,000 rad of local radiation given in 15 fractions of 200 rad each has been suggested (50). Swelling of the spinal cord and meninges can be treated with corticosteroids.

Severe neurologic complications can occur in leukemic patients treated with cytotoxic drugs. Intrathecal methotrexate has caused acute paraplegia and even death (53) and acute paraplegia with partial recovery 6 weeks (54) were observed. Permanent paralysis has followed the use of cytosine arabinoside (55). Intrathecal therapy must be immediately discontinued in such cases.

SPINAL LYMPHOMA

Spinal lymphomas can be intramedullary or extramedullary. Both are very uncommon in children.

Primary spinal intramedullary lymphomas are confined to a few isolated cases, all in adults, with the youngest being 26 years old. The most reliable diagnostic signs include increased cellularity of the CSF and segmental swelling of the cord on myelography. Clinical features are mainly motor deficits with pyramidal involvement and multisegmental impairment of upper and lower motor neurons, sensory changes, and sphincter dysfunction. Only two well-documented cases of malignant lymphoma involving only the spinal cord have been reported (56,57). Two other cases have been described in which lymphomatous involvement of the spinal cord was clearly secondary to diffuse meningeal invasion (58,59). Spinal cord lymphomas resulting from multifocal involvement or secondary meningeal spread and metastasis occur quite frequently; however, malignant lymphomas of the brain are far more common (60).

Prognosis is poor. Treatment consists of a combination of radiotherapy and chemotherapy. The longest survival is 4 years in a patient who, at this writing, is still alive (61).

Extramedullary lymphomas are generally a late manifestation of the illness. They are found most frequently in advanced stages of the disease, occurring in approximately 6% of patients. Reticulum cell sarcoma is the most frequent variety, followed by Hodgkin's disease and lymphosarcoma. Very few cases are seen among young people. Only two patients between 0 and 19 years were observed in a series of 81 cases of spinal cord compression (62). The most commonly compressed segments are the dorsal and lumbar areas. The cervical cord is compressed less commonly, especially in Hodgkin's disease. However, a 23-year-old patient with Hodgkin's disease affecting the scalp, skull, and epidural cervical cord was described by Tomaszek et al. (63). It is assumed that early detection of the illness in the neck in non-Hodgkin malignant lymphomas and irradiation of neck nodes in Hodgkin's disease, as well as difficulty in detecting signs of deep-seated lesions, may account for differences in the probability of cord compression. Pain is the most common symptom, either alone or in combination with other symptoms, followed by weakness, paresthesia, and alteration of sphincteric function. Examination of the spinal fluid shows protein elevation in more than two-thirds of patients. Concomitant vertebral bone involvement is present in about one-third of the patients, the dorsal vertebrae being the most frequently involved.

Histologic diagnosis may be difficult, and sometimes lymphoma is misdiagnosed (64). In the early stages, the bone may appear completely normal on X-ray despite widespread infiltration because lymphomas have a permissive growth pattern (65).

Myelography is abnormal in the majority of patients, revealing a complete or partial block. Correspondence between clinical and radiologic findings is often good, but discrepancies occur. For example, a normal myelogram does not exclude spinal lymphoma. In cases of complete block, lumbar and upper cervical instillation of contrast material may be required to define the lower and upper extent of the tumor. CT may provide information about paraspinal extension of the tumor and generally permits visualization of the contents of the spinal canal, especially if the study is combined with metrizamide myelography. MR, using a high field strength magnet and surface coil technique is superior to other imaging modalities currently in use to visualize the extent of tumor growth inside and outside the spinal canal (66–68). Inversion recovery (IR) permits better visualization of spinal lymphoma than spin echo (SE) (67).

Radiotherapy delivered in the early phases of the cord compression is often successful in reversing neurologic symptoms. A minimum dose of 2,500 rad appears to be necessary for local control of the disease. Early detection of disease in the deep-seated areas along the spinal cord and irradiation of these areas may prevent spread of the tumor to the epidural space.

Chemotherapy must be applied concomitantly or following radiotherapy. Nitrogen mustard gives the best results (62), either alone or in combination with other agents, such as steroids, vincristine, and other frequently used agents.

FIBROUS HISTIOCYTOMA

The term benign and malignant fibrous histiocytoma is applied to a group of benign and malignant lesions believed to be of histiocytic origin. Benign tumors are also known by the terms sclerosing hemangioma and fibrous xanthoma. Biologically malignant tumors are known by the terms malignant fibrous xanthoma, xanthosarcoma, and malignant fibrous histiocytoma. Other benign and malignant conditions may also have a histiocytic origin. In addition to those already described, Fu et al. (69) included among benign tumors dermatofibroma, nevoid histiocytoma (also known as nevo-xanthoendothelioma), and "atypical fibrous xanthoma"; and as tumorlike lesions xanthoma, villo-nodular synovitis, xanthogranuloma, giant cell tumor of tendon sheaths, and xanthomatous pseudotumor of the lung. Malignant tumors include malignant histiocytoma, malignant giant cell tumor of soft tissues, "reticulum cell sarcoma of soft tissues," and "malignant xanthogranuloma." From 158 cases of fibrosarcoma of bone and 962 cases of osteosarcoma of bone on file at the Mayo Clinic, 35 tumors were found to be properly designated as malignant fibrous histiocytomas (70).

These tumors are quite common in soft tissues, and they may also be found in bones. The spine is very seldom affected. Malignant fibrous histiocytoma may originate in the sacrum (70), cauda equina (71), lumbar (72), thoracic (73–75) and cervical spine (73,76). One case arose in a thoracolumbar myelomeningocele (77). Malignant fibrous histiocytoma of the dorsal spine was found in a 14-year-old boy (74) who presented with midthoracic pain, leg weakness, and bladder dysfunction. Both plain X-rays and bone scan studies were normal even though myelography demonstrated an extradural mass extending from T2 to T5. The tumor adhered to dura and bone. Other cases showed a lytic lesion in the body of a vertebra with a pathologic fracture through the inferior vertebral endplate (76) and a metastatic lesion in the posterior elements of a vertebra (73).

These tumors can occur at any age, but they are extremely rare in the first decade (70). They appear slightly more frequently in males than in females (70).

The main histologic features of the atypical fibrous histiocytoma incorporate most of the following features (78): histiocytic-like (epithelioid) cells, spindle cells (facultative fibroblasts), multinucleated benign giant cells, neoplastic giant cells (often bizarre), foam cells, inflammatory cells (usually lymphocytes), anaplasia of stromal cells, mitotic figures (normal and atypical), and "granulomatous" features. Metaplastic osteoid or chondroid tissue is present in some tumors (79). Electron microscopic study demonstrates fibroblast-like, histiocyte-like, and xanthomatous cells (69). Many differentiated chondrosarcomas, osteosarcomas, and fibrosarcomas of bone present histologic areas similar to those observed in malignant fibrous histiocytoma. Therefore, a careful differential diagnosis is necessary with those tumors. Any malignant tumor in which tumor cells unequivocally produce osteoid changes should be classified as an osteogenic sarcoma (80,81).

Radical removal must be carried out if possible. Decompression of the spinal cord and roots is urgently needed. Radiation therapy has been curative in some tumors outside the spine (70). Prognosis is usually poor because of the highly aggressive nature of this tumor and because of widespread metastatic disease at the time of presentation (73). In cases with tumors outside the spine, approximately one-third of patients alive at 5-year follow-up were long-term, symptom-free survivors (70).

ROSAI-DORFMAN DISEASE

Rosai and Dorfman (82) described a benign clinicopathologic entity consisting of histiocytosis of the sinuses with massive lymphadenopathy. Extranodal involvement was observed in 28% of the patients (83). When it is located in the orbit, eyelid, salivary glands, skin, bone, testes, and upper respiratory tract, the disease may also be found in the epidural space and the vertebral canal (83–86).

The involved lymph nodes are located bilaterally in the cervical region in 95% of patients and are painless. When the process is located in the epidural or subdural space, it can produce progressive quadriparesis or paraparesis, as well as compression of spinal nerve roots and dorsal root ganglia. In the series of Foucar et al. (86) of eight patients with involvement of the CNS, two had both cord compression and intracranial disease; one of them died 10 years after diagnosis. Spinal involvement is found in children as well as in adults.

Radiographs of the spine show an enlarged intervertebral foramen and partial loss of the pedicle adjacent to the lymphadenopathy. Myelography discloses an extramedullary block with a lobulated filling defect. CT scan reveals a localized vertebral defect with neighboring lymphadenopathy. Laboratory investigations may reveal an elevated erythrocyte sedimentation rate.

Histologically, the nodules show a mixture of histiocytes (large cells), plasma cells, lymphocytes, lymphoblasts, neutrophils, and eosinophils. The nuclei of the large cells appear ovoid, elongated, or indented, sometimes containing one or several small nucleoli, and they can have a loose chromatin network. The large macrophages may contain a large or moderate amount of eosinophilic or pale foamy cytoplasm.

The differential diagnosis of Rosai-Dorfman disease includes tumors such as neurofibroma or neurilemmoma, neuroblastoma, meningioma, histiocytosis X, lymphoma, Hodgkin's disease, as well as other types of adenopathies.

The nature of the disease is unknown. Treatment includes surgery with the early removal of the nodules, chemotherapy, or a combination of both.

REFERENCES

1. Lichtenstein L. Histiocytosis X. Integration of eosinophilic granuloma of bone, "Letterer-Siwe disease" and "Schüller-Christian disease" as related manifestations of a single nosologic entity. *Arch Pathol* 1953;56:84–102.
2. Oberman HA. Idiopathic histiocytosis. A clinicopathological study of 40 cases and review of the literature on eosinophilic granuloma of bone, Hand-Schüller-Christian disease and Letterer-Siwe disease. *Pediatrics* 1961;28:307–327.
3. Ekert H, Campbell PE. Histiocytosis X. *Aust Paediatr J* 1966;2:139–145.
4. Bökkerink JPM, de Vaan GAM. Histiocytosis X. *Eur J Pediatr* 1980;135:129–146.
5. Saloman M, Quest DO, Mount LA. Histiocytosis X of the spinal cord. *J Neurosurg* 1974;41:383–386.
6. Eli C, Adornato BT. Radicular compression in multifocal eosinophilic granuloma. Successful treatment with radiotherapy. *Arch Neurol* 1977;34:786–787.
7. Hewlett RH, Ganz JC. Histiocytosis X of the cauda equina. *Neurology* 1976;26:472–476.
8. Lucaya J. Histiocytosis X. *Am J Dis Child* 1971;121:289–295.
9. Newton WA, Hamoudi AB. Histiocytosis. A histological classification with clinical correlation. In: *Perspectives in pediatric pathology*, vol. 1. Chicago: Year Book Medical Publisher, 1973;251–283.
10. Lahey ME. Histiocytosis X—an analysis of prognostic factors. *J Pediatr* 1975;87:184–189.
11. Nezelof C, Frileux-Herbet F, Cronier-Sachot J. Disseminated histiocytosis X. Analysis of prognostic factors based on a retrospective study of 50 cases. *Cancer* 1979;44:1824–1838.
12. Cheyne C. Histiocytosis X. *J Bone Joint Surg* 1971;53B:366–382.
13. Yabsley RH, Harris WR. Solitary eosinophilic granuloma of a vertebral body causing paraplegia. Report of a case. *J Bone Joint Surg* 1966;48A:1570–1574.
14. Schajowicz F, Slullitel J. Eosinophilic granuloma of bone and its relationship to Hand-Schüller-Christian disease and Letterer-Siwe syndrome. *J Bone Joint Surg* 1973;55B:545–565.
15. Hewell GM, Alexanian R. Multiple myeloma in young persons. *Ann Intern Med* 1976;84:441–443.
16. Bernstein SC, Parez-Atayde AR, Weinstein HJ. Multiple myeloma in a child. *Cancer* 1985;56:2143–2147.
17. Jacoby P. Myelomatosis in a child of 8 years. *Acta Radiol* 1930;11:224–232.
18. Woodruff RK, Malpas JS, White FE. Solitary plasmacytoma. II. Solitary plasmacytoma of bone. *Cancer* 1979;43:2344–2347.

19. Lesoin F, Bonneterre J, Lesoin A, Jomin M. Plasmocytomes rachidiens à expression neurologique. *Neurochirurgie* 1982;28:401–407.
20. Svien HJ, Price RD, Bayrd ED. Neurosurgical treatment of compression of the spinal cord caused by myeloma. *JAMA* 1953;153:784–786.
21. Cohen DM, Svien HJ, Dahlin DC. Long-term survival of patients with solitary myeloma of the vertebral column. *JAMA* 1964;187:914–917.
22. Clarke E. Spinal cord involvement in multiple myelomatosis. *Brain* 1956;79:332–348.
23. Benson WJ, Scarffe JH, Todd IDH, Palmer M, Crowther D. Spinal-cord compression in myeloma. *Br Med J* 1979;1:1541–1544.
24. Loftus CM, Michelsen CB, Rapoport F, Lobo Antunes J. Management of plasmacytoma of the spine. *Neurosurgery* 1983;13:30–36.
25. Kyle RA. Multiple myeloma. Review of 869 cases. *Mayo Clin Proc* 1975;50:29–40.
26. Daffner RH, Lupetin AR, Dash N, et al. MRI in the detection of malignant infiltration of bone marrow. *Am J Roentgenol* 1986;146:353–358.
27. Valderrama JAF, Bullough PG. Solitary myeloma of the spine. *J Bone Joint Surg* 1968;50B:82–90.
28. Kyle RA. Long-term survival in multiple myeloma. *N Engl J Med* 1983;308:314–316.
29. Gilbert H, Apuzzo M, Marshall L, et al. Neoplastic epidural spinal cord compression: a current perspective. *JAMA* 1978;240:2771–2773.
30. Black P. Spinal metastasis: current status and recommended guidelines for management. *Neurosurgery* 1979;5:726–746.
31. Rodriguez M, Dinapoly RP. Spinal cord compression with special reference to metastatic epidural tumors. *Mayo Clin Proc* 1980;55:442–448.
32. Meyer JE, Schulz MD. "Solitary" myeloma of bone: a review of twelve cases. *Cancer* 1974;34:438–440.
33. Mill WB, Griffith R. The role of radiation therapy in the management of plasma cell tumors. *Cancer* 1980;45:647–652.
34. McIntyre OR. Current concepts in cancer: multiple myeloma. *N Engl J Med* 1979;301:193–196.
35. Early AP, Ozer H, Henderson ES. Multiple myeloma. *NY State J Med* 1981;81:883–893.
36. Longcope WT. Sarcoidosis or Bensier Boeck Schaumann disease. *JAMA* 1941;117:1321–1327.
37. Vighetto A, Fischer G, Collet P, et al. Intramedullary sarcoidosis of the cervical spinal cord. *J Neurol Neurosurg Psychiatry* 1985;48:477–479.
38. Snyder R, Towfighi J, Gonatas NK. Sarcoidosis of the spinal cord. Case report. *J Neurosurg* 1976;44:740–743.
39. Banerjee T, Hunt WE. Spinal cord sarcoidosis. *J Neurosurg* 1972;36:490–493.
40. Bloch S, Morison IJ, Seedat YK. Unusual skeletal manifestations in a case of sarcoidosis. *Clin Radiol* 1968;19:226–228.
41. Stump D, Spock A, Grossman H. Vertebral sarcoidosis in adolescents. *Radiology* 1976;121:153–155.
42. Moldover A. Sarcoidosis of the spinal cord. Report of a case with remission associated with cortisone therapy. *Arch Intern Med* 1958;102:414–417.
43. Wood EH, Bream CA. Spinal sarcoidosis. *Radiology* 1959;73:226–233.
44. Kirks DR, Newton TH. Sarcoidosis: a rare cause of spinal cord widening. *Radiology* 1972;102:643.
45. Magnet JL, Strauss J, Guard D. Localisation intramédullaire d'une sarcoïdose. *Nouv Presse Med* 1980;9:1518.
46. Viader F, Dairou R, Elghozi D, Bolgert F, Masson M. Myélopathie cervicale révélatrice d'une sarcoïdose. *Nouv Presse Med* 1982;11:1805.
47. Baruah JK, Glasauer FE, Sil R, Smith BH. Sarcoidosis of the cervical spinal canal: case report. *Neurosurgery* 1978;3:216–218.
48. Day AL, Sybert GW. Spinal cord sarcoidosis. *Ann Neurol* 1977;1:79–85.
49. Buge A, Escourolle R, Poisson M, Rancurel G, Gray F. Sarcoïdose médullaire. *Ann Med Interne (Paris)* 1975;126:1–16.
50. Lo WD, Matthay KK, Kushner J. Spinal cord compression in a child with acute lymphoblastic leukemia. *Am J Pediatr Hematol Oncol* 1985;7:373–376.
51. Krepler P, Jentzsch K, Mayer-Obiditisch J, Salah S. Lymphoblastic extramedullary spinal tumor during remission of acute lymphoblastic leukemia. *Acta Neuropathol (Berlin)* 1975;6(Suppl.):213–215.

52. Petursson SR, Boggs DR. Spinal cord involvement in leukemia: a review of the literature and a case of pH1+ acute myeloid leukemia presenting with a conus medullaris syndrome. *Cancer* 1981;47:346–350.
53. Back EH. Death after intrathecal methotrexate. *Lancet* 1969;ii:1005.
54. Gangliano RG, Costanzi JJ. Paraplegia following intrathecal methotrexate. Report of a case and review of the literature. *Cancer* 1976;37:1663–1668.
55. Saiki JH, Thomson S, Smith F, Atkinson R. Paraplegia following intrathecal chemotherapy. *Cancer* 1972;29:370–374.
56. Hautzer NW, Aiyesimoju A, Robitaille Y. "Primary" spinal intramedullary lymphomas: a review. *Ann Neurol* 1983;14:62–66.
57. Bruni J, Bilbao JM, Gray T. Primary intramedullary malignant lymphoma of the spinal cord. *Neurology* 1977;27:896–898.
58. Reznik M. Pathology of primary reticulum cell sarcoma of the human central nervous system. *Acta Neuropathol (Berlin)* 1975;6(Suppl.):91–94.
59. Slager UT, Kaufman RL, Cohen KL, Tuddenham WJ. Primary lymphoma of the spinal cord. *Neuropathol Exp Neurol* 1982;41:437–445.
60. Henry JM, Heffner RR Jr, Dillard SH, et al. Primary malignant lymphomas of the central nervous system. *Cancer* 1974;34:1293–1302.
61. Herbst DK, Corder MP, Justice GR. Successful therapy with methotrexate of a multicentric mixed lymphoma of the central nervous system. *Cancer* 1976;38:1476–1478.
62. Friedman M, Kim TH, Panahon AM. Spinal cord compression in malignant lymphoma. Treatment and results. *Cancer* 1976;37:1485–1491.
63. Tomaszek DE, Tyson GW, Stang P, Boulding T. Contiguous scalp, skull, and epidural Hodgkin's disease. *Surg Neurol* 1984;21:182–184.
64. Kozlowski K, Beluffi G, Masel J, et al. Primary vertebral tumours in children. Report of 20 cases with brief literature review. *Pediatr Radiol* 1984;14:129–139.
65. Pear BL. Skeletal manifestations of the lymphomas and leukemias. *Semin Roentgenol* 1974;9:229–240.
66. Holtas SL, Kido DK, Simon JH. MR imaging of spinal lymphoma. *J Comput Assist Tomogr* 1986;10:111–115.
67. Bydder GM, Young IR. MR imaging: clinical use of the inversion recovery imaging of lymphomas in children. *J Comput Assist Tomogr* 1985;9:659–675.
68. Cohen MD, Klatte EC, Smith JA, et al. Magnetic resonance imaging of lymphomas in children. *Pediatr Radiol* 1985;15:179–183.
69. Fu Y-S, Gabbiani G, Kaye GI, Lattes R. Malignant soft tissue tumors of probable histiocytic origin (malignant fibrous histiocytomas): general considerations and electron microscopic and tissue culture studies. *Cancer* 1975;35:176–198.
70. Dahlin DC, Unni KK, Matsuno T. Malignant fibrous histiocytoma of bone—fact or fancy? *Cancer* 1977;39:1508–1516.
71. Kellet RJ, Dearnaley JN. Malignant fibrous histiocytoma with diffuse spinal nerve involvement. *J Clin Pathol* 1976;29:910–915.
72. Kepes JJ. "Xanthomatous" lesions of the central nervous system: definition, classification and some recent observations. In: Zimmerman HM, ed. *Progress in neuropathology*, vol. 4. New York: Raven Press, 1979;179–213.
73. Feldman F, Lattes R. Primary malignant fibrous histiocytoma (fibrous xanthoma) of bone. *Skeletal Radiol* 1977;1:145–160.
74. Guarnaschelli JJ, Wehry SM, Serratoni FT, Ozenitis AJ. Atypical fibrous histiocytoma of the thoracic spine. Case report. *J Neurosurg* 1979;51:415–416.
75. Teddy PJ, Erisi MM. Malignant fibrous histiocytoma producing spinal cord compression. *J Neurol Neurosurg Psychiatry* 1979;42:838–842.
76. Rechtine GR, Hassan MO, Bohlman DH. Malignant fibrous histiocytoma of the cervical spine. Report of an unusual case and description of light and electron microscopy. *Spine* 1984;9:824–830.
77. Helle TL, Hanbery JW, Becker DH. Meningeal malignant fibrous histiocytoma arising from a thoracolumbar myelomeningocele. Case report. *J Neurosurg* 1983;58:593–597.
78. Soule EH, Enriquez P. Atypical fibrous histiocytoma, malignant fibrous histiocytoma, malignant histiocytoma, and epithelioid sarcoma. A comparative study of 65 tumors. *Cancer* 1972;30:128–143.

79. Weiss SW, Enzinger FM. Malignant fibrous histiocytoma. An analysis of 200 cases. *Cancer* 1978;41:2250–2266.
80. Spanier SS, Enneking WF, Enriquez P. Primary malignant fibrous histiocytoma of bone. *Cancer* 1975;36:2084–2098.
81. Spanier SS. Malignant fibrous histiocytoma of bone. *Orthop Clin N Am* 1977;8:941–961.
82. Rosai J, Dorfman RF. Sinus histiocytosis with massive lymphadenopathy. A newly recognized benign clinicopathological entity. *Arch Pathol* 1969;87:63–70.
83. Chan KW, Chow YYN, Ghadially FN, et al. Rosai-Dorfman disease presenting as spinal tumor. A case report with ultrastructural and immunohistochemical studies. *J Bone Joint Surg* 1985; 67A:1427–1431.
84. Kessler E, Srulijes C, Toledo Z, Shalit M. Sinus histiocytosis with massive lymphadenopathy and spinal epidural involvement. A case report and review of the literature. *Cancer* 1976;38:1614–1618.
85. Hass RJ, Helming MSE, Prechtel K. Sinus histiocytosis with massive lymphadenopathy and paraparesis: remission with chemotherapy. A case report. *Cancer* 1978;42:77–80.
86. Foucar E, Rosai J, Dorfman RF, Brynes RK. The neurologic manifestations of sinus histiocytosis with massive lymphadenopathy. *Neurology* 1982;32:365–371.

13

Vascular Tumors and Arteriovenous Malformations

Ignacio Pascual-Castroviejo

HEMANGIOPERICYTOMA

Hemangiopericytoma is a rare tumor that was first described by Stout and Murray in 1942 (1). It is now generally accepted that this tumor originates from pericytes, cells found around the reticular sheath of capillaries and postcapillary venules. The tumor can be found in many locations, though most frequently in the lower extremities. Involvement of the spine is uncommon. The majority of the nearly thirty reported cases were extradural.

The tumor affects both sexes with the same frequency and occurs at all ages. The prevalance of hemangiopericytoma affecting the central nervous system (CNS) varies in different published series. Clinically, it presents as a single mass which is asymptomatic and painless until it invades or compresses neighboring structures. Its manifestations depend on the organ affected, for instance hydronephrosis, urinary retention, constipation, thoracic scoliosis, congestive heart failure, telangiectasias, varicose veins, hemorrhoids, hypertension, etc. (2–8). Metastases occur in 15% (3) to 57% (9) of cases. A 10-year survival rate of 70% has been reported (3). Although metastases may appear as late as 26 years after diagnosis of the tumor (3,10,11), they usually occur within 5 years. This neoplasm has a hematogenous dissemination, often involving the lungs and skeleton (11,12).

Spinal involvement is accompanied by corresponding neurologic symptomatology, such as uni- or bilateral lower extremity weakness, paraparesis, decreased sensation over some dermatomes, paresthesias, difficulty in walking, back pain, radicular deficits, and scoliosis. On examination, the most frequent findings are hyperreflexia and Babinski toe signs.

Spine films reveal thinning of pedicles and scalloping of the affected vertebrae. Bone scan with ^{99m}Tc shows markedly increased uptake in the region of the tumor (13). Ultrasound reveals retroperitoneal and thoracic masses and their relationship with adjacent organs. Computerized tomography (CT) and nuclear magnetic resonance (MR) should be performed, if possible, because they show not only destruction of the body and pedicles by the tumor but also growth into the spinal canal that displaces the dural sac, and into the prevertebral space and paraspinal muscles. CT shows speckled calcifications in malignant hemangiopericytomas (14). Myelography commonly shows a partial or complete block by an epidural mass which may spread over several segments. Angiography usually reveals a highly vascular, multilobular mass receiving its blood from one or several arteries (7,15).

Microscopically, this tumor is a vascular neoplasm with sheets of round or ovoid cells (1,16,17) ensnared by reticulum and collagen fibers. The basement membrane, as well as the endothelial lining of the tumor vessels, appears normal. The tumor cells proliferate outside the basement membrane, which is helpful for making a differential diagnosis with hemangioendotheliomas. However, transitional forms between both types occur (16,17), and other tumors of mesenchymal origin, especially some types of sarcomas, must also be considered (16,18–20). Distinguishing hemangiopericytoma from angioblastic meningioma may be difficult. Some authors have considered both as the same neoplasm (16,18,19) while others differentiate them on the basis of electron microscopic features (16,21,22). Popoff et al. (21) pointed out that hemangiopericytomas have prominent basal laminar intercellular material with glycogen, cytoplasmic filaments 60 to 80 Å thick, and focal cytoplasmic condensations, whereas meningiomas lack basement membranes but have prominent desmosomes, thicker cytoplasmic filaments, and no condensations. Prognosis is poorer in patients with a lesser degree of lymphocytic infiltration, fewer vascular spaces, and little desmoplasia (3). These findings have limited prognostic value (3,4,11).

The treatment of choice for this tumor is surgical ablation, although its invasive nature and high vascularity make complete removal quite difficult. Consequently, embolization through selective catheterization of the feeding vessels may facilitate surgical excision (7), although removal must be carried out promptly, since a preexisting neurologic deficit often increases after embolization, probably as a result of swelling of the neoplasm after embolization (7).

Response to radiotherapy requires a high dose (from 7,500 to 9,000 rad) (23). This occurred in 26 of 29 patients described by Mira et al. (24), although the role of this therapy in the management of these tumors is controversial (23–25). Preoperative radiation may be helpful (7,20).

Chemotherapy attempts with several drugs (nitrogen mustard, methotrexate, chlorambucil, actinomycin D, 5-fluorouracil, fluorometholone, Adriamycin, and cyclophosphamide) have yielded poor results (3,11).

Tumors affecting the CNS have a higher recurrence rate than purely musculoskeletal ones. Incomplete removal plays an important role in recurrence and local spread (20,26).

HEMANGIOBLASTOMA

Spinal hemangioblastoma is a benign vascular tumor of the CNS. It occurs at any age and is quite frequent in children and adolescents. In one of the more recent reviews of the literature (27) encompassing 138 cases, 34 (25%) were children below 21 years of age. There is no predilection for either sex. The most common location of hemangioblastoma is the cerebellum, followed by the cerebral hemispheres and spinal cord. The tumor is usually well circumscribed and varies in size. The most common type, especially when the tumor is intramedullary, is a large cyst with a small mural nodule. Neither light nor electron microscopy has provided definitive evidence regarding the cell of origin of this tumor. It arises from the vascular mesenchyme as a dysgenetic abnormality, often accompanied by multiple tumors in other organs. It frequently arises in the context of von Hippel-Lindau disease, one of the phakomatoses (28,29). The spinal cord is probably involved in almost all cases of von Hippel-Lindau disease. This phakomatosis most likely arises at the end of the first month of gestation. Hemangioblastoma has been called hemangioma, capillary angioma, angioreticuloma, angiomatosis, hemangioendothelioma, and, occasionally, hemangiopericytoma and angioblastic meningioma. Very few cases in the literature are histologically confirmed as genuine hemangioblastomas (30). Most (88%) are located in the subdural space, with approximately 12% extradural (27), the latter always being solitary. Intramedullary tumors are most frequently located in the cervicodorsal and dorsolumbar regions. They occur mainly in the posterior half of the spinal cord, behind the central canal near the posterior columns. They may also be found in the intradural portion of the nerve roots and in the cauda equina.

Perhaps 25% of cases have a family history of CNS hemangioblastoma, and a positive family history is most common in patients with multiple tumors. Familial occurrence of an isolated spinal hemangioblastoma has seldom been reported (27,31). Three of Otanasek's (31) six patients with spinal hemangioblastoma also had a tumor in the posterior fossa.

The clinical features of spinal hemangioblastoma are nonspecific. As the tumor grows, symptoms of gradual cord compression appear with posterior column signs. Sphincter disturbance occurs late (31).

Radiology

Plain X-rays and tomography of the spine show alterations in 40% of cases (27). The main findings include widening of the spinal canal, lytic defects or even destruction of the pedicles, and scalloping of the vertebral bodies. Enlarged intervertebral foramina occur when tumors are located in nerve roots. Scoliosis is frequent in children and adolescents.

Myelography shows the combination of an expanded cord and serpiginous defects. These findings can be seen in other tumors and do not differentiate hemangioblastoma from an arteriovenous malformation (AVM) of the spinal cord. Arteriography is often diagnostic (32). A diffuse, homogeneous stain is characteristic of the hemangioblastoma tumor nodule, a feature not observed in any other mass of the spinal cord. Occasionally, hemangioblastomas may produce displacement of large vessels without a stain. Capillary hemangioblastoma of bone may resemble spinal hemangioma (33). With subtraction angiography it is possible to define individual vessels in AVM. The feeding vessels of hemangioblastoma arise from the posterior arterial system in almost two-thirds of patients, and from the anterior system in the rest (27). CT scanning may not show the lesion since the spinal cord itself is not sharply defined unless hydrosoluble contrast medium is introduced into the spinal canal. On the other hand, a highly vascularized lesion is always apparent when intravenous contrast is administered (34,35). Because of perfect correlation between CT images and spinal arteriography, CT is the method of choice because it is less invasive. MR imaging is a less sensitive method, although it may demonstrate an image suggestive of the abnormality (36,37).

Treatment and Prognosis

Complete removal of the tumor is the only effective therapy for spinal hemangioblastoma. Removal is possible when spinal angiography has provided accurate location of feeding arteries and venous drainage. Microsurgical techniques and preoperative embolization improve the surgical results. Although total removal of intramedullary tumors is more difficult, it is possible in most patients (27,38), and partial removal is possible in the remainder. Minimal to severe neurologic sequelae may result in a significant number of patients. Hemangioblastomas located extradurally and those of spinal roots and the cauda equina are usually well-circumscribed and without bony or meningeal adherences. This facilitates their complete removal with a favorable outcome. Only partial removal is feasible in some patients, most of whom will eventually develop a recurrence.

VERTEBRAL HEMANGIOMA

Generalities

Vertebral hemangioma is a benign slow-growing tumor that rarely causes compression of the nerve roots or spinal cord. In most cases the hemangioma is an incidental radiographic finding. The prevalence of these hemangiomas increases with age and is greater in females. They can occur anywhere along the spine, including the sacrum, but are most frequent in the thoracic region. Although hemangiomas of vertebral bodies are found in 10% of spines at autopsy (39), most patients are asymptomatic. However, local symptoms such as pain and tenderness may occur. Compression of the spinal cord, nerve roots, or the cauda equina occurs occasionally. Slight trauma may precipitate symptoms. These may be the result of (a) expansion of an involved vertebra leading to narrowing and deformity of the spinal canal, (b) extension of the tumor into the epidural space, (c) compression fracture of an involved vertebra (very uncommon), or (d) extradural hematoma secondary to the hemangioma (40).

Radiology

Although plain X-rays may be normal, they often show pathognomonic changes. These are axial sclerotic strands, produced by vertical trabeculae buttressed by new bone, between areas of rarefaction representing tumor tissue, occasionally mingled with fat. These alterations usually involve the vertebral body, but they may also spread to all other parts of the vertebra and, rarely, to surrounding structures. These radiologic findings can simulate several other bone diseases such as metastases (41), lymphoma, myeloma, blood dyscrasia, and Paget's disease. Myelography shows the extradural spinal compression, when it exists, but gives no specific evidence on the nature of the lesion. CT scan may show the abnormal texture of the vertebral body affected by a hemangioma, with its thickened bony trabeculae (42). Myelography and CT help document the extent of cord involvement. Spinal angiography may confirm the diagnosis of vertebral hemangioma and provide the opportunity to embolize it prior to surgical excision.

Treatment

When the arteries feeding the tumor are located by arteriography and they do not also supply an anterior spinal artery, they can be occluded to reduce vascularity by either embolism (43–46) or ligation (47) before surgical resection. Occasionally, the lesion is apparently cured after embolization of the hemangioma. Radiotherapy alone has produced good results in vertebral hemangioma, although there are no recent references regarding this method of therapy.

GLOMUS TUMORS OF THE COCCYGEAL REGION

Glomus tumors are benign neoplasms (48) originating from the body of the glomus, which has an arterial segment, the Sucquet-Hoyer canal, and a venous segment. They are composed of small vascular spaces, each lined by a single layer of endothelial cells surrounded by glomus cells. Glomera are found most often in the dermis of the hands and feet but also in several other locations, one of which is the coccygeal body. Ultrastructural studies have shown that glomus cells derive from pericytes (49). Their location in the coccygeal region has rarely been described (50,51). This tumor may appear at any age, but has a predilection for children and adolescents. Girls are more often affected than boys.

The glomus tumor is an encapsulated nodule measuring a few millimeters in diameter (52). Occasionally, it may be very small and difficult to see with the naked eye. It does not produce neurologic deficits. Its main symptom is coccygeal pain of insidious onset and varying intensity. Pain may be severe. Patients often describe the pain as burning or throbbing in character. Because of the unusual and deep location of the tumor in the coccyx and the absence of trigger-point sensitivity, the patient of Ho and Pak (50) had been labeled a neurotic for several months. Similarly, patients with glomus tumors in other locations have been called neurotic (53). Local pressure on the tip of the coccyx produces severe, sharp, stabbing pain (51). Some patients with coccydynia who failed to respond to conservative treatment were relieved by excision of the coccyx and the periococcygeal soft tissues (51). Failure to remove the glomus tumor may explain why symptoms persisted in some patients after coccygectomy. In order to diagnose this lesion, the bone as well as the soft tissues around the tip of the coccyx must be carefully examined.

ARTERIOVENOUS MALFORMATIONS

Generalities

Spinal cord AVM may be classified into three types (54,55):

Type I, the dorsal extramedullary AVM. These lesions are diagnosed most frequently in men between ages 40 and 70 years. Pregnancy and Valsalva maneuvers may exacerbate their symptoms.

Type II, the compact, usually intramedullary AVM with multiple feeders. This is also an adult disease. These lesions are frequently associated with large aneurysmal varicosities which may cause clinically significant cord compression.

Type III, the extensive juvenile malformation. This type of AVM occurs most frequently in adolescents and young adults, is predominantly intramedullary, and has several feeders that sometimes involve more than one vertebral segment. Extramedullary and paraspinal extension of the AVM is rare.

Recently, Heros et al. (56) proposed a new category, *Type IV*, a direct arteriovenous fistula involving the normal arterial supply of the cord. This type is characterized by a very distended venous outflow.

Spinal cord AVM may present at any age, including neonates (57), within the first year of life (58–60), childhood (61–64), youth, and adulthood. They may be located anywhere along the spinal cord. Angiography is required to define the type of AVM. Over 80% of spinal cord AVMs are predominantly extramedullary (65). In the largest series of AVM in children (66), they were thoracolumbar in 51% of the cases, cervical in 28%, and thoracic in 21%.

Clinical Findings

Clinical manifestations of AVM differ with age. The neonate described by Park et al. (57) developed severe paraparesis with abrupt neurologic deterioration, not due to hemorrhage or aneurysmal dilatation, but to ischemic damage of the spinal cord. In children of all ages, spinal cord AVM often presents acutely. In a series of 38 children (66), 84% experienced sudden onset of symptoms, often as a result of a physical effort. Neurologic signs may regress, but may also become permanent after several repeated attacks. Bleeding from an AVM is frequent in children (66). Delayed motor development of the legs in very young children (60), progressive spasticity and weakness of the legs (6), and even lower motor weakness are the main presenting symptoms in more than half of the patients (66), whereas in adults, a slowly progressive course is the rule (67,68). Pain, often low back pain, is almost always present, followed by impaired leg use, bladder and bowel dysfunction, less often numbness and tingling, and, occasionally, sexual dysfunction. Classic neurologic syndromes such as the Brown-Séquard syndrome, incomplete transverse cord section, or the cauda equina syndrome, are less frequent. Occasionally AVM produces only subarachnoid hemorrhage. In the series of Riché et al. (66), 13 cases (34%) also presented a deep or cutaneous angiodysplasia, in some but not all cases with a segmental distribution. These angiodysplasias include port-wine angiomas, Weber-Rendu-Osler disease, Klippel-Trenaunay disease, and Cobb syndrome. The association of a cutaneous hemangioma with a spinal AVM has been reported (63,69,70). Djindjian et al. (69) found five spinal AVM associated with Klippel-Trenaunay disease among 150 spinal AVM.

Isolated spinal aneurysms are very rare (71–73). They mostly present in association with an AVM (60,74,75). Most patients have bloody CSF with an increased protein content.

Radiology

Plain X-ray films show bony abnormalities in about 30% of patients (66). Most of these changes appear acquired. The most common vertebral alterations are erosion of the pedicles, scalloping of the vertebral body, widening of the vertebral canal, and kyphoscoliosis. A calcified intramedullary aneurysm in a spinal angioma is exceptional in children (76).

Myelography reveals enlarged vessels. When the AVM is intramedullary, the myelographic picture is that of spinal cord widening, suggesting an intraaxial neoplasm. CT scans show the enlarged spinal cord but give no indication of the nature of the mass (35). MR imaging may be diagnostic. Tortuous areas of low signal intensity surrounded by CSF, together with their appearance in T2-weighted images, help to define the extent of the AVM in the spinal canal (77).

Spinal arteriography is still the procedure of choice for diagnosis. Global aortic arteriography followed by selective arteriography is required in order to define the feeding and draining vessels of the AVM (Fig. 1A–C). MR is expected to be more informative in the near future. Detailed information about the AVM's blood supply is essential for planning the appropriate therapy (56,65,66).

Treatment

Type I AVM may improve by excision of the dural fistula (65), by intrathecal ligation of its arterial supply (65,78,79), or by embolization of the fistula (80–82).

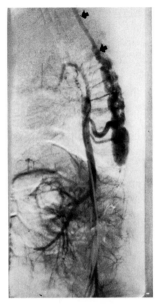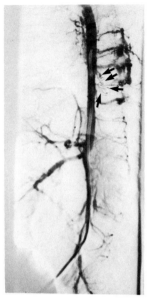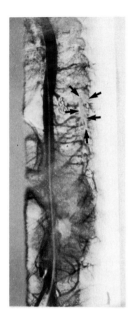

A-C

FIG. 1. A 4-month-old child with an extradural spinal arteriovenous malformation (SAVM) studied by selective angiography. The subtraction angiograms in lateral projection show the complete SAVM with feeders and a long, large draining vein (*arrows*) **(A)**; an important reduction of the SAVM size after intra-arterial clipping of the largest feeding artery (*arrows*) **(B)**; and complete disappearance of the SAVM after surgical clipping (*arrows*) **(C)**. (Courtesy of Dr. A. Perez-Higueras.)

Type II AVM are difficult to treat owing to their intramedullary location and the abundant feeders arising from the anterior spinal arterial system. Nonetheless, successful microsurgical removal (65,83,84), feeder ligation (55,85), or embolization has been achieved (81,82,86).

Type III AVM have been even more difficult to treat. Partial reduction in the volume of the lesion by embolization, feeder ligation, or partial surgical removal may be attempted (54,55). In any case, outcome is usually poor.

Type IV AVM has been reported only once (56), and the patient, a young man, was treated by surgical ligation of the fistula through an anterior transthoracic approach with relatively mild complications.

LYMPHANGIOMATOSIS OF THE SPINE

Lymphangiomatosis of the spine producing neurologic symptomatology is very rare. This soft tissue tumor occurs most frequently in the neck, axilla, and other organs but not the CNS (87). Primary lymphangiomatosis of bone is quite rare; metastasis in bone from a tumor located elsewhere in the body is more common.

Four types of lymphangiomas are known: (a) simple, (b) circumscribed, (c) cystic, and (d) diffuse. All are present since birth or appear in infancy. Hemangiomas and lymphangiomas are difficult to differentiate because of their similar clinical, radiographic, and histologic findings. Moreover, a mixture of the two conditions and even the association of a lymphangioma with an AVM of the CNS have been reported (88–90). Bone lesions may be single or multiple. Most cases occur in patients ranging from 3 months to 23 years of age (91).

The clinical manifestations vary depending on the site of involvement and the size of the lesion. The spinal cord, roots, or nerves may be compressed by deformed vertebrae. Despite impressive radiologic bony alterations, neurologic deficit is exceptional.

Radiographically, lymphangiomas are usually discrete, osteolytic, and involve both the cortex and spongiosa. In the vertebrae, an area of rarefaction may be traversed by thick bony trabeculae of variable size. The lesion may increase in size but may also be static or even shrink spontaneously. Lymphangiomas and hemangiomas of the spine have essentially the same radiologic appearance.

Their radiologic differential diagnosis includes aneurysmal bone cyst, hyperparathyroidism, histiocytosis X, and tumors (92,93). Lymphangiography may be helpful in the diagnosis (93–95), showing stasis and collateral formation with complete or partial obstruction of the lymphatics. Delayed films, as long as 6 days after injection, may be useful because contrast material is visible for many months.

Lymphangioma is a congenital tumor of lymph vessels. It is composed of endothelial cells and supporting connective tissue, both tissues participating in the neoplastic process. It arises from abnormal mesodermal rests that develop into isolated, imperfect lymph vessels with a slight tendency to abnormal growth. Microscopically, lymphangiomas consist of cystic structures and of vessels lined by a single layer of flat endothelial cells with a small amount of delicate fibrous tissue. Their exact vascular origin is difficult, if not impossible, to determine. Some authors doubt the neoplastic nature of lymphangiomas and prefer to call them lymphangiectasia, cystic lymphangioma, hamartomatous hemolymphangiomatosis, hemangiohamartoma, or cystic hamartomatous vascular malformation (96). Presentation of both hemangioma and lymphangioma in the same patient is not surprising since they have a common embryologic origin. Lewis (97) showed that the lymphatic sacs separate from the veins at the 16-mm to 20-mm embryologic stage but develop new connections with them toward the 30-mm stage.

Treatment of lymphangioma is usually symptomatic, but radiotherapy may play a role in the elimination of lymphangiomatosis from bone (98). We observed the disappearance of clinical and radiologic alterations after radiotherapy in a child who presented skull metastases from a primitive lymphangioma of the leg.

REFERENCES

1. Stout AP, Murray MR. Hemangiopericytoma: a vascular tumor featuring Zimmermann's pericytes. *Ann Surg* 1942;116:26–33.

2. Grode ML. Hemangiopericytoma of central nervous system. *NY State J Med* 1972;72:2557–2560.
3. Enzinger FM, Smith BH. Hemangiopericytoma: an analysis of 106 cases. *Hum Pathol* 1976;7:61–82.
4. Angervall L, Kindblom L-G, Nielsen JM, et al. Hemangiopericytoma: a clinicopathologic, angiographic and microangiographic study. *Cancer* 1978;42:2412–2427.
5. Harris DJ, Fornasier VL, Livingston KE. Hemangiopericytoma of the spinal canal: report of three cases. *J Neurosurg* 1978;49:914–920.
6. Pitluk HC, Conn J Jr. Hemangiopericytoma: literature review and clinical presentations. *Am J Surg* 1979;137:413–416.
7. Muraszko KM, Lobo Antunes J, Hilal SK, Michelsen WJ. Hemangiopericytoma of the spine. *Neurosurgery* 1982;10:473–479.
8. Krugliak KL, Barmeir E, Maroko I, et al. Un hémangiopéricytome rachidien malin, d'apparence radiologique bénigne. *J Radiol* 1984;65:485–487.
9. O'Brien P, Brasfield RD. Hemangiopericytoma. *Cancer* 1965;18:249–252.
10. Schirger A, Uihlein A, Parker HL, Kernohan JW. Hemangiopericytoma recurring after 26 years. Report of a case. *Mayo Clin Proc* 1958;33:347–352.
11. McMaster MJ, Soule EH, Ivins JC. Hemangiopericytoma: a clinicopathological study and long-term follow-up of 60 patients. *Cancer* 1975;36:2232–2244.
12. Palacios E, Azar-Kia B. Malignant metastasizing angioblastic meningiomas. *J Neurosurg* 1975; 42:185–188.
13. Stern MB, Grode ML, Goodman MD. Hemangiopericytoma of the cervical spine: report of an unusual case. *Clin Orthop* 1980;151:201–204.
14. Alpern MB, Thorsen MK, Kellman GM, et al. CT appearance of hemangiopericytoma. *J Comput Assist Tomogr* 1986;10:264–267.
15. Kriss FC, Kahn DR, Schneider RC. Value of angiography in intraspinal mediastinal hemangiopericytoma: case report. *J Neurosurg* 1968;29:535–539.
16. Ramsey HJ. Fine structure of hemangiopericytoma and hemangioendothelioma. *Cancer* 1966;19: 2005–2018.
17. Eddy RL, Sanchez SA. Renin-secreting renal neoplasm and hypertension with hypokalemia. *Ann Intern Med* 1971;75:725–729.
18. Pitkethly DT, Hardman JM, Kempe LG, Earle KM. Angioblastic meningiomas: clinicopathologic study of 81 cases. *J Neurosurg* 1970;32:539–544.
19. Lowden RG, Taylor HB. Angioblastic meningioma with metastasis to the breast. *Arch Pathol Lab Med* 1974;98:373–375.
20. Gerner RE, Moore GE, Pickren JW. Hemangiopericytoma. *Ann Surg* 1974;179:128–132.
21. Popoff NA, Malinin TI, Rosomoff HL. Fine structure of intracranial hemangiopericytoma and angiomatous meningioma. *Cancer* 1974;34:1187–1197.
22. Goellner JR, Laws ER Jr, Soule EH, Okazaki H. Hemangiopericytoma of the meninges: Mayo Clinic experience. *Am J Clin Pathol* 1978;70:375–380.
23. Friedman M, Egan JW. Irradiation of hemangiopericytoma of Stout. *Radiology* 1960;74:721–730.
24. Mira JG, Chu FCH, Fortner JG. The role of radiotherapy in the management of malignant hemangiopericytoma: report of eleven new cases and review of the literature. *Cancer* 1977;39:1254–1259.
25. Lal H, Sanyal B, Pant GC, et al. Hemangiopericytoma: report of three cases regarding role of radiation therapy. *Am J Roentgenol* 1976;126:887–891.
26. Kauffman SL, Stout AP. Hemangiopericytoma in children. *Cancer* 1960;13:695–710.
27. Hurt M, André JM, Djindjian R, et al. Les hémangioblastomes intrarachidiens. *Neurochirurgie* 1975;21(Suppl. 1):1–136.
28. Kinney TD, Fitzgeral PJ. Lindau von Hippel disease with hemangioblastomas of the spinal cord and syringomyelia. *Arch Pathol* 1947;43:439–455.
29. Kendall B, Russell J. Haemangioblastomas of the spinal cord. *Br J Radiol* 1966;39:817–823.
30. Iizuka J. Mikroämangioblastom des Rükenmarkes. In: *Forschritte auf dem Gebiet der Neurochirurgie*. Stuttgart: Hippokrates, 1970;294–300.
31. Otanasek FT, Silver ML. Spinal hemangioma (hemangioblastoma) in Lindau's disease. Report of six cases in a single family. *J Neurosurg* 1961;18:295–300.
32. Di Chiro C, Doppman JL. Differential angiographic features of haemangioblastomas and arteriovenous malformations of the spinal cord. *Radiology* 1969;93:25–30.

33. Stevens J, Love S, Davis C, Kendall BE. Capillary haemangioblastoma of bone resembling a vertebral haemangioma. *Br J Radiol* 1983;56:571–575.
34. Balériaux-Waha D, Retif J, Noterman J, et al. CT scanning for the diagnosis of the cerebellar and spinal lesions of von Hippel-Landau's disease. *Neuroradiology* 1978;14:214–244.
35. Di Chiro G, Doppman JL, Wener L. Computed tomography of spinal cord arteriovenous malformations. *Radiology* 1977;123:351–354.
36. Di Chiro G, Doppman JL, Dwyer AJ, et al. Tumors and arteriovenous malformations of the spinal cord: assessment using MR. *Radiology* 1985;156:689–697.
37. Masaryk TJ, Modic MT, Geisinger MA, et al. Cervical myelopathy: a comparison of magnetic resonance and myelography. *J Comput Assist Tomogr* 1986;10:184–194.
38. Yasargil MG, De Preux J. Expériences microchirurgicales dans 12 cas d'hémangioblastomes intramédullaires. *Neurochirurgie* 1978;21:425–434.
39. Schmorl G, Junghanns H. *The human spine in health and disease*, 2nd American ed. New York: Grune & Stratton, 1971;325.
40. McAllister VL, Kendall BE, Bull JWD. Symptomatic vertebral haemangioma. *Brain* 1975;98:71–80.
41. Zito G, Kadis GN. Multiple vertebral hemangiomas resembling metastases with spinal cord compression. *Arch Neurol* 1980;37:247–248.
42. Leehey, P, Naseem M, Every P, et al. Vertebral hemangioma with compression myelopathy: metrizamide CT demonstration. *J Comput Assist Tomogr* 1985;9:985–986.
43. Lepoire J, Montaut J, Picard L, et al. Embolisation préalable à l'exérèse d'un hémangiome du rachis dorsal. *Neurochirurgie* 1973;19:173–181.
44. Benati A, Da Pian R, Mazza C, et al. Preoperative embolization of a vertebral haemangioma compressing the spinal cord. *Neuroradiology* 1974;7:181–183.
45. Hekster REM, Luyendijk W, Tan TI. Spinal cord compression caused by vertebral haemangioma relieved by percutaneous catheter embolisation. *Neuroradiology* 1972;3:160–164.
46. Hemmy DC, McGee DM, Armbrust FH, Larson SJ. Resection of a vertebral haemangioma after preoperative embolization. Case report. *J Neurosurg* 1977;47:282–285.
47. Buckhill T, Jackson JW, Kemp HBS, Kendall BE. Haemangioma of a vertebral body treated by ligation of the segmental arteries: report of a case. *J Bone Joint Surg* 1973;55B:534–539.
48. Masson P. Le glomus neuromyo-artériel des régions tactiles et ses tumeurs. *Lyon Chir* 1924;21:257–280.
49. Tocker C. Glomangioma. An ultrastructural study. *Cancer* 1969;23:487–492.
50. Ho K-L, Pak MSY. Glomus tumor of the coccygeal region. *J Bone Joint Surg* 1980;62:141–142.
51. Pambakian H, Smith MA. Glomus tumours of the coccygeal body associated with coccydynia. A preliminary report. *J Bone Joint Surg* 1981;63B:424–426.
52. Shugart RR, Soule EH, Johnson EW Jr. Glomus tumor. *Surg Gynecol Obstet* 1963;117:334–340.
53. King ESJ. Glomus tumor. *Aust J Surg* 1954;23:280–295.
54. Malis LI. Arteriovenous malformations of the spinal cord. In: Youmans JR, ed. *Neurological surgery*, 2nd ed., vol. 3. Philadelphia: W.B. Saunders, 1982;1850–1874.
55. Ommaya AK. Spinal arteriovenous malformations. In: Wilkins RH, Rengachary SS, eds. *Neurosurgery*, vol. 2. New York: McGraw-Hill, 1985;1459–1499.
56. Heros RC, Debrun GM, Ojemann RG, et al. Direct spinal arteriovenous fistula: a new type of spinal AVM. *J Neurosurg* 1986;64:134–139.
57. Park TS, Cail WS, Delashaw JB, Kattwinkel J. Spinal cord arteriovenous malformation in a neonate. Case report. *J Neurosurg* 1986;64:322–324.
58. Béraud R, Meloche BR. A propos de deux cas de malformations médullaires. *Neurochirurgie* 1964;10:559–561.
59. Hoffman JH, Mohr G, Kusunohi T. Multiple arteriovenous malformations of spinal cord and brain in a child. Case report. *Childs Brain* 1976;2:317–324.
60. Binder B, Eng GD, Milhorat TH, Galioto F. Spinal arteriovenous malformations in an infant: unusual symptomatology and pathology. *Dev Med Child Neurol* 1982;24:380–385.
61. Odom GL, Woodhall B, Margolis G. Spontaneous hematomyelia and angiomas of the spinal cord. *J Neurosurg* 1957;14:192–202.
62. Sutton T, Murray PJ, Alexander WJ, Blundell JE. Arteriovenous malformations of the spinal cord in childhood. *Radiology* 1973;109:621–622.
63. Kaplan P, Hollenberg RD, Fraser FC. A spinal arteriovenous malformation with hereditary cutaneous hemangiomas. *Am J Dis Child* 1976;130:1329–1331.

64. Ouaknine GE, Godath N, Matz S, Shalit M. Congenital vascular malformation of the spinal cord simulating diastematomyelia. *Childs Brain* 1979;5:513–517.
65. Oldfield EH, Di Chiro G, Quindlen EA, et al. Successful treatment of a group of spinal cord arteriovenous malformations by interruption of dural fistula. *J Neurosurg* 1983;59:1019–1030.
66. Riché MC, Modenesi-Freitas J, Djindjian M, Merland JJ. Arteriovenous malformations (AVM) of the spinal cord in children. A review of 38 cases. *Neuroradiology* 1982;22:171–180.
67. Aminoff MJ, Logue V. Clinical features of spinal vascular malformations. *Brain* 1974;97:197–210.
68. Tobin WD, Layton DD Jr. The diagnosis and natural history of spinal cord arteriovenous malformations. *Mayo Clin Proc* 1976;51:637–646.
69. Djindjian M, Djindjian R, Hurth M, et al. Angiomes médullaires et syndrome de Klippel-Trénaunay-Weber. *Rev Neurol (Paris)* 1977;133:609–617.
70. Komatsu Y, Kuzhara S, Kanazawa I, Nakanishi T. Klippel-Trenaunay-Weber syndrome associated with spinal arteriovenous malformation. A case report. *Clin Neurol* 1985;25:830–836.
71. Leech PJ, Stokes BAR, Apsimon T, Harper C. Unruptured aneurysm of the anterior spinal artery presenting as paraparesis. Case report. *J Neurosurg* 1976;45:331–333.
72. García CA, Dulcey J. Ruptured aneurysm of the spinal artery of Adamkiewicz during pregnancy. *Neurology (NY)* 1979;29:394–398.
73. Vincent FM. Anterior spinal artery aneurysm presenting as a subarachnoid hemorrhage. *Stroke* 1981;12:230–232.
74. Caroscio JT, Brannan T, Budabin M, et al. Subarachnoid hemorrhage secondary to spinal arteriovenous malformation and aneurysm: report of a case and review of the literature. *Arch Neurol* 1980;37:101–103.
75. Smith BS, Penka CF, Erickson LVS, Matsuo F. Case report: subarachnoid hemorrhage due to anterior spinal artery aneurysm. *Neurosurgery* 1986;18:217–219.
76. Deeb ZL, Rosenbaum AE, Bensy JJ, Scarff TB. Calcified intramedullary aneurysm in spinal angioma. *Neuroradiology* 1977;14:1–3.
77. Kulkarni MV, Burks DD, Price AC, et al. Diagnosis of spinal arteriovenous malformations in a pregnant patient by MR imaging. *J Comput Assist Tomogr* 1985;9:171–173.
78. Ommaya AK, Di Chiro G, Doppman J. Ligation of arterial supply in the treatment of spinal cord arteriovenous malformations. *J Neurosurg* 1969;30:679–692.
79. Symon L, Kuyama H, Kendall B. Dural arteriovenous malformations of the spine. Clinical features and surgical results in 55 cases. *J Neurosurg* 1984;60:238–247.
80. Djindjian R. Embolization of angiomas of the spinal cord. *Surg Neurol* 1975;4:411–420.
81. Doppman JL, Di Chiro G, Ommaya AK. Percutaneous embolization of spinal cord arteriovenous malformations. *J Neurosurg* 1971;34:48–55.
82. Berenstein A, Young W, Ransohoff J, et al. Somatosensory evoked potentials during spinal angiography and therapeutic embolization. *J Neurosurg* 1984;60:777–785.
83. Krayenbühl H, Yasargil MG, McClintock HG. Treatment of spinal cord vascular malformations by surgical excision. *J Neurosurg* 1969;30:427–435.
84. Yasargil MG, DeLong WB, Guarnaschelli JJ. Complete microsurgical excision of cervical extra-medullary and intramedullary vascular malformations. *Surg Neurol* 1975;4:211–224.
85. Bailey WL, Sperl MP. Angiomas of the cervical spinal cord. *J Neurosurg* 1969;30:560–568.
86. Holgate RC, Lougheed WM. Global arteriovenous malformation of the cervical region. *Can J Neurol Sci* 1981;8:41–47.
87. Steinert GM, Farm J, Lawson JP. Lymphangiomatosis of bone. *Radiology* 1969;93:1093–1098.
88. Newton TH, Cronqvist S. Involvement of dural arteries in intracranial arteriovenous malformations. *Radiology* 1969;93:1071–1078.
89. Scavone C, Pascual-Castroviejo I, Tendero A, Villarejo F. Malformacion arteriovenosa intracraneal gigante (MAVG) y linfangioma facial. *An Esp Pediatr* 1980;13:589–592.
90. Pascual-Castroviejo I. The association of extracranial and intracranial vascular malformations in children. *Can J Neurol Sci* 1985;12:139–148.
91. Rogers HM, Chou SN. Lymphangioma of the craniocervical junction. Case report. *J Neurosurg* 1973;38:510–513.
92. Tucker AS. Lymphangiectasis—benign and malignant. *Am J Roentgenol* 1964;91:1104–1113.
93. Winterberger AR. Radiographic diagnosis of lymphangiomatosis of bone. *Radiology* 1972;102:321–324.

94. Nixon GW. Lymphangiomatosis of bone, demonstrated by lymphagiography. *Am J Roentgenol* 1970;110:582–586.
95. Sauvegrain J, Parsa G, Aicardi J, Manlot G. Lymphangiectasies intraosseuses et lymphoedème congénital. *Ann Radiol (Paris)* 1973;16:1–10.
96. Moseley JE, Starobin SG. Cystic angiomatosis of bone: manifestation of a hamartomatous disease entity. *Am J Roentgenol* 1964;91:1114–1120.
97. Lewis FT. The development of the lymphatic system in rabbits. *Am J Anat* 1905;5:95–111.
98. Edwards W Jr, Thompson RC, Varsa EW. Lymphangiomatosis and massive osteolysis of the cervical spine. A case report and review of the literature. *Clin Orthop* 1983;177:222–229.

14

Congenital Tumors or Malformations

Ignacio Pascual-Castroviejo

SACROCOCCYGEAL TERATOMA

Teratoma is a neoplasm that includes components of all three germinal layers and arises from the mesodermal streak and Hensen's node. These tumors occur in 1 of every 35,000 live births (1). Seventy-five percent are detected in the neonatal period; 9% require delivery by cesarean section. Sacroccocygeal teratomas are the most common neoplasms in the newborn (2–4). They are also the most common teratomas of the body. Most sacrococcygeal teratomas are found in girls, with a ratio of approximately 4 girls to 1 boy (1,5). These tumors are malignant in only one-third of cases (6). They may occur at any age, with the majority noted at birth or shortly thereafter. Congenital tumors are more likely to be malignant in boys than girls. In both sexes, tumors presenting before 6 months of age are likely to be malignant, while benign teratomas tend to present after 6 months (7). It is important not to delay the diagnosis, because the great majority of these tumors are benign in the neonate but undergo malignant degeneration during the first few months of life (1,5). At diagnosis, 5% will have metastases to the peritoneal cavity, lungs, brain, or liver (1). It is possible to detect these tumors antenatally by sonography (8–10).

Sacrococcygeal teratomas are divided into four types according to their location (1):

Type I: These tumors are mostly external. They may be eroded and produce various distortions and discolorations of the buttock. They have an abundant vascularization, and may bleed profusely. They may be associated with absence or destruction of the coccyx.

Type II: These tumors have an important intrapelvic component that can displace or invade pelvic structures. They also have a large external component (Fig. 1).

Type III: The intrapelvic and, in some cases, even the intraperitoneal component is larger than the external portion. The tumor displaces or invades surrounding structures.

Type IV: These tumors are presacral with no external mass in the newborn. The rectum and urinary bladder are displaced anteriorly. These tumors may be confused radiologically with several other presacral masses, such as abscesses, chordomas, neuroblastomas, anterior meningoceles, rectal duplications, and muscular hemangiomas.

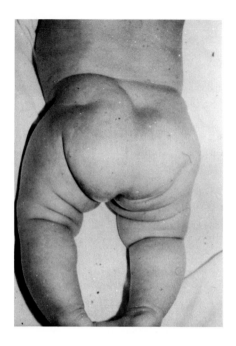

FIG. 1. An 8-month-old girl with sacrococcy-geal teratoma. Prominence of the buttock.

Types II, III, and IV tumors, if they grow extensively, may obstruct the bladder, rectum, or blood vessels. Sacrococcygeal teratomas with an intraspinal component may cause lower motor neuron signs and can be associated with congenital or acquired deformities of the sacrum and coccyx.

Teratomas may be cystic, solid, or mixed. Solid tumors are usually malignant. Most cystic and mixed teratomas are benign (6,11). There are exceptions, however (6,12). Calcification, which can be detected on plain radiographs, is found almost exclusively in benign tumors, although one of four patients with malignant tumors did have calcifications (6). The size of the mass is not correlated with malignancy. The biggest tumors have a high morbidity and mortality rate because large masses involving surrounding structures are difficult to remove, and have a tendency to bleed, a complication that can present during labor and surgical resection (8,9,13,14).

Children with sacrococcygeal teratomas have an increased prevalence of polyhydramnios and hydrops fetalis (14). In a series of 405 cases, 18% had additional congenital anomalies (1).

The term malignant teratoma is also used for related malignant tumors of germ cell derivation (yolk sac tumors or carcinomas, embryonal carcinomas or adenocarcinomas, papillary adenocarcinomas, chorioncarcinomas, papillary ependymomas, and germinomas or seminomas), one or more of which can occur in an otherwise benign or immature teratoma (12). Endodermal sinus tumors or yolk sac tumors were originally described by Teilum (15). Initially noted in the ovary and testicle, they may also occur in extragonadal sites such as the vulva, vagina, prostate, sacrococcygeal region, retroperitoneum, mediastinum, suprasellar region, and pineal gland. These malignant tumors are most common in young children (12). Peritoneal implants may arise from tumors in the ovary or testis, and following ventriculoperitoneal shunts for yolk sac tumors of the pineal gland. Alpha-fetoprotein is elevated in the serum of patients with these malignant tumors (16–18). Increased alpha-fetoprotein and acetylcholinesterase in amniotic fluid suggest the diagnosis of sacrococcygeal teratoma in the fetus (19). They are not always elevated, however (20), so that sonographic examination is advisable in all pregnancies.

Clinical Findings

Many present with an external mass of the buttock (Fig. 1). In addition to involving the bladder, rectum, and other pelvic structures, one of the most severe complications of these tumors is neurologic deficit resulting from spinal cord or cauda equina involvement. Unfortunately, at the time of diagnosis most affected children have already developed weakness or paralysis of the legs with sphincter disturbance. Permanent sequelae will result if the spinal cord and nerve roots are not decompressed expeditiously. Children recover better from such neurologic insults than adults (18). Sacrococcygeal teratomas seem to be particularly frequent in monozygotic twins (21). These tumors may be hereditary in some families. Ashcraft and Holder (22) described 17 patients in 6 kindreds with presacral teratoma and sacral defects, often associated with anorectal and other local anomalies. The tumor complex was inherited as an autosomal dominant characteristic.

Radiology

Sacrococcygeal teratoma may be diagnosed *in utero* by sonography. Not only can the tumor be detected (8,9) but also its solid and cystic components, as well as any areas of calcification (10).

Plain radiographs may show agenesis or destruction of the coccyx and calcifications in the teratoma, even in neonates (Fig. 2A). These calcifications can be any size, shape, or configuration. They are found in 50% of sacrococcygeal teratomas and are almost always a sign that the tumor is benign, although some calcification is present in about 13 to 25% of malignant ones (6,12). An important radiologic sign of yolk sac tumor is destruction of the affected vertebrae.

Other radiologic studies can show anterior narrowing or displacement of the rectum (Fig. 2B) and bladder, hydronephrosis, or vascular obstruction. Myelography shows partial or total block of the contrast medium by an extradural mass.

These tumors may be supplied by branches coming from the middle sacral, lateral sacral, hypogastric, and femoral arteries (23,24). Some authors have emphasized the value of conventional arteriography (24) and digital subtraction

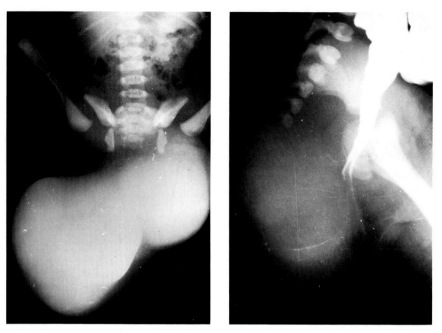

A,B

FIG. 2. A: Voluminous sacrococcygeal teratoma evident by plain X-ray. **B:** Important forward displacement of the rectum in the same case as in **A**.

angiography (DSA) (25) to delineate their vascular anatomy, which facilitates resection. Sagital computerized tomography (CT) is possible in neonates and provides more accurate information about the portion of the tumor located between the rectum and the sacrum (25). Magnetic resonance (MR) imaging provides the same information as CT.

Treatment

Treatment consists of a combination of surgery, radiotherapy, and chemotherapy (5,12,26). Large benign-appearing, external tumors in newborns are easily removed. Large, fixed, mostly internal tumors in infants over the age of 1 year are difficult or impossible to remove (12,26). The majority of malignant teratomas are not resectable because most fill the pelvis, obstructing the urinary tract and rectum. The coccyx must always be excised with the mass (1). Grossly apparent areas of necrosis or hemorrhage are strongly suggestive of malignancy. Since benign and malignant elements may be observed throughout the mass, the histologic study of all tissue components is important. Because a correct diagnosis is essential for appropriate treatment, the pathologist must search meticulously for malignant areas (3,4). Although very uncommon, intraspinal extension does occur

(12,22,24), especially in intrapelvic presacral tumors. Invasion of the spinal canal takes place from adjacent structures. Palliative decompression laminectomy must be performed. A missed cerebrospinal fluid (CSF) leak has a high morbidity and mortality.

Radiation therapy in doses ranging from 2,000 to 5,000 rad administered to the tumor, when indicated together with radiation of other structures (lung, thoracic or lumbar spine, etc.), has been used with good results (26).

Chemotherapy with actinomycin-D, vincristine, cyclophosphamide, methotrexate, associated with surgery and sometimes with radiotherapy, has given good responses even in cases with metastases and urinary or rectal obstruction (5,7,12,18,26–29). Although isolated cases, even some having metastases, have improved with chemotherapy (30), there is no satisfactory therapy for the endodermal sinus tumor, regardless of its location, when there are distant metastases at the time of diagnosis.

Prognosis

Patients with benign tumors and adequate surgical treatment usually have a normal outcome. Prognosis for infants with malignant sacrococcygeal teratoma is poor. Long-term disease-free survivors account for 6% (30) to 17% of cases (26).

SPINAL LIPOMA

Generalities

Intraspinal lipomas are masses of mature fat and connective tissue that are connected to the spinal cord and may be attached to the meninges. These tumors may be found extradurally, intradurally, and intra-extradurally. The intradural portion can be extramedullary or intramedullary. The intramedullary ones include two well-defined varieties, lipomyelomeningoceles and lipomas of the filum terminale. A variant of spinal lipoma is the angiolipoma. Myelolipoma is a benign tumor made up of mature fat cells and hematopoietic elements, commonly located in the adrenal gland. It has never been described in people less than 40 years of age and never causes neurologic disturbances.

All subtypes of lipomas can produce symptoms of spinal cord and radicular compression. Lipomeningoceles and lipomas of the filum terminale are complicated by tethering of the spinal cord, which causes stretching and ischemia of the spinal cord and nerve roots.

Originally, lipoma was an autopsy diagnosis (31). Clinical diagnosis became possible by X-ray, especially myelography. More modern techniques (CT and MR) have provided ease and rapidity of diagnosis, with high quality images, and they have eliminated the discomfort and danger of invasive presurgical studies.

The prevalence of spinal lipoma differs depending on the age of the patient and

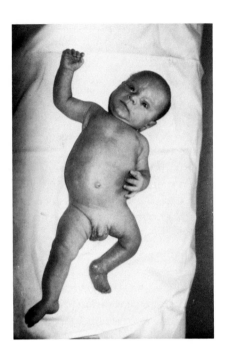

FIG. 3. A 4-month-old child with intra-extradural lumbosacral lipoma with more severe spread on the left side.

on whether one is concerned with isolated lipomas or those associated with spina bifida. Spinal lipomas are very rare in adults; the incidence may be 1% (32,33) to 1.5% (34) of all spinal cord tumors, while they account for 5% (35), 6% (36), or 47% (in our series) of all intraspinal masses in children. The association of lipomas with spina bifida, especially those of the lumbar and lumbosacral regions, has been reported in 56% (37), 78% (38), or 100% (39,40) of cases. It is nearly 100% in our series. Intra-extradural lipomas unassociated with meningocele were seen in 21 cases (39% of all lipomas). Meningolipomas were found in 19 patients (35%); some of them were extradural. Lipoma of the filum terminale was observed in 8 cases (15%), extradural lipoma in 6 cases (11%), and pure intramedullary lipoma in 1 case, in the cervical region.

Pure intramedullary lipomas are rare. Most childhood cases are intra-extradural. Purely extradural lipomas are less frequent in children than in adults. Lipomas of the filum terminale and lipomeningoceles associated with tethering of the spinal cord are very frequent in children.

Most spinal lipomas of all types located in the lumbosacral region are suspected at birth, although neurologic symptoms often do not appear until periods of rapid gain in height (41) or weight (42). Lumbosacral skin abnormalities such as tufts of hair, hemangiolipomas, lipomas, skin tags, or pigmented nevi, in conjunction with lower limb abnormalities (Fig. 3), deformity of the intergluteal crease, or anovaginal defects (Fig. 4) such as imperforate anus and rectovaginal fistula, should lead one to suspect the presence of a lipoma. Associated anomalies include clubfeet, progressive muscular atrophy in the lower limbs, sphincter disturbances,

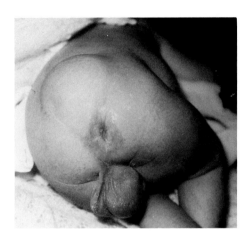

FIG. 4. Myelomeningolipoma. Asymmetry of the gluteal folds and buttocks. Skin angioma in the zone where the anus was surgically opened because of an imperforate anus.

as well as scoliosis, gait abnormalities, weakness, or decreased ankle-jerks. Any child with orthopedic deformities, bowel or bladder dysfunction, and neurologic abnormalities associated with lumbosacral skin lesions requires investigation by a child neurologist or neurosurgeon. Neuroradiologic studies, including plain films, myelography, CT, or MR, usually yield a correct diagnosis prior to removal of the mass.

This condition has an embryologic origin. Closure of the neural tube takes place between the third and fifth weeks of intrauterine life, when the ectoderm differentiates into the epithelial and neural tissues. Any error in this process may lead to abnormalities in the skin and the central nervous system (CNS). Depending on when the error happens, lipomas may be intramedullary, intra-extradural, or epidural. Intramedullary lipomas originate embryologically before the other types of lipomas, and epidural lipomas originate last.

There may be associated anomalies in organs or structures originating from the endoderm or the mesoderm. The most common are absent kidneys, Klippel-Feil syndrome, intracranial aneurysms, arteriovenous malformations, and anomalies of the fingers and toes. Lumbosacral agenesis is rare (43). Multiple intracranial lipomas were found at autopsy in a patient who showed a completely intradural lipoma of the thoracic cord (38). Spinal lipoma may also present as a mediastinal mass (44).

Treatment of spinal lipomas is controversial. Many patients are initially asymptomatic or minisymptomatic, and some patients remain so throughout life. Most patients develop progressive neurologic and sphincter dysfunction, so that excision is advisable. Most lipomas end up being removed sooner or later.

Histology

Congenital lipomas comprise normal adipose tissue, with additional connective tissue (45). Lipomas that are both intra- and extradural have the same intimate connection with neural tissue as do the completely intradural tumors. Although lipomas are rarely completely surrounded by neural tissue, they are firmly adherent and tightly attached to neural tissue by fibrous septa. Consequently, complete removal of the fat is difficult. There may be dense collagen in the root of the lipomatous mass (46). Walsh and Markesbery (47) found a variety of unusual ectopic neuroectodermal and mesodermal tissues in spinal lipomas. All were densely fibrous. An ependymal-lined canal resembling a terminal ventricle was encountered in a patient with an intradural lipoma. The subependymal layer was neuroglial, and smooth muscle fibers were scattered throughout the adjacent connective tissue and lipoma. In all cases of lipomeningocele, the lipoma tapered to a firm fibrous tract that blended into the conus medullaris. This fibrous tract consisted not only of a relatively acellular connective tissue stroma, but in one case, of sheets or islands of neuroglia and scattered nerve cells; another had an epithelial cyst with a smooth muscle and fibrous tissue wall; and, in a third patient, there was embryonic bone. These findings suggested to the investigators (47) that there is a second phase to caudal neural tube development and that congenital lipomas are formed by persistence and differentiation of ordinarily vestigial pluripotential embryonic cells.

Intraspinal Lipomas

Intramedullary lipomas are rare. For the most part, they are considered together with intraspinal subdural lipomas because of the intramedullary nature of a portion of the mass and the intra-extramedullary—but subdural—other portion of the lipoma. Intraspinal subdural lipomas are rare tumors of the spinal canal since they constitute only 1% of them (32). Occasionally, lipomas are observed in the thoracic and cervical regions. Only one case was found by Koos et al. (35) among 834 spinal tumors collected from several important series, including their own. Extension into the posterior fossa (48,49) and fourth ventricle is even less common. When the lipoma extends into the fourth ventricle, it may cause obstructive hydrocephalus (50–52). Most lipomas in children and adolescents are intradural extramedullary masses (48,50–56). Even in the intramedullary lipomas of the cervicothoracic region (57,58) their intramedullary location is uncertain because intradural lipomas originate in a dorsal, juxtamedullary position. Their growth flattens the anterior spinal cord, separates the posterior columns, and encases nerve roots. All these features give the tumor the appearance of being intramedullary at surgery (52). Nonetheless, its upper and lower margins are easily separable from the cord. In contrast, its midportion merges into the cord, and there is no cleavage plane between cord and tumor (58).

Clinical symptoms and signs consist of delayed motor milestones, hypotonia, weakness of the neck and limbs, loss of position sense, and gait disturbance. An inexpressive face, retrocollis, inability to elevate the arms to the level of the shoulders, hyperreflexia, Babinski signs, and sphincter disturbances may also occur. A typical mode of presentation is scapulohumeral atrophy without upper motor neuron signs. The clinical course is slowly progressive, and children ultimately present paraparesis or tetraparesis. Skin abnormalities are not common in cervicothoracic lipomas although a subcutaneous lipomatous mass may be present in the back of the neck (50).

Plain radiographs of the cervical and dorsal spine usually show significant widening of the spinal canal and thinning of the pedicles in the area involved by the tumor. The child we observed presented incomplete closure of the arches of several vertebrae (50,58). Myelography usually shows complete obstruction to contrast flow by an intradural extramedullary mass that is usually lobulated and asymmetric or intramedullary and symmetric (58). Some authors believe that they can differentiate subpial lipomas from intramedullary lesions on the basis of their radiographic features (59). Plain X-rays have been superseded by CT and MR. CT scans are characteristic and diagnostic because they show a mass of typical fatty tissue that in some cases appears to be inside the spinal cord. More often the spinal cord is thinned and flattened ventrally, compressed by the hypodense fatty mass (49,50,52,60,61). MR imaging is useful for delineating the anatomy of the lipoma and its relationship to adjacent structures. The characteristically short T1 of fat and the possibility of obtaining pictures in the sagittal plane, as well as inversion recovery ones, provide accurate localization of the tumor with its exact extension and size in cervical (61) and cervicobulbar (49) regions. MR also shows whether the lipoma is intramedullary or extramedullary. Total removal of even extramedullary lipomas is very difficult because of the infiltrative nature of the lesion. Simple decompressive laminectomy may be beneficial, but subtotal excision of the lipoma is a better form of therapy. Survival with good neurologic function following subtotal removal may last for many years, although death a short time after surgery may occur, especially in young infants (50).

Extradural Lipomas

Extradural or epidural spinal lipomas may or may not be associated with spinal dysraphism. Those with spinal dysraphism are mostly seen during the first decade of life and have virtually the same clinical presentation as any other spinal lipoma that penetrates into the dura.

Some investigators (62,63) believe that it is important to distinguish between two histologic types: true lipoma and angiolipoma. True lipoma is yellow, firmly adherent to adjacent tissues, and causes many problems for complete surgical removal. The angiolipoma (see Angiolipomas, below) is brown, elastic, soft, and barely adherent to adjacent tissues. This facilitates total removal and results in a better outcome. Angiolipomas are extradural, whereas pure lipomas can have both extradural and intradural components. Angiolipomas may be associated with other vascular malformations and are not associated with malformations of the spinal cord.

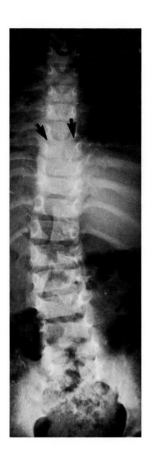

FIG. 5. Extradural lipoma. The X-ray film shows a widened spinal canal from D8 (*arrows*) to the sacrum. Almost all the vertebrae present deformities of the arch, especially along the trajectory of the spinous processes.

Clinical symptoms and signs may appear at any age. These tumors may be present at birth, but their discovery in adults is also common. Most patients have sphincteric disturbances from the onset. They may also have a clubfoot, usually unilateral, sensory disturbances, especially in the perineal region, sexual impotence, muscular atrophy in one or both lower limbs, and hyperreflexia. Lumbosacral skin abnormalities are often present.

Extradural lipomas unassociated with spinal dysraphism account for less than 1% of primary intraspinal tumors (32,34). They are mostly seen in adults, but a third of the cases have been reported to occur in the first two decades of life (63). Females are affected almost twice as often as males (63). These tumors are most often located in the thoracic region at all ages, although, in children and adolescents, lumbar and sacral lipomas predominate. Lipomas commonly extend along several spinal segments. They may occasionally present as a mediastinal mass that compresses the spinal cord and also distorts the trachea, esophagus, and blood vessels.

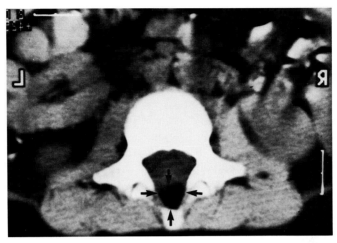

FIG. 6. Extradural lipoma. CT shows the low attenuation values of the lipoma located posteriorly in the spinal canal (*arrows*).

X-ray films and plain tomography show nonspecific changes. The most consistent findings are the presence of a paraspinal mass and bony erosion of the vertebral body, as well as of the pedicles (Fig. 5). Occasionally, extradural lipoma is associated with lumbosacral agenesis (43). Myelography shows an extradural mass displacing the spinal cord or blocking the column of contrast medium either totally or partially. CT, which shows the low attenuation values of the tumor (Fig. 6), provides a rapid and unequivocal diagnosis (44). MR imaging may be the most suitable method for determining the exact location, size, and extension of the lipoma.

Treatment is surgical. Complete removal of the lipoma is easier in angiolipomas than in pure lipomas. Outcome is variable, depending on whether total extirpation was possible.

Lipomeningocele

Lipomeningocele or lipomyelomeningocele (or meningolipoma or meningomyelolipoma) is a spinal intra-extradural lipoma, often associated with a lipoma of the filum terminale. It is a form of dysraphism (64) when associated with a meningocele or myelomeningocele and usually with a tethered cord as well. This association is quite common; in our series of 51 patients, we observed 19 cases with lipomas in the lumbosacral region. Almost all these lipomas are single, although they often extend along several spinal segments. Occasionally, they have been called double lipomyelomeningoceles (65) because the lipoma and the dysraphism exist at two separate levels. Sometimes the lipoma is extradural and associated with a meningeal diverticulum or meningocele, and does not penetrate the dura or involve the spinal cord directly. Such cases are properly meningolipomas or lipomeningolipomas. When the lipoma penetrates the meninges and there is a tethered spinal cord, frequently associated with extensive dysraphism, the tumor can be called meningomyelolipoma or lipomyelomeningocele. The tethered spinal cord produces a clinical syndrome characterized by progressive motor and sensory deficits in the legs, incontinence, back or leg pain, and scoliosis. Experimental studies suggest that the symptoms and signs of spinal cord tethering are indicative of lumbosacral neuronal dysfunction, and reflect impairment of mitochondrial oxidative metabolism under constant or intermittent cord stretching (66).

There are cases of spina bifida cystica with an associated malignant neoplasm. This can be seen in patients with lipomeningocele (67,68), as well as those with meningocele or myelomeningocele (69–75). These neoplasms can be located anywhere along the spine and occur mostly in young or middle-aged adults, but occasionally also in children (67). Wilms tumor (67), anaplastic carcinoma (69), adenocarcinoma (teratoma) (70), squamous cell carcinoma (68,71–74), and malignant fibrous histiocytoma have been reported, commonly with a short survival. Most patients present cutaneous defects at the level of the spinal lesion. The most frequent sign is gluteal asymmetry, with deviation of the midline toward one side, followed by the development of a more or less voluminous soft mass, generally exhibiting hemangiomatous nevi, pigmented or depigmented macules, or other types of discoloration of the skin, a dermal sinus, or hypertrichosis.

The tethered cord syndrome may also be seen in adults with a lipomyelomeningocele (76). They do not usually show cutaneous defects. Pain is their most common symptom; it is usually diffuse and bilateral, and the anal-perineal region is often involved. Musculoskeletal deformities, such as shortening of one or both lower limbs, and clubfeet, local lesions, and lipomas of the filum terminale are common (42,77,78). Numerous cases have been reported (79–84) in adults as well as children (76,85,86).

Those associated with a lipomeningocele have tethering of the spinal cord. Lipomeningocele associated with tethered spinal cord was common in our series, as it was in some others (64,76). Symptoms and signs are similar to those observed in lipomyelomeningocele. These features are, in approximate order of frequency: congenital dermal lesions (soft fatty tumor, nevi, hyperpigmented skin macules, asymmetrical buttocks, dimple, hair, skin appendages, and dermal sinus) at or below the level of the spinal tumor; sphincter incontinence; foot deformities; weakness or awkwardness of the feet and legs; diminished reflexes; numbness of legs; back or leg pain; imperforate anus; and toe deformities. Adherence of an extra-intradural lipoma to the conus is very common.

About 25% of patients with lipomeningocele show as their main clinical findings muscular atrophy of one or both legs, toe deformities, rectovaginal fistula with cloacal evacuation, imperforate anus, hypoplasia of the external genitalia, motor deficits, sensory disturbances, and osteotendinous hyporeflexia and sphincter disturbances, together with musculoskeletal deformities. A close relationship exists between cloacal exstrophy and lipomyelomeningocele, as well as with other forms of dysraphism. Cloacal exstrophy is believed to represent a defect in the embryogenesis of the cloacal membrane and of the trunk-tail bud. Lipomeningocele may represent a diffuse abnormality in the development of the distalmost conus medullaris and the filum terminale.

Radiology

The most frequent radiologic abnormalities are defects in the body and arches of the lumbar and sacral vertebrae. These findings include spina bifida occulta, a widened spinal canal, sacral deformities of several types (lateral deviation, partial absence or splitting or complete absence of the sacrum), and scalloping of the posterior aspect of one or several vertebral bodies, causing the radiologic image of "dog vertebrae" in the affected zone on lateral views.

Myelography is always pathologic. The main findings are the presence of a low conus medullaris, distortion of the lower end of the dural sac, a thickened filum terminale, a widened meningeal sac, block of the contrast by the tumor, and inverted roots which travel in an upward direction, a finding that is most pronounced at the lower end of the mass. Extension of a lipoma of the conus terminalis into the subcutaneous tissues is commonly seen on myelography (Fig. 7).

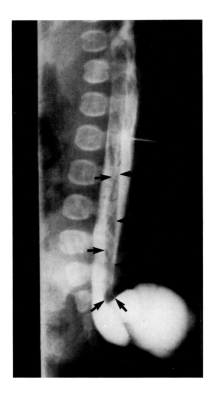

FIG. 7. Metrizamide myelography in a child with lipomyelomeningocele. Downward displacement of the conus medullaris (*arrows*) is obvious down to the level of the meningocele and subcutaneous tissues.

Myelography with tomography often shows the tethered spinal cord with focal cord widening, downward or lateral displacement of the spinal cord, and herniation of the cord out of the spinal canal at the level of the extraspinal mass. High-resolution metrizamide CT myelography is an excellent method for evaluating such lesions. It shows an area of decreased attenuation impinging on the subarachnoid space posteriorly, and demonstrates the relationship between the lipoma and the spinal canal and spinal cord (64,65,90).

CT shows that the lowest part of the spinal cord is constituted mainly of fatty tissue (64,65). Intrathecal metrizamide may be required in some cases to define the intramedullary location of the tumor. Currently, CT findings are somewhat more specific than those on MR (87).

MR can also show the tethered spinal cord associated with the lipoma of the filum terminale, especially on lateral views. MR using a spin-echo pulse sequence with short repetition times (TR) and echo delay times (TE) in T1 permits one to distinguish the high lipomatous signal of the lipoma, the middle signal of the spinal cord, and the absence of signal of the CSF (87–89). Multiplanar cuts are necessary to obtain a more complete delineation of the alterations at the lumbosacral level.

High-resolution spinal sonography seems to be a useful method for screening children for a possible tethered spinal cord (91,92). Digital myelography has also been considered a worthwhile technique (93). Untethering procedures in humans with tethered cords improve oxidative metabolism and probably facilitate repair mechanisms in injured neurons (66).

Treatment

Surgical treatment of lipomeningocele is generally recommended. It is believed that operation protects most of the patients from eventual neurologic deterioration. Patients should be operated on at the onset of neurologic symptoms. Some investigators recommend early intervention, even in the absence of any neurologic disturbance (79,80). Although some authors report successful results in more than 50% of their patients (79,85), the majority describe poorer results after operation and report improvement or cure in 4.6% (80), 33.3% (83), and 34.7% (84) of cases.

An operation to reduce the bulk of the fatty intracanalicular mass and to untether the cord is necessary. Surgical reconstruction of the dural and arachnoid tubes is required to restore the natural environment of the cord. Special care has to be taken with very vulnerable nerve roots in this zone, because they are intricately bound up with the adjacent tissues, and dissection is very difficult. Neurologic disturbances present prior to surgical treatment persist following the operation.

Lipomas of the Filum Terminale

Lipomas of the filum terminale are also known as lipomas of the conus medullaris. The first cases were described at autopsy as incidental findings in patients without signs of a spinal tumor. Today, neuroradiologic studies are regularly performed in patients with lumbosacral skin lesions and insidious impairment of bladder and bowel function (81).

Laser resection is recommended because it reduces the duration of the operation, intraoperative blood loss, and the amount of manipulation of the spinal cord and nerve roots (89). Surgery usually does not increase the neurologic deficit, but if the patient shows gradual deterioration over the following years, he or she may possibly need a second operation and should be reinvestigated.

Angiolipomas

Another variant of spinal lipomas has been variously labeled angiolipoma, hemangiolipoma, angiomyolipoma, and fibromyolipoma. In most of the cases, the term angiolipoma has been applied to lipomatous masses consisting of mature adipose elements with a substantial vascular component permeating the tumor stroma. Occasionally, the tumor may also present with a broader array of mesenchymal components (angiomyolipoma). This tumor is restricted to the epidural space. The first case was reported by Berenbruch in 1890 (94). A recent review of the literat:.re collected 35 cases published from 1928 to 1980 (95). Spinal angiolipoma is estimated to account for less than 0.14% of all spinal tumors (95), although they represent 35% of epidural lipomas (32,34,96). Most patients experience the onset of symptoms in the thoracic region at middle age. Very few patients were less than 20 years of age, although we know of a few cases aged 16 years (94), 17 years (98), and 20 years (99).

Spinal angiolipoma and spinal lipoma are considered to be the same entity by some autl,ors (32), and in the literature there are cases of typical angiolipoma described as lipoma (97). Miki et al. (62) specified the following differences between spinal angiolipomas and lipomas: (a) all angiolipomas have been located exclusively in the epidural space, whereas lipomas are found either epidurally or intradurally; (b) lipomas are often found associated with spina bifida, whereas angiolipomas are not associated with spina bifida; (c) histologically, angiolipoma is constituted of fatty and angioma-like tissues, whereas lipoma has only mature fatty tissue; and (d) angiolipoma is brown and elastic, soft, and well-demarcated from the surrounding tissues, whereas lipoma is yellow and soft, and infiltrates the surrounding tissues, making complete surgical removal difficult. Hemangiolipomas are considered true hamartomas, which stresses their congenital nature.

Clinical symptoms of extradural angiolipomas are similar to those of other spinal masses. Most patients present with lower extremity weakness or other signs of epidural cord compression. Pain and paresthesias in both legs are common when the cauda equina is compressed (100). Spinal hemangiolipomas become symptomatic under various conditions, especially pregnancy (32,96,99). Patients present after an average of 1 year of symptoms. Slow progression for 9 to 10 years and a relapsing course have been reported (96,99,101). Onset of symptoms is occasionally sudden.

Plain X-ray films are usually normal. Generalized severe osteoporosis and a pathologic fracture of a vertebral body at the level of the tumor have been described. Bony infiltration with direct extension of the angiolipoma (102–104) or angiomyolipoma (95,98) into a vertebral body may occur.

Myelography almost always shows a partial block of the contrast medium. Complete block is exceptional. CT scans show a soft tissue mass in the epidural space.

Treatment consists of radical excision. This is followed by complete neurologic recovery in most patients despite commonly extensive neurologic deterioration prior to surgery.

DERMOID AND EPIDERMOID SPINAL CORD TUMORS

Generalities

The term epidermoid comes from Böstroem (105), who based the name on the pathogenesis of these tumors. Previously, it had been named pearly tumor by Cruveilhier (106), because its gross appearance was similar to that of pearls. It also received the name cholesteatoma (107) because of its cholesterol content. Epidermoid cysts are lined only by stratified squamous epithelium, whereas the lining of dermoid cysts also includes skin appendages such as hair follicles, sebaceous glands, and sweat glands (108).

Dermal sinuses originate from an incomplete separation between the cutaneous ectoderm and the neuroectoderm, which occurs between the third and fifth week of embryogenesis (105,111–114). As a result, the neural tube carries behind it a narrow portion of invaginated skin, which will be the origin of a dermal or epidermoid tumor. The cause of this occult spinal dysraphism is unknown.

Cystic dermoids and epidermoids are some of the more frequent intraspinal expansive masses of children. They were second in prevalence in our series, immediately after lipomas. They appear at any age, but adults are clearly affected less often than infants and children. These tumors can be congenital (intrauterine or dysembryoplastic) or acquired.

Dysembryoplastic Dermoid

The dysembryoplastic type is commonly associated with an external defect of the skin, such as a dermal sinus, cutaneous angioma, and tuft of hair in the middle of the back or the lumbosacral region. The origin of dermal sinuses is an incomplete separation between the cutaneous ectoderm and the neuroectoderm, which occurs from the third to fifth week of embryogenesis (105). The association of sacrococcygeal and pontocerebellar dermoid cysts in the same patient has been reported (109).

Most cases are associated with sinuses communicating with the skin. These sinuses are most common in the lumbosacral region, followed by the occipital region, and less commonly, the cervical and dorsal regions. Several other tumors, such as teratomas, lipomas, chordomas, and myxopapillary ependyomomas, can also be associated with a pilonidal sinus (110).

Cystic dermoids or epidermoids with communicating sinuses are often associated with recurrent meningitis in childhood and even in young adults (115,116). Since Moise published the first case in 1926 (116), our experience suggests that the subject has been referred to less often than warranted by its numbers. Isolated patients or small series have been reported. The most common microorganism causing meningitis in these patients is *Staphylococcus* (*aureus* or *albus*) (111, 116,117); other reported infections were caused by Gram negative enterobacteria, such as *Escherichia coli* (114,118), probably because of its proximity to the anus, anaerobic Peptococcus (115), and *Proteus mirabilis* (111,114). We found descriptions of three children with recurrent meningitis, from all of whom *Proteus mirabilis* grew out of the cerebrospinal fluid (CSF) (119–121). Subdural or spinal abscesses and even intracranial abscesses can be associated with dermal sinuses (113,122).

Although the diagnosis of spinal epidermoid or dermoid is easy if attention is focused on the presence of a skin defect in the midline along the spine, patients can present neurologic symptoms or signs for a long time without being correctly diagnosed. Prognosis depends on the complete and total removal of the tumor and

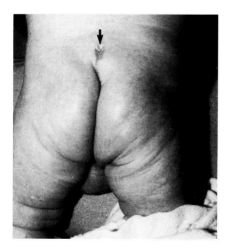

FIG. 8. Epidermoid tumor in the lumbosacral region in a 10-month-old child who shows moderate intergluteal deformity and a sinus with secreted material (*arrow*).

on the promptness of the diagnosis. Unfortunately, many patients present to the neuropediatrician and neurosurgeon too late (119), after having had meningitis and having had a lumbar puncture needle introduced into the tumor cyst. This causes not only an increase in symptomatology, but also fosters spread of the tumor which then involves nerve roots and the spinal cord. In such cases, more or less severe sequelae persist after removal of the tumor (112,114,115,119,123). One must suspect a spinal epidermoid or dermoid cyst in patients with recurrent meningitis, spinal compression, sphincter disturbances, paretic gait, clubfeet, and cutaneous angiomas in the midline of the spine with a pilonidal sinus. The sinus may sometimes communicate with the subarachnoid space and contain hairs or material secreted by the intraspinal cyst through the sinus opening (Fig. 8). Lumbar punctures at the affected level as well as fistulographies should be avoided.

Radiology

Plain X-ray films are usually abnormal, revealing spina bifida, widening of the canal, and erosion of one or several pedicles. Myelography may show an intramedullary tumor, as well as an extramedullary process with total or partial block. When the intraspinal mass is extramedullary, the contrast medium is displaced

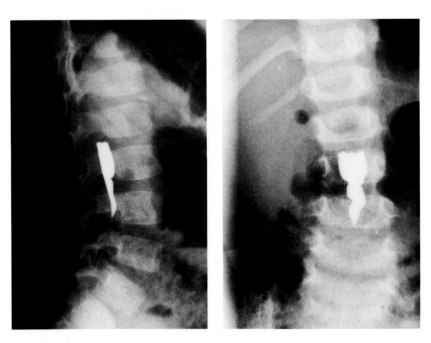

FIG. 9. Intraspinal extramedullary epidermoid in a 4-year-old child. Myelography in lateral and frontal projections shows a block and irregularities of the contrast medium and its forward displacement by the tumor, which is located posteriorly in the spinal canal.

forward, indicating the posterior location of the tumor in the spinal canal (Fig. 9). On CT, the lesion presents areas of different and abnormal densities; fat and more solid components of the tumor are well delineated, and the nature of the tissues that constitute the mass may be identified through their densities (124,125). MR can display the precise morphology and location of the mass as well as character- ize the heterogeneity of its contents. A spin-echo sequence with prolonged TR gives the best differentiation between its component tissues (124).

Acquired Epidermoids

Acquired epidermoids are late iatrogenic complications of a surgical operation on the spinal canal or of a lumbar puncture, particularly when it is carried out with a needle without a stylet (126–128). They result from implantation of skin frag- ments into the spinal canal. Symptoms may appear at any age between 1 and 23 years (129) or even 33 years (130). They illustrate the risk of a later intraspinal epidermoid when hollow needles or butterfly scalp-vein needles are used for lum- bar puncture in newborns, countering the statement that this technique presents no complications (131). Gibson and Norris (132) thrust hollow needles of various sizes through the skin into surgical and necropsy specimens and observed that coring of a fragment of skin occurred in two out of three times. Similar findings have been obtained experimentally in rats (133) and dogs (134). Because of these findings, some investigators (126) blame the use of needles with ill-fitting stylets or with no stylets at all for intraspinal epidermoids that occur several years after a lumbar puncture. Many of the published cases were attributed to intrathecal treat- ment of tuberculous meningitis many years earlier (130,135–137). Epidermoids secondary to spinal anesthesia (130,138) and myelography (139) have been re- ported in the past. Patients having a history of intrathecally treated meningitis may present progressive leg pain, sometimes sciatica, low back pain, lordosis, diffi- culty walking, and patellar or Achilles tendon hyporeflexia or areflexia. Occa- sionally, epidermoid have been found in patients with myelomeningocele months (140) to a few years (130) after operation.

Cervical Dermoids

A cervical dermal sinus communicating with an intraspinal dermoid is quite rare. Although dermoids and epidermoids are the second most frequent intraspinal tumors in our series, we observed only one case with a cervical location (141). We turned up few cases in our review of the literature (35,142–149). It occurs with equal frequency in males and females (143). Most patients were children, but age ranged from less than a year to 35 years (143). Clinical signs and symptoms were uniform in the majority of patients. A dermal sinus may have a tuft of hair or may be surrounded by a superficial hemangioma; it can even present a fistulous opening (144). Progressive motor difficulty with paraparesis, hemiparesis, or quadriparesis, neck rigidity, mild amyotrophy in one or both shoulders, hyper-reflexia, Babinski signs, episodes of irritability, neck pain, and abnormal twisting movements of the neck accompanied by stereotyped movements of hands have been reported. An infected cervical dermoid, like dermal sinuses in other locations, may be responsible for recurrent episodes of purulent meningitis (143) or an intramedullary abscess (145). Electromyography can show signs of chronic partial denervation in muscles of the upper limbs (141). The CSF is normal in some cases, but it may also show pleocytosis and increased protein. Radiographs of the cervical spine show defects of the laminas and a widened spinal canal. Myelography shows complete or incomplete obstruction with swelling of the cord and usually images of an intramedullary tumor. The reason for the rarity of cervical dermoid or epidermoid tumors is unknown. They may be related to a defect in closure of the neural tube.

Treatment

Surgical removal of the tumor must be performed as soon and as completely as possible. Only the removal of the entire tumor can ensure permanent cure. Remnants of the epidermoid regrow (112,114,119,121), and the possibility of destruction of the spinal cord or roots increases, as well as the difficulty of performing a complete and clean secondary exeresis. Sequelae affecting motricity, sensitivity, sphincters, and sexuality are much more frequent in patients with late removal, as well as in patients with an incorrect initial diagnosis or who had complications during clinical or radiologic studies (119), or during surgery (130).

ANTERIOR SACRAL MENINGOCELE

Generalities and Clinical Findings

Anterior sacral meningocele is a rare type of spinal dysraphism. It is caused by herniation of the thecal sac through a bony defect in the anterior sacral wall. The sac is composed of an external dural membrane and an internal arachnoid membrane; its contents are CSF, occasionally neural elements, and, rarely, congenital tumors, such as a dermoid tumor (150). Congenital tumors can also be located adjacent to an anterior meningocele (151–153). Such tumors are located outside the meningocele, and they are usually diagnosed at surgery (151). Several malformations may be associated with anterior sacral meningocele. The most common are bicornuate or double uterus, double vagina, atresia or imperforate anus or vagina, and double ureters and kidneys. More than 150 cases have been described (150,154,156). This anomaly has occasionally been found in Marfan's syndrome (157,158) and in neurofibromatosis (159–161).

Anterior meningocele may present at any age, from the newborn (155) to adult age, although most cases are diagnosed in the third decade. Their frequency is four times as high in females as in males. Patients commonly present with symptoms related to the pelvic mass, such as chronic constipation, urinary disturbances, dystocia, and dysmenorrhea. Headache and pain and numbness in the back or lower limbs are occasionally observed. Constipation is the most frequent symptom, and most patients have already been studied by the gastroenterologist when they come to the neurologist or neurosurgeon. A long history of use of laxatives or enemas prior to diagnosis of an anterior spinal meningocele is quite common. All these symptoms are caused by pressure of the anterior sacral meningocele on the rectum, urinary bladder, female genital organs, and sacral roots. Headache is produced when CSF in the meningocele is displaced into the spinal canal and head. The meningocele may present as an abdominal, pelvic, or gluteal mass. Dystocia may be avoided if a good prenatal examination, especially with echographic study, is performed. However, cesarean section has been necessary in some cases (162). Males are often asymptomatic. The meningocele is commonly a soft mass situated between the sacrum and the rectum, which in most instances can be palpated by rectal examination. The size of the cystic mass varies from a centimeter to more than fifteen cm in diameter. Familial anterior sacral meningocele has been reported as a dominant sex-linked trait (163), and also without specific gender predominance (164,165).

Radiology

Plain X-ray films of the sacrum and the soft tissues usually show a scimitar-shaped sacrum (Fig. 10A). This deformity is caused by the pressure of the meningocele. The rectum, bladder, and uterus are commonly displaced forward or laterally when the meningocele is large. Conventional radiologic studies allow the differentiation of anterior sacral meningocele from teratoma, lipoma, chordoma, chondroma, glioma, plasmacytoma, neurofibroma, or other tumors of this region. Metrizamide myelography demonstrates the malformation, although maneuvers may be necessary to introduce the contrast medium into the meningocele if it has a narrow pedicle. CT and MR are the diagnostic radiologic procedures of choice; these updated techniques clearly demonstrate the characteristics of the anterior sacral meningocele, which appears as a homogeneous liquid mass with a density similar to CSF (Fig. 10B), while the rectum presents gas density, and other tumors appear as solid masses. These studies provide exact information on the size and extent of the meningocele in the pelvis and the shape of its pedicle, and the relationship of the malformation to the other intrapelvic structures (166).

Treatment and Evolution

Currently, most authors use sacral laminectomy and ligation or suture of the pedicle. With this posterior approach, it is highly unlikely that an associated mass, if it exists, will be identified. CT or MR studies enable preoperative detection of a

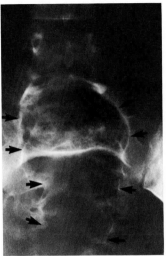
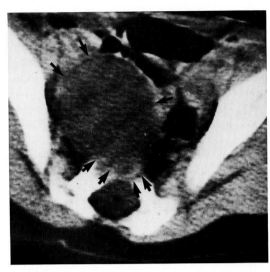

A,B

FIG. 10. A: Anterior sacral meningocele in a 10-year-old girl. Plain X-ray in frontal projection showing a severe defect of the anterior part of sacrum (*arrows*). **B:** Anterior sacral meningocele in a 7-year-old girl complaining of severe and persistent constipation. CT shows the meningocele (*large arrows*) protruding through a defect in the anterior portion of the sacrum (*small arrows*). The presacral fat, rectum, and bladder are displaced forward and laterally to the right.

congenital tumor and provide the indication for its removal. The abdominal route has been used successfully in the past, but this approach had more risks, and the neck of the meningocele cannot always be closed. Bacterial meningitis may be a complication of transabdominal surgical approaches.

CT and MR are indicated to follow the evolution of the meningocele after occlusion of its pedicle. When this has been correctly performed, the patient is symptom free, although constipation usually persists. There are no abnormal neurologic findings, and radiologic studies commonly show absence of the anterior sacral meningocele.

Spontaneous regression does not occur. Patients not treated surgically have a 30% mortality owing to pelvic obstruction at the time of labor or to erosion into the rectum followed by meningitis (167).

HYDROMYELIA AND SYRINGOMYELIA

Generalities

Hydromyelia is the widening of the central canal of the spinal cord. Syringomyelia consists of glial intramedullary degeneration with a pathologic cavity in the spinal cord. Since the two conditions frequently occur together, and in most cases probably have a common pathogenesis, this condition is often referred to as hydrosyringomyelia. Hydromyelia is commonly observed in children with a lumbar meningomyelocele and Chiari II malformation.

There are other circumstances which may be associated with an intramedullary cavity. It occurs in posttraumatic cystic myelopathy, also known as posttraumatic syringomyelia and posttraumatic spinal cord cyst (168–172). Myelomalacia may develop in a region of the trauma. Several theories to explain its pathogenesis include ischemia, release of cellular enzymes, vasoactive chemicals, or the immediate concussive effects of trauma (169). Acquired syringomyelic cavities have also been occasionally described after tuberculous meningitis (173,174). Syringomyelia may be associated with spinal tumors, especially gliomas (175) and ependymomas (176), usually in the cervicothoracic region, although they have occasionally been associated with cauda equina tumors (176,177). Congenital tumors such as teratomas and other types of tumors associated with hereditary diseases (von Hippel-Lindau and von Recklinghausen diseases) can also be associated with spinal cord syringomyelic cavities (177–180). The cavitations appearing in spinal cord tumors have sometimes been very suitably termed pseudosyringomyelias (181). Some authors exclude spinal cord tumors and significant spinal cord injury from the definition of syringomyelia (182).

Clinical Symptomatology

According to our experience with children, the first clinical signs and symptoms affect the neck and shoulders. The neck may appear short, hyperlordotic, and wide, as is commonly found in basilar impression and platybasia. Other cases show a long neck, with progressive muscular atrophy affecting all muscles of the neck and shoulders. Flaccid paresis of the arms is also one of the earlier symptoms of syringomyelia in children. Kyphoscoliosis, kyphosis, and other alterations of the spine are already apparent in early childhood, particularly in patients with dysraphism and may be the presenting signs of the disease. Progression of spinal deformities probably is related to spreading of the syringomyelic cavity to the ventral and dorsomedial regions of the spinal cord (183,184). Pain in the back, abdomen, or head is often the first subjective manifestation of the disease in children. The dissociated sensory disturbance, which is characteristic of adults who have impairment of pain and temperature sensation due to damage to the decussating pathways, is demonstrable in older children who can cooperate with the sensory examination. Spasticity of the legs is a late symptom in children. Some patients present trophic and vasomotor alterations caused by destruction of the intermediolateral tract. Involvement of the laryngeal musculature produces aphonia. Symptoms more likely related to syringobulbia than hydrosyringomyelia include bradycardia and inspiratory stridor with apneic spells. Children with hydromyelia who have been operated for myelomeningocele with an associated Chiari II malformation may experience neurologic deterioration several years following neonatal repair of the dysraphism.

According to the literature, the disease may follow three main courses (184): (a) 50% to 70% of cases undergo slow progression; (b) 30% to 40% of cases have an episodic course which persists over many years, with or without subsequent rapid deterioration; and (c) 6% to 8% of cases experience rapid progression.

Rapidly progressive forms may lead to death within a few weeks to months, yet survival for longer than 20 years has been described.

Radiology

X-ray films may show widening of the spinal canal at the level of the syringomyelic cavity. Most often, however, radiographies are normal. Basilar impression with or without platybasia is found in some cases.

Myelography shows a widened spinal cord (185–187). Contrast medium injected into the syringomyelic cavity shows it to have a tubular or scalloped appearance (188).

Today myelography and spinal CT are the most widely used neuroradiologic methods to confirm the clinical diagnosis of syringomyelia. However, even with high resolution contrast enhancement CT, about 20% of syrinx cavities are not detected (189). MR is currently the best method for diagnosing syringomyelia. Sagittal MR images show a tubular CSF-containing central cavity within the spinal cord with low proton signal intensity (Fig. 11). Very clear visualization of large portions of the spinal cord is possible with sagittal slices (Fig. 12A,B), although

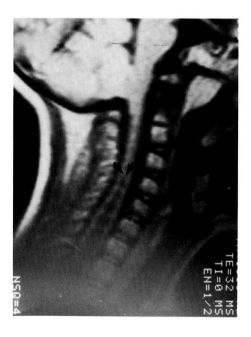

FIG. 11. Hydrosyringomyelia in a 13-year-old girl. MR shows intramedullary cavities from C5 (*arrows*) downward, a Chiari I malformation, and basilar impression.

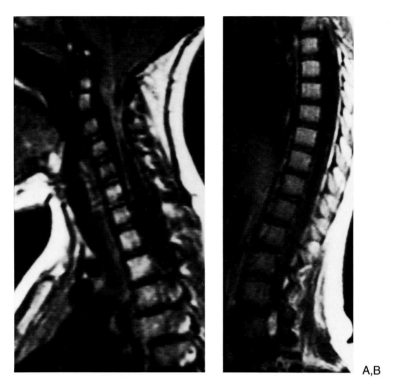

FIG. 12. A,B: A 5-year-old girl operated on for lumbosacral myelomeningocele at 1 month. MR in T1 and lateral projections show a Chiari II malformation and a syringomyelic cavity that extends along the cervical and cervico-dorsal spinal cord.

this is not always feasible in patients with spinal deformities. Several papers illustrate the appearance of typical syringo- and hydromyelia (90,190–193). The Chiari malformation, location of the fourth ventricle, basilar impression, and syringomyelic cavities were easily visualized in our patients. Optimal contrast between the syrinx cavity and spinal cord tissue was provided by using TR values of about 1,600 msec and TE values of about 34 msec (193). Higher TR and TE values led to increased CSF intensity, making the contrast between cavity and cord less sharp. If the cysts are not clearly seen with either of these pulse sequences, intrathecal metrizamide with delayed CT scanning or gas myelography is indicated (192).

Pathogenesis

There are several theories concerning the pathogenesis of syringomyelia. Gardner (194) believed that impaired outflow from the fourth ventricle resulted in transmission of arterial pulsations of CSF to the cervical cord. Ball and Dayan (195) thought CSF pressure waves force CSF into the syrinx along Virchow-Robin spaces. Williams (196–199) postulated that defective intracranial drainage may cause partial obstruction of the free flow of CSF from the cranium into distensible spinal subarachnoid spaces and provokes the introduction of fluid into the syrinx from the floor of the fourth ventricle. Zaragozá (200) found a narrow and long vallecula in the patients with syringomyelia of his series, which would confirm Williams' theory. Taylor (201) found that impaired venous drainage leads to central cord necrosis. Aboulker (202) suggested that the syringomyelic cavity is due to obstruction of the cisterna magna which, associated with high venous pressure, causes transmedullary passage of CSF. Welch et al. (203) reported that the spinal canal absorbs a disproportionate amount of CSF, thus creating a negative gradient of pressure and the development of an acquired Chiari malformation; secondarily, this results in foraminal obstruction and the formation of a syrinx. Experimental studies of Marin-Padilla and Marin-Padilla (204) showed that the cartilagineous basicranium of fetuses with Chiari malformations types I and II is shorter than normal and lordotic in relation to the axis of the spine. This underdevelopment of the occipital bone is especially noticeable in its basal component and results in a short and small posterior fossa, which is inadequate to its contents. The developing cerebellum is displaced downward to an anomalous position just above the foramen magnum, and the developing medulla is compressed or crowded into the small posterior fossa. Protrusion of the odontoid peg into the cranial cavity was also found in these fetuses. Hydrosyringomyelia would be secondary to the malformation of the base of the skull. Some investigators report that this theory fits with their data (205,206).

Experimental syringomyelia may be due to ischemic lesions produced by adhesive arachnoiditis as a complication of the associated hydrocephalus (207). Each of these theories has several weaknesses and none is universally accepted.

Treatment

Surgical approaches to syringomyelia depend on which of these theories individual neurosurgeons endorse. Suboccipital craniectomy and plugging of the obex, craniovertebral decompression to alleviate craniospinal pressure dissociation, and surgery to enlarge the cisterna magna are the main surgical approaches in current use. Surgical treatment of the Chiari malformation unassociated with syringomyelia usually relieves increased intracranial pressure and may improve cerebellar dysfunction (182,208,209). Placement of a shunt tube into the syringomyelic cyst, frequently performed in the past, has fallen into disrepute. Occlusion of the central canal has no greater influence on the progression of the disease than simple decompression (210). The longer the postoperative follow-up, the higher the incidence of recurrence of symptoms (202).

NEURENTERIC CYST

Generalities and Embryology

The terms neurenteric, enterogenous, enteric, gastroenteric, gastrocytoma, bronchogenic, and teratomatous cysts have been used for masses that occur from the brainstem to the conus (211). They are most frequent in the posterior mediastinum and abdominal and pelvic regions. These masses are distinct from the esophagus and bowels and may be connected to the spinal contents through a defect in the vertebral body. Neurenteric cysts occur with the "split notochord" syndrome. They may be found at any age and have been described in newborns (212,213) and from a few weeks (214) to 54 years of age (215,216). We have seen a single case in a 3-year-old child. Males are somewhat more numerous than females. Most patients have a single cyst, although occasionally multiple cysts have been found in the same patient (217). Neurenteric cysts are occasionally associated with a myelomeningocele (212,218).

The names given to embryonic cysts relate to the timing of their formation (219–221).

Neurenteric cysts are characterized by an intra- and extraspinal mass associated with vertebral defects. The intrathoracic or intra-abdominal mass is a cystic structure containing esophageal or gastric mucosa, which is separate from the esophagus and is attached to the dura or to a vertebral body. The cyst arises early in embryonal development, within the first 3 weeks when the notochord (which gives rise to the vertebrae) and the endoderm (which gives rise to the primitive digestive tube) are in close contact. At this time of embryogenesis, the neurenteric canal of Kovalevsky provides an evanescent connection between the notochord and the endoderm. The notochord can draw a pedicle of endoderm into the forming neural tube. Mesodermal masses, which usually surround the tube, are therefore prevented from complete closure, resulting in butterfly vertebrae or anterior spina bifida as the mesenchymal masses differentiate into vertebral bodies (222). The later differential growth of the spine and cord results in caudal placement of the cord lesions with respect to the vertebral anomalies (222). Autopsies of patients with a neurenteric cyst have occasionally shown an Arnold-Chiari malformation associated with hydrocephalus, microgyria, congenital heart disease (212), intestinal duplication (213), and mediastinal enterogenous cyst and intestinal abnormalities (223).

Bronchogenic cysts result from abnormal isolation of part of a lung bud that develops into a cyst in close association with the central bronchial tree. They are not associated with vertebral malformations because the defect occurs between the third and sixth embryonal weeks, after the notochord and endoderm have separated. Enteric cysts are produced after the sixth embryonal week. At that time, an embryological anomaly of the digestive tract will only affect it.

Neurenteric cysts are classified into three groups based on their histology (216,224): Type I consists of simple or pseudostratified, columnar or cuboidal epithelium, with or without cilia, lying on a basement membrane; Type II is similar to Type I plus mucus glands, smooth muscle, fat, cartilage, bone, elastic fibers, lymphoid tissues, or ganglion cells; and Type III is similar to Type II plus ependymal or glial tissue.

Clinical Findings

Neurenteric cysts may produce symptoms and signs of spinal cord compression. They may be associated with external anomalies such as meningomyelocele with hydrocephalus, or dorsal dermal sinus. Children who are symptomatic during the neonatal period (212,213,218) usually have associated malformations that are incompatible with survival. The intraspinal disease may go unsuspected despite its early clinical symptoms and signs. Klump (214) described an infant who was brought to the emergency room at 6 weeks of age because of irritability and crying whenever he was picked up. By 10 weeks of age his mother noted that he was particularly irritable when his neck or back was touched or moved; he preferred to keep his head turned to the left and had not been moving his left arm normally in the weeks prior to diagnosis. Our patient, a 3-year-old boy, had been taken to several pediatricians before consulting us. His mother reported symptoms similar to those of Klump's patient. For a year, the child had been considered hysterical and had been treated by a psychiatrist because of irritability that was exacerbated every time he was obliged to move his head, neck, and shoulders to get in or out of a car. Finally, he was noted to have muscular atrophy in both shoulders, almost complete immobility of the left arm, and a left Horner's sign. Delayed gross motor function may be detected at 1 year of age (222). Most patients have signs of spinal cord compression with paraparesis or quadriparesis, spasticity, Babinski signs, hyperreflexia, and occasionally a sensory level. Neurenteric cysts affecting the cauda equina may present with chronic low back pain and sciatica (225). The CSF protein is usually elevated. Neurenteric cysts are difficult to suspect without radiologic studies.

Radiology

Plain radiographs must include the chest and abdomen as well as the spine. Vertebral defects affecting several vertebral bodies and arches are common. Spina bifida occulta, eroded pedicles with a widened spinal canal, spondylolisthesis, hemivertebrae, butterfly vertebrae, fused vertebrae, erosion of the posterior aspect of the vertebral bodies at the level of the cyst, and rib malformations are common findings. Films of the chest and abdomen may show a parahilar, paratracheal, or paraesophageal mass. The esophagus may be greatly displaced by an intrathoracic cyst (226). Metrizamide myelography shows an intradural-extradural space-occupying lesion; sometimes, it may have the false appearance of an intramedullary mass causing an incomplete or complete block. CT images in axial projection may show a pulmonary mass, and the "tunnel" in the affected vertebral body through which a band of soft tissue connects the intraspinal component of the neurenteric cyst to the trachea and esophagus (222). MR images in sagittal view show the neurenteric cyst located behind the dysplastic vertebral bodies. The cyst appears as an intraspinal mass which has excavated a niche into the cord (222,227). The soft tissue band extending between the intraspinal neurenteric cyst and esophagus and trachea can also be visualized with MR (222).

Treatment

Total removal of the cyst is necessary to cure this disease. If some remnants of the capsule remain in the spinal canal, recurrence is likely a few months to several years after the operation (211).

ARACHNOIDAL CYSTS

Generalities and Clinical Findings

Arachnoidal cysts are benign leptomeningeal diverticuli lined by arachnoid and collagen tissue. They usually communicate with the subarachnoid space through a narrow neck. They may occur in the intradural, (228–235), extradural (229,231,236–240), or perineural (241–243) spaces. Cysts usually present as isolated lesions, but multiple lesions in the same patient can also occur (244). These rare intraspinal processes may be located anywhere along the spinal canal, either posteriorly or anteriorly to the spinal cord, or in both locations (245). The cysts, mostly of congenital origin, can cause symptoms at any age. Symptoms and signs depend on their location. Cervical cysts can cause quadriparesis and respiratory problems (228,231). Dorsal and lumbar cysts produce paraparesis. Spasticity, paresthesias, sphincter disturbances, and local pain are common symptoms in any location. Spontaneous exacerbation or remission of symptoms are frequent. Congenital arachnoidal cyst should be suspected in a child who presents progressive paraparesis or quadriparesis with normal spine films and normal CSF.

Familial extradural arachnoidal cysts associated with distichiasis (double row of eyelashes) and lymphedema (237,239,240), as well as familial intradural arachnoidal cysts (235), have been reported. Inheritance is autosomal dominant in both types. These familial cysts are always midthoracic. Posttraumatic (246,247) and postinfectious (248) spinal arachnoidal cysts may also occur. How arachnoidal cysts arise is not well understood.

Radiology

Plain X-ray films are usually normal, without widening of the canal or erosion of the pedicles. Extradural arachnoidal cysts, in contrast to intradural ones, may increase the interpedicular distance (237,239,240). Myelography usually reveals a block of the contrast medium at the level of the cyst. A very complete study with the patient in several positions is required because of the different possible locations of the cyst (243,249). Metrizamide CT myelography shows displacement of the spinal cord and the space occupied by the cyst (234,249).

MR reveals the cyst which has a long T1 and a long T2 (243,250). MR imaging, because of the three-dimensional views it provides, is almost always diagnostic.

Treatment

Removal of the cyst is necessary as soon as the diagnosis is made. This usually results in cure of the patient. Recurrent intraspinal arachnoidal cyst requiring treatment by shunting has been reported (233).

SPINAL INTRADURAL EPENDYMAL CYST

Intradural extramedullary ependymal cysts of the spinal cord are very rare. A recent review of the literature (251) found only six cases with ages ranging from 6 to 58 years. Three of the patients were between 6 and 7 years old. Spinal ependymal cysts were found in several locations along the spinal canal but preferentially in the cervical region and at the thoraco-lumbar junction. In all but one of the reported cases, the cyst was situated ventrally to the spinal canal, compressing the spinal cord which was severely displaced backward against the dura mater. The cyst contained either clear cerebrospinal-like or turbid, cloudy fluid. This fluid was thought to be secreted by the nonciliated cells which constitute the cyst wall.

Histologic features vary. Some authors describe nonciliated cuboidal or columnar epithelial cells (228,252,253), whereas others report a mixture of ciliated and nonciliated cells (251,254–256) resting directly on connective tissue. None of the cysts had a direct connection with the central ependymal canal of the spinal cord. How ependymal cells arise in the extramedullary area is unknown. An embryonal connection between the cyst and the central canal, which later becomes obliterated, has been suggested (254). The cyst could be the result of either evagination of cells from the central canal or the migration of primitive cells coming from the embryonal neural plate of the spinal cord.

Symptoms may have a sudden onset, sometimes precipitated by trauma or straining, or they may run a slowly progressive course. Pain is a constant finding and of radicular type in some patients, especially adults. Spastic paraparesis, reduced sensation on both sides of the body, and loss of bowel and bladder sphincter function may occur. The neurologic manifestations reflect the anterior or anterolateral location of the cyst. Severity and mode of presentation depend on the active production of fluid by the secreting cells of the cystic wall.

Plain films of the spine almost always show some abnormality at the level of the affected area, such as a widened spinal canal, thinned pedicles, sometimes a congenital anomaly such as fused laminae or bifid vertebrae. Diagnosis and accurate localization of the intradural extramedullary mass is established by myelography combined with spinal CT scanning. It is often necessary to introduce the contrast medium through both the lumbar and the cisternal regions to define the lower and upper extent of the mass. MR may show the mass noninvasively. Rapid deterioration in neurologic symptoms may occur after myelography (251).

The only treatment is surgical removal of the cyst. Recovery of neurologic function is rapid when the operation is done in time. Total removal of the cyst is difficult because of lack of cleavage between the wall of the cyst and the spinal cord. Recurrence is uncommon.

SPINAL PSEUDOCYST

Spinal pseudocyst is a rare lesion with a wall composed of dense connective tissue without epithelial or neoplastic cells. It does not communicate with the surrounding spaces. Pseudocysts contain a collection of fluid that arises from the loculation of hemorrhage, necrosis, or an inflammatory process. Most pseudocysts have been described in organs outside the CNS, such as the liver, pancreas, spleen, parotid gland, ureter, lung, and perineal area. Pseudocysts seldom occur in the CNS. We know of two intraspinal cases: a meningeal one in the cervical region (257) and a spinal intramedullary pseudocyst at the level of T1 (258). This latter patient had sustained a direct contusion of the anterior upper chest wall with severe chest pain following a fall 2 years earlier, which may have been the cause of the intramedullary pseudocyst. Clinical examination showed alterations of motricity, sensitivity, and sphincter control that were appropriate to the level of the pseudocyst.

Plain films of the spine show no evidence of a destructive lesion. The lesion can be demonstrated by CT, myelography, and MR.

The differential diagnosis of spinal intramedullary cystic lesions includes dermoid, epidermoid, neurenteric, and ependymal cysts, and different types of tumors with cystic intramedullary components such as astrocytomas, ependymomas, spongioblastomas, glioblastomas, and hemangioblastomas. Some characteristics help in the differential diagnosis. Dermoid cysts contain a yellowish, thick, and cheesy fluid (259); moreover, they contain skin appendages, hair follicles, and sweat glands. Ependymal cysts have single or multiple layers of cuboidal and cylindrical epithelial cells. Neurenteric cysts include among their histologic findings a single layer of connective tissue.

Treatment is laminectomy for removal of the cyst. The postoperative course is usually without complications and recovery usually occurs (258).

DIASTEMATOMYELIA

Generalities and Clinical Findings

Diastematomyelia is a dysraphic myelodysplasia in which the spinal cord is divided into a variable number of segments along the sagittal plane. Median bony, cartilaginous, or fibrous septae are found in approximately one-half of the cases. The cleft in the spinal cord is located between D_9 and S_1 in 85% of cases and is exclusively thoracic in 20% of cases (260). Cervical diastematomyelia has seldom been described (261–263).

This condition may be recognized by chance in patients who are symptom-free, usually because of the presence of cutaneous abnormalities such as a hairy patch on the back, a nevus, a skin dimple, or a small meningocele. Diastematomyelia is said to account for about 5% of cases of congenital scoliosis (264).

The neurologic and orthopedic syndrome of diastematomyelia in children consists of sensory impairment, muscular weakness, impaired sphincter control, back deformity, and a hypoplastic foot and leg. The lesion is rarely evident at birth, the growing child is referred because of an abnormal gait or poor posture, or because one leg and foot have been noticed to be shorter or thinner than the other. The ankle-jerk is usually absent and the plantar response extensor, with pain in the neck and arm when the malformation is cervical (265). Diastematomyelia with scoliosis may lead to paraplegia (266,267). Most adults with diastematomyelia have other lesions that may account for their clinical symptomatology. There are descriptions of cases associated with a herniated disc (268), with a large coccygeal cyst tethered to a tight filum terminale containing a lipoma (269,270), with fused vertebrae and narrow intervertebral foramina (265).

Diastematomyelia is a dysraphic disorder involving all embryonic layers. It includes not only the ectodermic neural tube but also the mesodermic notochord and entoderm, as well as the persistence of the neurenteric canal. This explains the frequent congenital spine deformities (264–267,270–276) and other dysraphisms associated with it.

Several mechanisms may contribute to progressive neural damage by diastematomyelia. The bone spur fixes the contents of the spinal canal and precludes the normal differential rate of growth between the spinal cord and the spine. It also impales the cord in the vicinity of a spinal curvature. Minor traumas and traction during repeated movements of the head may increase late neurologic damage.

Radiology

Plain X-ray films show anomalies of both vertebral body segmentation and closure of the posterior arch. Scoliosis, fused laminae, hemivertebrae, spinous process hypertrophy, widened interpedicular distance, narrowing of the spinal canal in the lateral view, and a calcified spur are the radiologic features of diastematomyelia. Myelography shows a persistent central filling defect at the level of the median septum (Fig. 13). CT myelography shows the divided spinal cord, which appears as two small hemicords with a commisural band of tissue between them. MR not only shows the divided spinal cord and median septum, but also the nature of the tissue as well as the vertebral and paravertebral abnormalities.

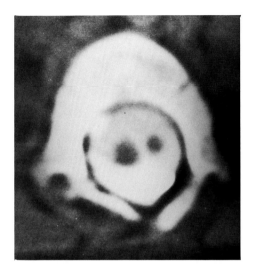

FIG. 13. Diastematomyelia. CT myelogram at the thoracolumbar level reveals two discrete hemicords.

Treatment and Prognosis

Treatment is surgical. The fused laminar block and spur are resected, which enables the opening of the duplicated spinal canal. An adjacent laminectomy may be required. Removal of the spur is recommended at all ages; ideally it should be performed as early as possible. Prophylactic removal of the septum stabilizes but does not reverse existing neurologic deficits (271). Lipomas, myelomeningoceles, and other associated congenital malformations should also be removed. Orthopedic correction is recommended for scoliosis, clubfeet, and other congenital anomalies of the spine and lower limbs.

REFERENCES

1. Altman RP, Randolph JG, Lilly JR. Sacrococcygeal teratomas: American Academy of Pediatrics surgical section survey, 1973. *J Pediatr Surg* 1974;9:389–398.
2. Dillard BM, Mayer JH, McAllister WH, et al. Sacrococcygeal teratoma in children. *J Pediatr Surg* 1970;5:53–59.
3. Mahour HG, Wooley MM, Trivedi SN, et al. Sacrococcygeal teratoma. A 33 year experience. *J Pediatr Surg* 1975;10:183–188.
4. Carney JA, Thomson DP, Johnson CL, et al. Teratomas in children: clinical and pathological aspects. *J Pediatr Surg* 1971;7:271–282.
5. Grosfeld JL, Ballantine TVN, Lowe D, Baehner RL. Benign and malignant teratomas in children: analysis of 85 patients. *Surgery* 1976;80:297–305.
6. Schey WL, Shkolnik A, White H. Clinical and radiographic considerations of sacrococcygeal teratomas: an analysis of 26 new cases and review of the literature. *Radiology* 1977;125:189–195.
7. Ghazali S. Presacral teratomas in children. *J Pediatr Surg* 1973;8:915–918.
8. Sand H, Bock JE. Prenatal diagnosis of soft-tissue malformations by ultrasound and X-ray. *Acta Obstet Gynecol Scand* 1976;55:191–199.
9. Hodek B, Pavlakovic I, Pirkic A. Antenatal diagnosis by means of ultrasound in the rare case of foetal parasitic tumor. *Z Geburtshilfe Perinatol* 1976;180:91–94.

10. Less RF, Williamson BRJ, Brenbridge NAG, et al. Sonography of benign sacral teratoma in utero. *Radiology* 1980;134:717–718.

11. Hunt PL, Davidson KC, Ashcraft KW, Holder TM. Radiography of hereditary presacral teratoma. *Radiology* 1977;122:187–191.

12. Ein SH, Mancer K, Adeyemi SD. Malignant sacrococcygeal teratoma—endodermal sinus yolk sac tumor—in infants and children: a 32-year review. *J Pediatr Surg* 1985;20:473–477.

13. Schiffer MA, Greenberg E. Sacrococcygeal teratoma in labor and the newborn. *Am J Obstet Gynecol* 1956;72:1054–1062.

14. Kohler HG. Sacrococcygeal teratoma and "non-immunological" hydrops fetalis. *Br Med J* 1976; 2:422–423.

15. Teilum G. Endodermal sinus tumor of the ovary and testis. *Cancer* 1959;12:1092–1105.

16. Tsuchida Y, Kaneko M, Yokomori K, et al. Alpha-fetoprotein, prealbumin, albumin, alpha-1-antitrypsin and transferrin as diagnostic and therapeutic markers for endodermal sinus tumors. *J Pediatr Surg* 1978;13:25–29.

17. Jukes AW, Fraser MM, Dexter D. Endodermal sinus (yolk sac) tumors in infants and children. *J Pediatr Surg* 1979;14:520–524.

18. Weinblatt ME, Kenigsberg K. Paraplegia in children with malignant teratoma. *Cancer* 1985;56: 2140–2142.

19. Hecht F, Hecht BK, O'Keefe D. Sacrococcygeal teratoma: prenatal diagnosis with elevated alpha-fetoprotein and acetylcholinesterase in amniotic fluid. *Prenat Diag* 1982;2:229–231.

20. Szabó M, Verga P, Zalatnai A, et al. Sacrococcygeal teratoma and normal alphafetoprotein concentration in amniotic fluid. *J Med Genet* 1985;22:405–408.

21. Smith DW, Jones KL. *Recognizable patterns of human malformation*, 3rd ed. Philadelphia: W.B. Saunders, 1982;506.

22. Ashcraft KW, Holder TM. Hereditary presacral teratoma. *J Pediatr Surg* 1974;9:691–697.

23. McDonald P. Malignant sacrococcygeal teratoma. A report of 4 cases. *Am J Roentgenol Rad Ther Nucl Med* 1973;118:444–449.

24. Smith WL, Stokka C, Franken EA. Arteriography of sacrococcygeal teratomas. *Radiology* 1980; 137:653–655.

25. Keller MS, Wagner DK, Lee YJ. Evaluation of neonatal sacrococcygeal teratoma by DSA and direct sagittal CT. *Br J Radiol* 1985;58:1120–1122.

26. Raney RB Jr, Chatten J, Littman P, et al. Treatment strategies for infants with malignant sacrococcygeal teratoma. *J Pediatr Surg* 1981;16:573–577.

27. Donnellan WA, Swanson O. Benign and malignant sacrococcygeal teratoma. *Surgery* 1968;64: 834–846.

28. Chretien PB, Mylam JD, Foote FW, et al. Embryonal adenocarcinomas (a type of malignant teratoma) of the sacrococcygeal region, clinical and pathologic aspects of 21 cases. *Cancer* 1970; 26:522–535.

29. Applebaum H, Exelby PR, Wollner N. Malignant presacral teratoma in children. *J Pediatr Surg* 1979;14:352–355.

30. Olsen MM. Raffensperger JG, Gonzalez-Crussi F, et al. Endodermal sinus tumor: a clinical and pathological correlation. *J Pediatr Surg* 1982;17:832–840.

31. Roberts HP. Case of disease of the spinal cord with observations. *London Med Gaz* 1834;13:946–950.

32. Ehni G, Love JG. Intraspinal lipomas. Report of cases; review of the literature and clinical and pathological study. *Arch Neurol Psychiatry* 1945;53:1–28.

33. Rand RW, Rand CW. *Intraspinal tumors of childhood*. Springfield, Ill.: Charles C Thomas, 1960;415.

34. Giuffré R. Spinal lipomas. In: Vinken PJ, Bruyn GN, eds. *Handbook of clinical neurology*, vol. 20, pt. 2. Amsterdam: North-Holland, 1976;389–414.

35. Koos W, Laubichler W, Sorgo G. Statistische Untersuchungen bei spinalen Tumoren im Kindes- und Jugendalter. *Neuropädiatrie* 1973;4:273–303.

36. Matson DD. Intraspinal tumors in children. In: *Neurosurgery of infancy and childhood*, 2nd ed. Springfield, Ill.: Charles C Thomas, 1969.

37. Obrador S. Villarejo F. Displasias raquimedulares de la region lumbosacra. *Rev Clin Esp* 1975; 115:17–25.

38. Rogers HM, Long DM, Chou SN, French LA. Lipomas of the spinal cord and cauda equina. *J Neurosurg* 1971;34:349–354.

39. Swanson HS, Barnett JC. Intradural lipomas in children. *Pediatrics* 1962;29:911–926.
40. Lassman LP, James CC. Lumbosacral lipomas: critical survey of 26 cases submitted to laminectomy. *J Neurol Neurosurg Psychiatry* 1967;30:174–181.
41. Love JG, Daly DD, Harris LE. Tight filum terminale: report of condition in three siblings. *JAMA* 1961;176:61.
42. Bassett RC. The neurologic deficit associated with lipoma of the cauda equina. *Ann Surg* 1950; 131:109–116.
43. Hafeez M, Tihansky DP. Intraspinal tumor with lumbosacral agenesis. *AJNR* 1984;5:481–482.
44. Quinn SF, Monson M, Paling M. Spinal lipoma presenting as a mediastinal mass: diagnosis by CT. *J Comput Assist Tomogr* 1983;7:1087–1089.
45. Dubowitz V, Lorber J, Zachary RB. Lipoma of the cauda equina. *Arch Dis Child* 1965;40:207–213.
46. Emery JL, Lendon RG. Lipomas of the cauda equina and other fatty tumours related to neurospinal dysraphism. *Dev Med Child Neurol* 1969;(Suppl. 20):62–70.
47. Walsh JW, Markesbery WR. Histological features of congenital lipomas of the lower spinal canal. *J Neurosurg* 1980;52:564–569.
48. Drapkin AJ. High cervical intradural lipoma. *J Neurosurg* 1974;41:699–704.
49. Mori K, Kamimura Y, Uchida Y, et al. Large intramedullary lipoma of the cervical cord and posterior fossa. Case report. *J Neurosurg* 1986;64:974–976.
50. Rappaport ZH, Tadmor B, Brand N. Spinal intradural lipoma with intracranial extension. *Child's Brain* 1982;9:411–418.
51. White WR, Fraser RAR. Cervical spinal cord lipoma with extension into the posterior fossa. *Neurosurgery* 1983;12:460–462.
52. Wood BP, Harwood-Nash DC, Berger P, Goske M. Intradural spinal lipoma of the cervical cord. *AJR* 1985;145:174–176.
53. Bucy PC, Gustafson WA. Intradural lipoma of the spinal cord. *Zentralbl Neurochir* 1938;6:341–349.
54. Jabotinski J. Fibrolipome intradural de la moelle. *Rev Neurol (Paris)* 1939;72:15–31.
55. Beaudoing A, Butin LP, Fischer G, et al. Les lipomes spinaux sousduraux chez l'enfant. *Pediatrie* 1966;21:909–916.
56. Hubert JP, Monseu G, Stoupel N, et al. Lipome spinal. Observation anatomoclinique. *Acta Neurol Belg* 1972;72:338–346.
57. Ammerman BJ, Henry JM, De Girolami U, Earle KM. Intradural lipomas of the spinal cord. A clinicopathological correlation. *J Neurosurg* 1976;44:331–336.
58. De la Cruz M, Pascual-Castroviejo I. Lipoma intramedular cervical en una niña de catorce meses. *An Esp Pediatr* 1985;23:211–214.
59. Johnson RE, Roberson GH. Subpial lipoma of the spinal cord. *Radiology* 1974;111:121–125.
60. Bertolino GC, Cusmano F, Pichezzi P, et al. Computed tomography of intradural cervical lipoma. *Neuroradiology* 1985;27:184.
61. Kean DM, Smith MA, Douglas RHB, Martyn CN, Best JJK. Two examples of CNS lipomas demonstrated by computed tomography and low field (0.08T) MR imaging. *J Comput Assist Tomogr* 1985;9:494–496.
62. Miki T, Oka M, Shima M, et al. Spinal angiolipoma. A case report. *Acta Neurochir (Wien)* 1981;58:115–119.
63. Butti G, Gaetani P, Scelsi M, Pezzotta S. Extradural spinal lipomas. Report of two cases and review of the literature. *Neurochirurgia (Stuttg)* 1984;27:28–30.
64. Naidich TP, McLone DG, Mutluer S. A new understanding of dorsal dysraphism with lipoma (lipomyeloschisis): radiologic evaluation and surgical correction. *Am J Roentgenol* 1983;140: 1065–1078.
65. Gorey MT, Naidich TP, McLone DG. Double discontinuous lipomyelomeningocele: CT findings. *J Comput Assist Tomogr* 1985;9:584–591.
66. Yamada S, Zinke DE, Saunders D. Pathophysiology of "tethered cord syndrome." *J Neurosurg* 1981;54:494–503.
67. Mickle JP, McLennan JE. Malignant teratoma arising within lipomeningocele. Case report. *J Neurosurg* 1975;43:761–763.
68. Marini G, Bollati A, Galli G, et al. Carcinoma associated with lipomeningocele: case report. *Neurosurgery* 1979;5:268–269.
69. Thorp RH. Carcinoma associated with myelomeningocele. Case report. *J Neurosurg* 1967;27:446–448.

70. Love JG. Delayed congenital teratoma with spina bifida. Case report. *J Neurosurg* 1968;29:532–534.
71. Pope M, Todorov A. Cutaneous squamous cell carcinoma as a rare complication of cervical meningocele. *Birth Defects* 1975;11:336–337.
72. Benarjee T. Nonhealing myelomeningocele in an adult. *South Med J* 1977;70:367–368.
73. Saksun JM, Fisher BK. Squamous cell carcinoma arising in a meningomyelocele. *Can Med Assoc J* 1978;119:739–741.
74. Van Tintelen JFM, Buchan AC, Shaw JF, Sclare G. Carcinoma associated with myelomeningocele. *Dev Med Child Neurol* 1980;22:512–514.
75. Helle TL, Hanbery JW, Becker DH. Meningeal malignant fibrous histiocytoma arising from a thoracolumbar myelomeningocele. Case report. *J Neurosurg* 1983;58:593–597.
76. Pang D, Wilberger JE Jr. Tethered cord syndrome in adults. *J Neurosurg* 1982;57:32–47.
77. Pascual-Castroviejo I. *Diagnostico clínico-radiologico en neurología infantil.* Barcelona; Cientifico-Médica, 1971;615–624.
78. Pascual-Castroviejo I. *Neurolgía infantil.* Barcelona: Científico-Médica, 1983;1259–1266.
79. Lapras C, Patet JD, Huppert J, Bret P. Syndrome de traction du cône terminal ou syndrome de la moelle attachée. Lipomes lombo-sacrés. *Rev Neurol (Paris)* 1985;141:207–215.
80. Pierre-Kahn A, Reiner D, Sainte-Rose C, Hirsch JF. Les lipomes lombo-sacrés avec spina bifida. Corrélations anatomo-cliniques. Résultats thérapeutiques. *Neurochirurgie* 1983;29:359–363.
81. Anderson FM. Occult spinal dysraphism: a series of 73 cases. *Pediatrics* 1975;55:826–835.
82. Villarejo FJ, Blazquez MG, Gutierrez-Diaz JA. Intraspinal lipomas in children. *Child's Brain* 1976;2:361–370.
83. Chapman PH. Congenital intraspinal lipomas. Anatomic correlations and surgical treatment. *Child's Brain* 1982;9:37–47.
84. Bruce DA, Schut L. Spinal lipomas in infancy and childhood. *Child's Brain* 1979;5:192–203.
85. Petit H, Jomin M, Julliot JP, et al. Dysraphie lombo-sacrée et "moelle longue" de révélation tardive (neuf observations). *Rev Neurol (Paris)* 1979;135:427–438.
86. Kaplan OF, Quencer RM. The occult tethered conus syndrome in adult. *Radiology* 1980;137:387–391.
87. Barnes PD, Lester PD, Yamanshi WS, Prince JR. MRI in infants and children with spinal dysraphism. *Am J Roentgenol* 1986;147:339–346.
88. Awada A, Chatta G, Majdalani A, Gautier JC. Moelle épinière attachée et lipome. Apport de l'imagerie par résonance magnétique. *Rev Neurol (Paris)* 1986;142:553–555.
89. McLone DG, Naidich TP. Laser resection of fifty spinal lipomas. *Neurosurgery* 1986;18:611–615.
90. Modic MT, Weinstein MA, Pavlicek W, et al. Nuclear magnetic resonance imaging of the spine. *Radiology* 1983;148:757–762.
91. Naidich TP, Fernbach SK, McLone DG, Shkolnik A. Sonography of the caudal spine and back: congenital anomalies in children. *Am J Roentgenol* 1984;142:1229–1242.
92. Kangarloo H, Goild RH, Diament MJ, et al. High-resolution spinal sonography in children. *Am J Roentgenol* 1984;142:1243–1247.
93. Barnes PD, Reynolds AF, Galloway DC, et al. Digital myelography of spinal dysraphism in infancy. Preliminary results. *Am J Roentgenol* 1984;142:1249–1252.
94. Berenbruch K. Ein Fall von multiplen Angiolipomen kombiniert mit einem Angiom des Rückenmarks. Tübingen, 1890.
95. Von Hanwehr R, Apuzzo MLJ, Ahmadi J, Chandrasoma P. Thoracic spinal angiomyolipoma: case report and literature review. *Neurosurgery* 1985;16:406–411.
96. Cull DJ, Endohazi M, Symon L. Extradural haemangiolipoma of the spinal canal: two cases presenting during pregnancy. *Acta Neurochir (Wien)* 1978;45:187–193.
97. Bender JL, Van Landingham JH, Manno NJ. Epidural lipoma producing spinal cord compression: report of two cases. *J Neurosurg* 1974;41:100–103.
98. Pearson J, Stellar S, Feigin I. Angiomyolipoma: long-term cure following radical approach to malignant-appearing benign intraspinal tumor. Report of three cases. *J Neurosurg* 1970;33:466–470.
99. Balado M, Morea R. Hemangioma extramedular produciendo paraplegias durante al embarazo. *Arch Argent Neurol* 1928;1:345–351.
100. Schiffer J, Gilboa Y, Ariazoroff A. Epidural angiolipoma producing compression of the cauda equina. *Neurochirurgia (Stuttg)* 1980;23:117–120.

101. Taylor J, Harries BJ, Schurr PH. Extrathecal haemangiolipomas of the spinal canal. *Br J Surg* 1951;39:1–7.
102. Gonzalez-Crussi F, Enneking WF, Arean VM. Infiltrating angiolipoma. *J Bone Joint Surg* 1966; 48A:1111–1124.
103. Obrador S, Villarejo F, Deblas A. Angiolipoma extradural: causa infrecuente de compresión medular. *Rev Clin Esp* 1977;146:395–396.
104. Padovani R, Tognetti F, Speranza S, Pozzati E. Spinal extrathecal hemangiolipomas: report of two cases and review of the literature. *Neurosurgery* 1982;11:674–677.
105. Böstroem E. Über die pialem Epidermoide, Dermoide und Lipoma und durale Dermoide. *Zentralbl Allg Pathol* 1897;8:1–98.
106. Cruveilhier J. *Anatomie pathologique du corps humain*, vol. 1. Paris: Bailliere Masson, 1929.
107. Müller J. *Über den feiner Bau und die Formen der krankhaften Geschwülste*. Berlin: G. Reimer, 1838;60.
108. Rubinstein LJ. Tumors of the central nervous system. In: *Atlas of tumor pathology*, 2nd series, fascicle 6. Washington, DC: Armed Forces Institute of Pathology, 1972;288–292.
109. Arias MJ. Asociación de un quiste dermoide sacrocoxigeo y un epidermoide intracraneal. *Actas Luso Esp Neurol Psinquiatr* 1984;12:171–174.
110. Ciraldo AV, Platt MS, Agamanolis DP, Boeckman CR. Sacrococcygeal myxopapillary ependymomas and ependymal rests in infants and children. *J Pediatr Surg* 1986;21:49–52.
111. Walker AE, Bucy PC. Congenital dermal sinuses: a source of spinal meningeal infection and subdural abscesses. *Brain* 1934;57:401–421.
112. Mount LA. Congenital dermal sinuses as a cause of meningitis, intraspinal abscess and intracranial abscess. *JAMA* 1948;139:1263–1268.
113. Matson DD, Ingraham FD. Intracranial complications of congenital dermal sinuses. *Pediatrics* 1951;8:463–474.
114. Matson DD, Jerva MJ. Recurrent meningitis associated with congenital lumbosacral dermal sinus tract. *J Neurosurg* 1966;25:288–297.
115. Schnegg JF, Glauser M, de Tribolet N. Infection of lumbar dermoid cyst by an anaerobic peptococcus. *Acta Neurochir* 1981;58:127–129.
116. Moise TS. Staphylococcus meningitis secondary to a congenital sacral sinus. *Surg Gynecol Obstet* 1926;42:394–397.
117. Ripley W, Thompson DC. Pilonidal sinus as a route of infection in a case of staphylococcus meningitis. *Am J Dis Child* 1928;36:785–788.
118. Wright RL. Congenital dermal sinuses. *Prog Neurol Surg* 1971;4:175–191.
119. Román Riechmann E, Verdú Perez A, Alvarez-Coca J, Pascual-Castroviejo I. Meningitis asociada a seno dérmico congénito. *An Esp Pediatr* 1983;18:243–247.
120. Woltman HW, Adson AW. Abscess of the spinal cord. Report of a case with function recovery after operation. *Brain* 1926;49:193–206.
121. El Gindi S, Fairfurn B. Intramedullary spinal abscess as a complication of a congenital dermal sinus. *J Neurosurg* 1969;30:494–497.
122. Probst FP, Brun A. Recurrent meningoencephalitis and ascending myelitis caused by dermal sinus tract of extraordinary length. *Neuroradiology* 1980;19:161–165.
123. Guidetti B, Gagliardi FM. Epidermoid and dermoid cysts. Clinical evaluation and late surgical results. *J Neurosurg* 1977;47:12–18.
124. Monojati A, Spitzer RM, Wiley JLR, Heggeness L. MR imaging of a spinal teratoma. *J Comput Assist Tomogr* 1986;10:307–310.
125. Buge A. Chamouard JM, Schadeck B, et al. Kyste épidermoide congénital médullaire (un cas dorsal). *Rev Neurol (Paris)* 1985;141:810–813.
126. Batniksy S, Keucher TR, Mealey J Jr, Campbell RL. Iatrogenic intraspinal epidermoid tumors. *JAMA* 1977;237:148–150.
127. Shaywitz BA. Epidermoid spinal cord tumors and previous lumbar puncture. *J Pediatr* 1972;80: 638–640.
128. Halcrow SJ, Crawford PJ, Craft AW. Epidermoid spinal cord tumour after lumbar puncture. *Arch Dis Child* 1985;60:978–979.
129. Manno NJ, Uhlein A, Kernohan JW. Intraspinal epidermoids. *J Neurosurg* 1962;19:754–756.
130. Blazquez MG, Oliver B. Epidermoides intrarraquídeos de inclusion yatrogénica. *Arch Neurobiol* 1980;43:217–228.

131. Greensher J, Mofenson HC, Borofsky LG, Sharma R. Lumbar puncture in the neonate: a simplified technique. *J Pediatr* 1971;78:1034–1035.
132. Gibson T, Norris W. Skin fragments removed by injection needles. *Lancet* 1958;ii:983–985.
133. Van Gilder JC, Schwartz HG. Growth of dermoids from skin implants to the nervous system and surrounding spaces of the newborn rat. *J Neurosurg* 1967;26:15–20.
134. Oblu N, Wasserman L, Sandulescu G, Onofrei T. Experimental investigation of the origin of intraspinal epidermoid cysts. *Acta Neurol Scand* 1967;43:78–86.
135. Choremis C, Economos D, Papadatos C, Garcoulas A. Intraspinal epidermoid tumors (cholesteatomas) in patients treated for tuberculous meningitis. *Lancet* 1956;ii:437–439.
136. Economus D, Caracalos A. Cholestéatomes intrarachidiens multiples, complication tardive d'injections intrarachidiennes pour méningite tuberculeuse de l'enfance. *Rev Neurol (Paris)* 1957;97:81–101.
137. Canlorbe PJ, Dalloz C, Turquet J. Les kyste épidermoïdes intrarachidiens postméningés de l'enfant (cholestéatomes). *Arch Fr Pediatr* 1964;21:1153–1178.
138. Michelsen J. Cholesteatom des Rückenmarks. *Dtsch Z Nerveheilk* 1932;127:123–130.
139. Boyd HR. Iatrogenic intraspinal epidermoids. *J Neurosurg* 1966;24:105–107.
140. Bryant H, Dayan AD. Spinal inclusion dermoid cyst in a patient with a treated myelocystocoele. *J Neurol Neurosurg Psychiatry* 1967;30:182–184.
141. Verdu A, De la Cruz M, Pascual-Castroviejo I, Villarejo F. Intramedullary dermoid of the cervical spinal cord in a child. *J Neurol Neurosurg Psychiatry* 1986;49:462–463.
142. Takeuchi J, Ohta T, Kajikawa H. Congenital tumours of the spinal cord. In: Vinken PJ, Bruyn GN, eds. *Handbook of clinical neurology*, vol. 32. Amsterdam: North-Holland, 1978;355–392.
143. Nagahiro S, Matsukado Y, Miura M, Yoshioka S. Cervical dermal sinus associated with meningitis and motor paralysis. *Brain Dev* 1985;7:504–507.
144. Schiffer J, Till K. Spinal dysraphism in the cervical and dorsal regions in childhood. *Child's Brain* 1982;9:73–84.
145. Been JR, Walsh JW, Blacker HM. Cervical dermal sinus and intramedullary spinal cord abscess: case report. *Neurosurgery* 1975;5:60–62.
146. Sachs E, Horrax G. A cervical and a lumbar pilonidal sinus communicating with intraspinal dermoids. Report of 2 cases and review of the literature. *J Neurosurg* 1949;6:97–112.
147. Thieffry S, Lepintre L, Masselin S, Fauré C. Fistules dermoïdes congénitales communiquant avec le système nerveux central. *Semain Hop Paris* 1958;34:1178–1187.
148. Higazi I. Intraspinal epidermoids. Report of two cases. *J Neurosurg* 1963;20:805–808.
149. Arseni C, Danaila L, Constantinescu AI, Carp N. Spinal dermoid tumours. *Neurochirurgia (Stuttg)* 1977;20:108–116.
150. Quigley MR, Schinco F, Brown JT. Anterior sacral meningocele with an unusual presentation. Case report. *J Neurosurg* 1984;61:790–792.
151. Leibowitz E, Barton W, Sadighi P, Ross JS. Anterior sacral meningocele contiguous with a pelvic hamartoma. Case report. *J Neurosurg* 1984;61:188–190.
152. Smith HP, Davis CH. Anterior sacral meningocele: two case reports and discussion of surgical approach. *Neurosurgery* 1980;7:61–67.
153. Klerk DJJ, McCusker I, Loubser JS. Anterior sacral meningocele. *S Afr Med J* 1978;54:361–365.
154. Villarejo F, Scavone C, Blazquez MG, et al. Anterior sacral meningocele: review of the literature. *Surg Neurol* 1983;19:57–71.
155. Kaufmann HI. Anterior sacral meningocele. *Ann Radiol (Paris)* 1967;10:121–128.
156. Werner JL, Taybi H. Presacral mass in childhood. *Am J Roentgenol* 1970;109:403–410.
157. Le Mercier Y, Decazes JM, Mechali D, et al. Méningite purulente par inoculation chirurgicale d'une méningocèle sacrée antérieure. Une complication rare de la maladie de Marfan. *Ann Med Interne (Paris)* 1980;131:289–290.
158. Strand RD, Eisenberg HM. Anterior sacral meningocele in association with Marfan's syndrome. *Radiology* 1971;99:653–654.
159. Gutierrez Maxwell V, Gil R. Meningocele sacro anterior. *Bol Soc Cor B Aires* 1964;48:286–297.
160. Meigs JV. Anterior meningocele as a gynecologic problem. *Prog Gynecol* 1963;4:365–392.
161. Oren M, Laber B, Lee SH, et al. Anterior sacral meningocele. Report of five cases and review of the literature. *Dis Colon Rectum* 1977;20:492–505.

162. Johnson LH. Pregnancy associated with an anterior sacral meningocele: case report. *South Med J* 1970;63:432–434.
163. Cohn J, Bay-Nielsen E. Hereditary defect of the sacrum and coccyx with anterior sacral meningocele. *Acta Paediatr Scand* 1969;58:268–274.
164. Aaronson I. Anterior sacral meningocele, anal canal duplication cyst and covered anus occurring in one family. *J Pediatr Surg* 1970;5:559–563.
165. Klenerman L, Merrick MW. Anterior sacral meningocele occurring in a family. *J Bone Joint Surg* 1973;55B:331–334.
166. Balériaux-Waha D, Osteaux M, Terwinghe G, et al. The management of anterior sacral meningocele with computed tomography. *Neuroradiology* 1977;14:45–46.
167. Amacher AL, Drake CG, McLachlin AD. Anterior sacral meningocele. *Surg Gynecol Obstet* 1968;126:986–994.
168. McLean DR, Miller JDR, Allen PBR, Ezzeddin SA. Posttraumatic syringomyelia. *J Neurosurg* 1973;39:485–492.
169. Quencer RM, Green BA, Eismont FJ. Posttraumatic spinal cord cysts: clinical features and characterizations with metrizamide computed tomography. *Radiology* 1983;146:415–423.
170. Seibert CE, Dreisbach JN, Swanson WB, et al. Progressive posttraumatic cystic myelopathy: neuroradiologic evaluation. *Am J Roentgenol* 1981;136:1161–1165.
171. Vernon JD, Chir B, Silver JR, Ohry A. Posttraumatic syringomyelia. *Paraplegia* 1982;20:339–364.
172. Gebarski SS, Maynard FW, Gabrielsen TO, et al. Posttraumatic progressive myelopathy. Clinical and radiologic correlation employing MR imaging, delayed CT metrizamide myelography, and intraoperative sonography. *Radiology* 1985;157:379–385.
173. Giménez Roldán S, Esteban A, Benito C. Communicating syringomyelia following cured tuberculous meningitis. *J Neurol Sci* 1974;23:185–197.
174. Papin B, Frenay J, Goldstein B, et al. Syndrome syringomyélique après méningite tuberculeuse (à propos de quatre observations). *Rev Neurol (Paris)* 1977;133:697–708.
175. Kiwak KJ, Deray MJ, Shields WD. Torticollis in three children with syringomyelia and spinal cord tumor. *Neurology* 1983;33:946–948.
176. Nagahiro S, Matsukado Y, Kuratsu J, et al. Syringomyelia and syringobulbia associated with an ependymoma of the cauda equina involving the conus medullaris: case report. *Neurosurgery* 1986;18:357–360.
177. Barnett HJM, Rewcastle NB. Syringomyelia and tumor of the nervous system. In: Barnett HJM, Foster JB, Hudgson P, eds. *Syringomyelia*. London: W.B. Saunders, 1973;261–301.
178. Wolk A, Wilens SL. Multiple hemangioblastoma of the spinal cord with syringomyelia: a case of Lindau's disease. *Am J Pathol* 1934;10:545–567.
179. Sloof JL, Kernohan TW, MacCarthy CS. *Primary intramedullary tumors of the spinal cord and filum terminale*. Philadelphia: W.B. Saunders, 1964;180–189.
180. Ferry MDJ, Hardman CJM, Earle KM. Syringomyelia and intramedullary neoplasms. *Med Ann DC* 1969;38:363–365.
181. Lichtenstein BW, Zeitlin H. Ganglioglioneuroma of the spinal cord associated with pseudosyringomyelia: a histologic study. *Arch Neurol Psychiatry* 1949;62:1356–1370.
182. Cahan LD, Bentson JR. Considerations in the diagnosis and treatment of syringomyelia and the Chiari malformation. *J Neurosurg* 1982;57:24–31.
183. Huebert HT, McKinnon WB. Syringomyelia and scoliosis. *J Bone Joint Surg* 1969;51B:338–343.
184. Eggers C, Hamer J. Hydrosyringomyelia in childhood: clinical aspects, pathogenesis, and therapy. *Neuropadiatrie* 1979;10:87–99.
185. Resjo IM, Harwood-Nash DC, Fitz CR, Chuang S. Computed tomographic metrizamide myelography in syringomyelia. *Radiology* 1979;131:405–407.
186. Bonafé A, Manelfe C, Espagno J, et al. Evaluation of syringomyelia with metrizamide computed tomography myelography. *J Comput Assist Tomogr* 1980;4:797–802.
187. Aubin ML, Vignaud J, Jardin C, Bar D. Computed tomography in 75 clinical cases of syringomyelia. *AJNR* 1981;2:199–204.
188. Stanley P, Senac MC Jr, Seagall HD, Parks TS. Syringomyelia following meningomyelocele surgery—role of metrizamide myelography and computed tomography. *Pediatr Radiol* 1984;14:278–283.

189. Sotaniemi KA, Pythienen J, Myllylä VV. Computed tomography in the diagnosis of sy-
     ringomyelia. *Acta Neurol Scand* 1983;68:121–127.
190. De la Paz RL, Brady TJ, Buananno FS, et al. Nuclear magnetic resonance (NMR) imaging of
     Arnold-Chiari type I malformation with hydromyelia. *J Comput Assist Tomogr* 1983;7:126–129.
191. Yeates A, Brant-Zawadski M, Norman D, et al. Nuclear magnetic resonance imaging of sy-
     ringomyelia. *AJNR* 1983;4:234–237.
192. Pojunas K, Williams AL, Daniels DL, Haughton VM. Syringomyelia and hydromyelia: magnetic
     resonance evaluation. *Radiology* 1984;153:679–683.
193. Aichner F, Poewe W, Rogalsky W, et al. Magnetic resonance imaging in the diagnosis of spinal
     cord diseases. *J Neurol Neurosurg Psychiatry* 1985;48:1220–1229.
194. Gardner WJ. Hydrodynamic mechanism of syringomyelia: its relationship to myelocele. *J Neurol
     Neurosurg Psychiatry* 1965;28:247–259.
195. Ball MJ, Dayan AD. Pathogenesis of syringomyelia. *Lancet* 1972;ii:799–801.
196. Williams B. A critical appraisal of posterior fossa surgery for communicating syringomyelia.
     Brain 1978;101:223–250.
197. Williams B. The distending force in the production of communicating syringomyelia. *Lancet*
     1970;ii:41–42.
198. Williams B. Pathogenesis of syringomyelia (letter). *Lancet* 1972;ii:969–970.
199. Williams B. On the pathogenesis of syringomyelia: a review. *J R Soc Med* 1980;73:798–806.
200. Zaragozá E. Malformaciones de la charnela occipito-cervical y sus correlaciones clínicas. Tesis
     doctoral. *Monografía (Madrid)* 1974.
201. Taylor AR. Another theory of the aetiology of the syringomyelia cavity. *J Neurol Neurosurg
     Psychiatry* 1975;38:825 (Abstr.).
202. Aboulker J. La syringomyélie et les liquides intra-rachidiens. *Neurochirurgie* 1975;25(Suppl. 1):
     1–144.
203. Welch K, Shillito J, Strand R, et al. Chiari I malformation—an acquired disorder? *J Neurosurg*
     1981;55:604–609.
204. Marin-Padilla M, Marin-Padilla T. Morphogenesis of experimentally induced Arnold-Chiari mal-
     formation. *J Neurol Sci* 1981;50:29–55.
205. Coria F, Quintana F, Rebollo M, et al. Occipital dysplasia and Chiari type I deformity in a
     family. Clinical and radiological study of three generations. *J Neurol Sci* 1983;62:147–158.
206. Coria F, Berciano J. La displasia occipito-cervical. *Med Clin (Barc)* 1985;84:199–205.
207. Hall PV, Muller J, Campbell RL. Experimental hydrosyringomyelia, ischemic myelopathy, and
     syringomyelia. *J Neurosurg* 1975;43:464–470.
208. Saez RJ, Onofrio BM, Yanagihara T. Experience with Arnold-Chiari malformation, 1960 to
     1970. *J Neurosurg* 1976;45:416–422.
209. Banerji NK, Millar JHD. Chiari malformation presenting in adult life. Its relationship to sy-
     ringomyelia. *Brain* 1974;97:157–168.
210. Logue V, Edwards MR. Syringomyelia and its surgical treatment—an analysis of 75 patients. *J
     Neurol Neurosurg Psychiatry* 1981;44:273–284.
211. Chavda SV, Davies AM, Cassar-Pullicino VN. Enterogenous cysts of the central nervous system:
     a report of eight cases. *Clin Radiol* 1985;36:245–251.
212. Rhaney K, Barclay GPT. Enterogenous cysts and congenital diverticula of the alimentary canal
     with abnormalities of the vertebral column and spinal cord. *J Pathol Bacteriol* 1959;77:457–471.
213. Millis RR, Holmes AE. Enterogenous cyst of the spinal cord with associated intestinal duplica-
     tion, vertebral anomalies, and dorsal dermal sinus. Case report. *J Neurosurg* 1973;38:73–77.
214. Klump TE. Neurenteric cyst in the cervical spinal cord of a 10-week-old boy. Case report. *J
     Neurosurg* 1971;35:472–476.
215. Fabinyi GCA, Adams JE. High cervical spinal cord compression by an enterogenous cyst. *J
     Neurosurg* 1979;51:556–559.
216. Kwok DMF, Jeffreys RV. Intramedullary enterogenous cyst of the spinal cord. Case report. *J
     Neurosurg* 1982;56:270–274.
217. Kahn AP, Hirsch KF, De Lange C, et al. Les kystes entériques intrarachidiens. A propos de trois
     observations. *Neurochirurgie* 1971;17:33–44.
218. Odake G, Yamaki T, Naruse S. Neurenteric cyst with meningomyelocele. Case report. *J Neuro-
     surg* 1976;45:352–356.
219. Fallon M, Gordon ARG, Lendrum AC. Mediastinal cysts of fore-gut origin associated with
     vertebral abnormalities. *Br J Surg* 1954;41:520–533.

220. Gimeno A, Lopez F, Figuera D, Rodrigo L. Neurenteric cyst. *Neuroradiology* 1972;3:167–172.
221. Kirwan WO, Walbaum PR, McCormack RJM. Cystic intrathoracic derivatives of the foregut and their complications. *Thorax* 1973;28:424–428.
222. Kantrowitz LR, Pais MJ, Burnett K, et al. Intraspinal neurenteric cyst containing gastric mucosa: CT and MRI findings. *Pediatr Radiol* 1986;16:324–327.
223. Rewcastle NB, Francouer J. Teratomatous cysts of the spinal canal. With sex chromatin studies. *Arch Neurol* 1964;11:91–99.
224. Wilkins RH, Odom GL. Spinal intradural cysts. In: Vinken PJ, Bruyn GW, eds. *Handbook of clinical neurology*, vol. 20, part 2: *Tumors of the spine and spinal cord.* New York: Elsevier, 1976;55–102.
225. Page RE. Intraspinal enterogenous cyst associated with spondylolisthesis and spina bifida occulta. Report of a case. *J Bone Joint Surg* 1974;56B:541–544.
226. Piramoon AM, Abbassioun K. Mediastinal enterogenous cyst with spinal cord compression. *J Pediatr Surg* 1974;9:543–545.
227. Di Chiro G, Doppman JL, Dwyer AJ, et al. Tumors and arteriovenous malformations of the spinal cord: assessment using MR. *Radiology* 1985;156:689–697.
228. Hoffmann GT. Cervical arachnoidal cyst. Report of a 6-year-old negro male with recovery from quadriplegia. *J Neurosurg* 1960;17:327–330.
229. Raja IA, Hankinson J. Congenital spinal arachnoid cysts. Report of two cases and review of the literature. *J Neurol Neurosurg Psychiatry* 1970;30:105–110.
230. Stewart DH Jr, Red DE. Spinal arachnoid diverticula. *J Neurosurg* 1971;35:65–70.
231. Palmer JJ. Spinal arachnoid cysts. Report of six cases. *J Neurosurg* 1974;41:728–735.
232. Fortuna A, Latorre E, Ciappetta P. Arachnoid diverticula: a unitary approach to spinal cysts communicating with the subarachnoid space. *Acta Neurochir (Wien)* 1977;39:259–268.
233. Jensen F, Knudsen V, Troelsen S. Recurrent intraspinal arachnoid cyst treated with a shunt procedure. *Acta Neurochir (Wien)* 1977;39:127–129.
234. Camras LR, Van Doornick S, Krettek JE. Metrizamide CT myelography in the evaluation of spinal arachnoid diverticula. *J Comput Assist Tomogr* 1983;7:1084–1086.
235. Aarabi B, Pasternak G, Hurko O, Long DM. Familial intradural arachnoid cysts. Report of two cases. *J Neurosurg* 1971;50:826–829.
236. Nugent GR, Odom GL, Woodhall S. Spinal extradural cysts. *Neurology* 1959;9:397–406.
237. Robinow M, Johnson GF, Verhagen AD. Distichiasis-lymphedema. A hereditary syndrome of multiple congenital defects. *Am J Dis Child* 1970;119:343–347.
238. Weir B. Leptomeningeal cysts in congenital ectopia lentis. Case report. *J Neurosurg* 1973;38:650–653.
239. Chynn K-Y. Congenital spine extradural cyst in two siblings. *Am J Roentgenol* 1967;101:204–215.
240. Bergland RM. Congenital intraspinal extradural cyst. Report of three cases in one family. *J Neurosurg* 1968;28:495–499.
241. Tarlov IM. Perineurial cysts of the spinal nerve roots. *Arch Neurol Psychiatry* 1938;40:1067–1074.
242. Rengachary SS, Boynick PO, Karlin CA, et al. Intrasacral extradural communicating arachnoid cysts: case report. *Neurosurgery* 1981;3:236–240.
243. Sundaram M, Awward EA. Magnetic resonance imaging of arachnoid cysts destroying the sacrum. *Am J Roentgenol* 1986;146:359–360.
244. Teng P, Rudner N. Multiple arachnoid diverticula. *Arch Neurol* 1960;2:348–365.
245. Herskowitz J, Bielawski MA, Venna N, Sabien TD. Anterior cervical arachnoid cyst stimulating syringomyelia. A case with preceding posterior arachnoid cysts. *Arch Neurol* 1978;35:57–58.
246. Hoffman EP, Garner JT, Johnson D, Sheldon CH. Traumatic arachnoidal diverticulum associated with paraplegia. Case report. *J Neurosurg* 1973;38:81–85.
247. El Mahdi MA. Arachnoid cyst and cord compression in association with tangential shrapnel injuries of the spine. *Neurochirurgia (Stuttg)* 1977;20:1–7.
248. Jelsma F. Cervical intramedullary cyst due to corynebacterium diphtheriae gravis. Case report. *J Neurosurg* 1973;38:78–80.
249. Kendall BE, Valentine AR, Keis B. Spinal arachnoid cyst: clinical and radiological correlation with prognosis. *Neuroradiology* 1982;22:225–234.
250. Kjos BO, Brant-Zawadski M, Kucharczyk W, et al. Cystic intracranial lesions: magnetic resonance imaging. *Radiology* 1985;155:363–369.

251. Findler G, Hadani M, Tadmor R, et al. Spinal intradural ependymal cyst: a case report and review of the literature. *Neurosurgery* 1985;17:484–486.
252. Morello G, Lombardi G. Choroido-ependymal cysts of the spinal roots. *J Neurosurg* 1964;21: 1103–1107.
253. Moore MT, Book MH. Congenital cervical ependymal cyst. *J Neurosurg* 1966;24:558–561.
254. Hayman I, Hamby WB, Sanes S. Ependymal cyst of the cervicodorsal region of the spinal cord. *Arch Neurol Psychiatry* 1938;40:1005–1012.
255. Wisoff HS, Ghatak NR. Ependymal cyst of the spinal cord. Case report. *J Neurol Neurosurg Psychiatry* 1971;34:546–550.
256. Mosso JA, Verity MA. Ependymal cyst of the spinal cord. Case report. *J Neurosurg* 1975;43: 757–760.
257. Sakae T, Bourke J, Bedbrook GM, et al. Fifty years survival after cervical fracture and fusion. *Paraplegia* 1983;21:249–257.
258. Chuang K-S, Wang Y-C, Tsai S-H, Liu M-Y. Spinal intramedullary pseudocyst. Case report. *J Neurosurg* 1985;63:453–455.
259. Baecque C, Snyder DH, Suzuki K. Congenital intramedullary spinal cyst associated with an Arnold-Chiari malformation. *Acta Neuropathol (Berl)* 1977;38:239–242.
260. Hilal SK, Marton D, Pollack E. Diastematomyelia in children. *Radiology* 1974;112:609–621.
261. Herren RY, Edwards JE. Diplomyelia (duplication of the spinal cord). *Arch Pathol* 1940;30: 1203–1214.
262. Giordano GB, Davidotis P, Cerisoli M, Giulioni M. Cervical diplomyelia revealed by computed tomography. *Neuropediatrics* 1982;13:93–94.
263. Levine RS, Geremia GK, McNeill TW. CT demonstration of cervical diastematomyelia. *J Comput Assist Tomogr* 1985;9:592–594.
264. Winter RB, Haren JJ, Moe JH, Lagaard SM. Diastematomyelia and congenital spine deformities. *J Bone Joint Surg* 1974;56A:27–39.
265. Roosen N, De Moor J. Cervicobrachialgia with congenital vertebral anomalies and diastematomyelia. *Surg Neurol* 1984;21:493–496.
266. Shorey WD. Diastematomyelia associated with dorsal kyphosis producing paraplegia. *J Neurosurg* 1955;12:300–305.
267. Keim HA, Greene AF. Diastematomyelia and scoliosis. *J Bone Joint Surg* 1973;55A:1425–1435.
268. Garcia FA, Kranzler LI, Siqueria EB, et al. Diastematomyelia in an adult. *Surg Neurol* 1980;14: 93–94.
269. Maroun FB, Jacob JC, Heneghan WD. La diastématomyélie. Ses manifestations cliniques et son traitement chirurgical. *Neurochirurgie* 1972;18:285–316.
270. Maroun FB, Jacob IC, Mangan MA, Hardjasudarma M. Adult diastematomyelia: a complex dysraphic state. *Surg Neurol* 1982;18:289–294.
271. Guthkelch AN, Hoffman GT. Diastematomyelia with median septum. *Brain* 1974;97:729–742.
272. Faithfull DK. Diastematomyelia complicating congenital scoliosis. *J Bone Joint Surg* 1973;55B: 431(Abstr.).
273. Leonard MA. Diastematomyelia and scoliosis. *J Bone Joint Surg* 1975;57B:403–404.
274. Hood RW, Risenborough EJ, Nehme AM, et al Diastematomyelia and structural spinal deformities. *J Bone Joint Surg* 1980;62A:520–528.
275. Mathieu JP, Decaire M, Pube J, Marton D. La diastématomyélie. Etude de 96 cas. *Chir Pediatr* 1982;23:29–35.
276. Frerebeau P, Dimeglio A, Gras M, Harbi H. Diastematomyelia: report of 21 cases surgically treated by a neurosurgical and orthopedic team. *Child's Brain* 1983;10:328–339.

15

Inflammatory and Parasitic Processes

Ignacio Pascual-Castroviejo

POTT'S DISEASE

Generalities

Tuberculous spondylitis is on the decline, and today cases with neurologic symptomatology are rare. The nonspecific presenting symptoms of this illness make early diagnosis difficult. Months or years may elapse before the correct diagnosis is made. Previous lung or bowel tuberculosis is common, although sometimes overlooked, before vertebral tuberculosis appears, usually via the hematogenous route. Commonly, infection starts in the superior or inferior surface of the vertebral body, adjacent to the articular cartilaginous tissue which is very vascularized. These areas are destroyed, with resultant narrowing or destruction of the disc. Fusion of contiguous vertebral bodies is frequent. Destruction of the anterior aspect of the affected vertebral bodies causes kyphosis. The infected disc may be located anywhere along the spine, most commonly in the dorsal and lumbar regions (1).

Tuberculosis of the cervical spine is uncommon (2,3). Wang (4) found only 15 cases of atlanto-axial involvement in 5,393 cases of tuberculous spondylitis. Prominent features of upper cervical tuberculosis include pain and stiffness, paralysis, swelling of the retropharyngeal soft tissues, osteolytic erosion, and atlanto-axial subluxation (3). The spinal cord at the spinomedullary junction is threatened by atlanto-axial subluxation or upward translocation of the dens, by compression from a tuberculous abscess or by direct tuberculous invasion. Neurologic involvement may include monoparesis, hemiparesis, tetraparesis, and sensory and sphincteric dysfunctions. Children under 10 years of age have more extensive and diffuse involvement, with formation of larger abscesses. Patients above 10 years of age tend to have a more localized process with less pus, but they present a much higher incidence of Pott's paraplegia. The overall incidence of cord compression is 42.5% (2). Torticollis, gibbus or kyphosis, and lymphadenopathy may occur at the beginning or during the course of the disease. Pressure on the cord from a cold abscess and from a gibbus are responsible for neurologic symptoms in patients with tuberculosis of the lower cervical spine. Some patients may have a second turberculous lesion farther down the spine. The onset of cord compression is gradual in cervical disease, usually occurring over a period of 4 to 8 weeks after the onset of pain (2). Besides compressing the spinal cord, a large retropharyngeal abscess may cause acute dysphagia and asphyxia, inspiratory stridor, attacks of cyanosis, and discomfort in the throat when swallowing. Most patients have a short history before being diagnosed.

Destruction of the disc affects contiguous vertebrae in approximately half the cases of tuberculous spondylitis. Involvement of noncontiguous vertebral bodies may occur via the hematogenous route or by spread of the infection beneath the anterior longitudinal ligament. Paraspinal infection is typical and may spread to mediastinal, abdominal, retropharyngeal, and epidural spaces. Intradural and intramedullary tuberculomas are uncommon. Differential diagnosis with spinal metastases has to be considered, especially in older people. A gradual onset of neurologic involvement with bilateral symmetrical symptomatology is common. There may be systemic symptoms and signs of tuberculosis such as fever, pallor, profuse sweating, leukocytosis, elevated sedimentation rate, and a positive Mantoux test. Conversely, metastatic disease often presents with acute paraplegia and asymmetrical neurologic involvement.

Radiology

The typical aspect of tuberculous spondylitis on plain films of the spine consists of destruction of the anterior part of the vertebral body associated with narrowing of the disc space (Fig. 1). Kyphosis was frequent in the past but is rarely seen

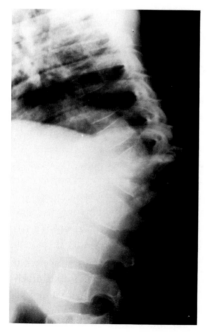

FIG. 1. A 6-year-old girl with Pott's disease. X-ray film in lateral projection shows severe kyphosis, narrowing of the intervertebral space, and partial destruction of the vertebral bodies.

today. There is often a soft tissue mass adjacent to the affected vertebrae. Chest films are abnormal in 75% of patients. Other radiologic findings, such as compression of a single vertebral body without disc space involvement, osteoporosis, and joint sclerosis, can occasionally be observed. Computerized tomography (CT) always shows vertebral body destruction or compression (1). Psoas, paraspinous, or retropharyngeal abscesses are seen clearly. Epidural compression may be visible with or without metrizamide enhancement. CT-guided aspiration can be performed successfully.

Treatment

Antituberculous chemotherapy is the preferred treatment. Several drugs are used in combinations of two or three at a time. The dose of streptomycin sulfate is 20 mg/kg/day; max, 1 g in a single intramuscular injection for 3 to 9 months. Para-aminosalicylic acid (PAS) in doses of 0.2 g/kg/day (max, 10 g) given in two daily doses plus isoniazid 10 mg/kg/day (max, 500 mg) are commonly prescribed for 15 to 24 months. Another combination is rifampicin and isoniazid prescribed for 12 to 15 months. Patients who are resistant to these drugs may receive additional courses of ethionamide, pyrazinamide, or both for 3 to 6 months (2).

The Medical Research Council (5), in its prospective trial on thoracic and lumbar tuberculosis, has shown that the best surgical adjunct is excision of the diseased bone via anterior spinal surgery and filling of the gap with a bone graft. With this operation, pain, upper respiratory obstruction, and cord compression are effectively and rapidly relieved. Neurologic signs disappear within a few weeks or months, and kyphosis does not progress. Cases have presented neither reactivation nor development of a new focus in the spine for a period of 5 years (5). In small children with extensive disease in the cervical region, anterior spinal debridement without fusion may suffice.

SPINAL ARACHNOIDITIS

Generalities

Spinal arachnoiditis consists of focal inflammation of the spinal leptomeninges. Other names for this disease include chronic spinal meningitis, adhesive arachnoiditis, and meningitis serosa circumscripta spinalis. Spinal arachnoiditis rarely occurs today. Within the past 20 years, we observed only one case in a 4-year-old child who presented neurologic symptoms. The disease is much more prevalent in adults than in children (6,12). Shaw et al. (6) found 80 cases of spinal arachnoiditis among 7,600 myelographies. It may be caused by infection with a number of different agents, by reaction to agents introduced into the subarachnoid space, and by spinal trauma. The leptomeninges also present a reactional inflammation when they are compressed or invaded by tumors, herniated intervertebral discs, spinal cysticercosis, or bony lesions, and after surgical intraspinal interventions.

Infectious agents, especially tuberculosis and syphilis, were the most frequent causes of arachnoiditis several decades ago. Chemical substances injected intrathecally for the study and treatment of a neurologic disorder are the main agents today. Other causes include subarachnoid hemorrhage, lymphocytic meningitis, and spinal anesthetics. Thoracic spinal arachnoiditis caused by fungi such as Cryptococcus (7,8) and Blastomyces (9) has been described recently in children and adolescents. Intraspinal arachnoiditis caused by contrast media used for myelography is located in the lumbosacral region in more than 70% of cases, with only 20% involving the thoracic region (6). Removal of oily positive contrast media immediately on completion of myelography does not necessarily protect the patient from the risk of developing arachnoiditis. Water-soluble contrast media are not entirely free of the complication, although modern contrast media such as metrizamide rarely cause arachnoiditis (10,11). Many authors have suggested that hyperosmolarity of water-soluble myelographic contrast agents plays an important role in the causation of toxic reactions, but other factors may be involved as well.

The time interval between the precipitating factor and the onset of symptoms arising from the arachnoiditis varies. Fifty percent develop symptoms in less than 1 year, but symptoms can appear after more than 10 years (6).

Laboratory

Lumbar puncture may yield only a small amount of xanthochromic cerebrospinal fluid (CSF) with a more or less elevated protein content. Serum for cryptococcal antigen, rheumatoid factor, and serology should be drawn. CSF culture for bacteria, mycobacteria, and fungi will confirm the presence of infection, if it exists.

Clinical Findings

A transverse spinal cord syndrome is the main presentation in cases of thoracic arachnoiditis. Lumbosacral involvement causes bilateral sciatica, severe pain with evidence of multiple root lesions, paresthesias, and occasionally difficulty voiding. Spinal arachnoiditis rarely progresses to paraplegia unless the thoracic or cervical regions are involved.

Radiology

Plain X-ray films are usually normal. Myelography shows an irregular distribution or blocks of the contrast medium (Fig. 2A,B), and, occasionally, thickened nerve roots. Similar myelographic findings are seen in cases of intraspinal metastases.

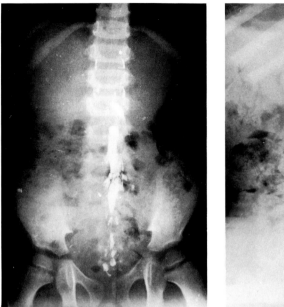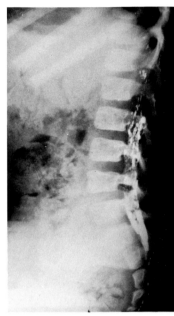

A,B

FIG. 2. A,B: Spinal arachnoiditis. Irregular distribution of the contrast medium with lateral displacement and discontinuity of the contrast column.

Treatment

Corticosteroids or other antiinflammatory drugs may be indicated in the acute phase of the disease, but their benefit is uncertain (6). Although radiotherapy was earlier said to be beneficial (13), most authors disagree (6). Treatment of bacterial or fungal infections depends on the organism identified. If cryptococcosis is suggested by the initial studies, systemic treatment with 5-fluorocytosine (100–150 mg/day) and amphotericin B (0.3–0.6 mg/kg/day) is the indicated therapy (8). The role of surgery in the treatment of spinal arachnoiditis remains in question, which is understandable since the disease is often caused by the combination of surgery and contrast medium myelography. No more than 25% to 30% of patients show improvement after surgery. Prognosis is usually poor. More or less severe neurologic sequelae remain depending on how much time has elapsed since the onset of the disease.

Conversely, pachymeningitis hypertrophica responds favorably to surgery (14). This rare condition may cause radiculopathy and spinal cord compression. Its main symptoms and signs are pain, weakness, and numbness of limbs. The process can occur at any level along the spine. Its etiology is not clear, although infections, toxins, trauma, metabolic disease, and rheumatoid arthritis have been implicated, usually in adults.

DISC SPACE INFECTIONS (DISCITIS)

Clinical Findings

The pathology of disc space infections is not well known in children. Various terms describing disc space infections include discitis, nonspecific spondylitis, intervertebral disc space inflammation, and spondylarthritis.

Discitis may be classified as "nonspecific" or pyogenic. More than 250 cases in children have been reported (15). Clinical symptomatology usually occurs well before radiographic findings. Abdominal pain, refusal to walk or sit, low back pain, irritability, general malaise, paraspinal spasm, and spinous process tenderness are common findings. Localization of the site of maximum pain may often be difficult, and findings may suggest disease of the hip joint. A febrile illness, most commonly a respiratory infection, often precedes the spinal disease. Discitis commonly occurs in early childhood. Trauma may be a precipitating cause (16,17). The early stages of discitis often mimick abdominal disease or a lower lumbar disc hernia. Tenacity and a high degree of suspicion are necessary to make a diagnosis of discitis.

Laboratory

A very high sedimentation rate and a high white count with a shift to the left are usually found. The most common organism cultured is coagulase-positive *Staphylococcus aureus* (17–20). Others include *Streptococcus alpha*- and *beta-hemoliticus, Escherichia coli, Proteus, Moraxella, Diplococcus pneumoniae*, microbacteria, fungi, and others (21). Success in isolating the pathogenic organism is higher if the culture or biopsy studies are performed at the beginning of the illness.

Radiology

Plain X-ray films may be normal during the first weeks of the disease (15). Tomography, especially with isotope bone scanning, or perhaps in conjunction with magnetic resonance (MR) imaging, can show narrowing or even destruction of the disc space (22–24).

Myelography is usually normal. Radiologic alterations may persist for a long time, sometimes several years.

Treatment

The treatment is controversial. Appropriate antibiotic therapy is the treatment of choice. Immobilization for at least 2 to 3 months has been recommended. Prognosis is usually good, although narrowing of the disc remains for a long time.

INTRASPINAL SYNOVIAL CYST

Synovial cyst is a disease that usually occurs in damaged joints. Although the pathogenesis of the lesion is unclear, it is believed to be an inflammatory, proliferative reaction of synovial tissues. Gortvai (25) suggested that most extradural synovial cysts are congenital in origin, although some could be the result of trauma. In 1941, Jaffe et al. (26) suggested the term pigmented villonodular synovitis. Other terms have been used, such as synovial cyst and ganglion cyst.

Synovial cyst is rare in the spinal canal. Most of these cysts have been reported in the age group 11 to 15 years. The majority of the 61 extradural cysts, collected by Gortvai in 1963 (25), were located in the lower thoracic area. About half of them were associated with kyphosis. Clinical symptomatology is that of a rheumatoid disease with systemic involvement, back or radicular pain, sciatica, claudication, kyphosis, and other less frequent findings.

The cyst wall is lined with synovial cells forming villous fronds that have a cellular stroma and that often contain multinucleated giant cells. Electron microscopy shows two populations of cells in the stroma: fibroblasts and macrophages which often contain hemosiderin (27,28). Villonodular synovitis is a benign process, but its cellularity and occasional mitotic activity may be confused with some malignant lesions (29).

Plain spine films commonly show erosion of the pedicles or scalloping of the vertebral bodies (25,27,29,30). Most adults present signs of arthrosis and intervertebral disc narrowing at the level of the synovial cyst. Occasionally, pseudospondylolisthesis may be observed (31). Myelography shows nonspecific findings of an expansive process. CT is diagnostic (31,32). The cyst presents intraspinally, usually in a lateral location, with variable density depending on its size; calcifications, most often at the periphery of the cyst, less often inside it, are common. The differential diagnosis includes herniated disc and arachnoidal cyst.

When cysts are symptomatic, removal after laminectomy is the recommended treatment. Although synovial cysts are benign, they may recur if incompletely excised (33). Surgery may be difficult, because the cyst may collapse during laminectomy (32). Before surgery is recommended, conservative treatment should be considered if there are no signs of spinal cord or root compression.

ABSCESSES

Generalities and Clinical Findings

Spinal epidural abscesses are infections in the space between the dura mater and the surrounding vertebral bodies. They may contain liquid pus or granulation tissue and are commonly located in the posterior part of the epidural space of the thoracic or lumbar spine. These abscesses often have a length of three to six vertebrae (34). They may be caused by bacterial (34–36) and nonbacterial (37) agents.

Bacterial abscesses are uncommon in children (37–39). Tuberculous abscesses tend to present in young or middle-aged adults (37). The main findings are paraparesis, fever, and back pain that has a radicular component. Back pain may have been present for a few days or weeks in bacterial abscesses (37). Paraparesis occurs within a week in bacterial abscesses and is delayed more than 3 weeks in tuberculous abscesses. Over 70% to 80% of patients with bacterial abscesses are febrile and have a leukocytosis (34,37,40). Both fever and leukocytosis are uncommon in tuberculous abscesses.

The CSF protein is usually increased, markedly so in patients with a complete block. Hypoglycorrhachia may be found in patients with bacterial or tuberculous abscesses. Pleocytosis is inconsistent.

Intramedullary spinal cord abscesses are very rare. In 1944, Arzt (41) reported 3 cases and reviewed 37 previously published cases. Menezes et al. (42) located 54 reports in 1977. Only 7 additional cases have been reported since 1977 (43), 6 of them in persons between the ages of 15 years (44) and 32 years (45), most between 18 and 21 years of age (46–48). Primary infection was most often associated with a dermal sinus or an intramedullary epidermoid tumor. The disease can be found anywhere along the spinal cord but is most frequent in the cervical segments. It is more common in males than females. Duration of symptoms varies between a few days and 2 months. Intramedullary abscess should be considered in cases of spinal disease with rapid deterioration. Neck pain occurs in most cases of cervical intramedullary abscess. CSF and blood findings are similar to those observed in patients with epidural abscess.

Etiology

Intramedullary spinal cord abscesses are caused by the same infectious agents as epidural abscesses (43). Mild, blunt spinal trauma (34,35,39,40) and illicit drug use (49–51) seem to increase susceptibility to transient bacteremia. *Staphylococcus aureus* is the most common agent in spinal epidural abscess. Hematogenous spinal abscesses can result from remote infections located anywhere in the body, such as skin, subcutaneous tissues, lung, heart, teeth, and sinuses (34,35,37,40). Other infectious agents include *S. aureus, S. pneumoniae*, and most Gram-positive and Gram-negative cocci, anaerobic organisms, and Gram-negative bacilli (*E. coli, Serratia marcescens, Enterobacter cloacae*, and *Pseudomonas aeruginosa*), these latter agents especially in drug addicts (37). Actinomycosis (52,53), cryptococcosis (54), brucellosis (55), and nocardiosis (56) are causes of spinal epidural abscess. Tuberculous abscesses are usually a solitary and small infectious focus. Active tuberculous infection at another site besides the lung has been reported in between 9% (57) and more than 50% (37) of cases.

Radiology

Plain spine X-rays are usually normal in intramedullary abscesses. They may also be normal in epidural abscesses, especially in cases with a brief course. Vertebral osteomyelitis, contiguous to a bacterial or tuberculous epidural abscess, can often be seen. X-ray changes are usually evident in tuberculous spondylitis. The radiologic findings in spinal abscess are easily differentiated from those of spinal tumors (widening of the canal, eroded pedicles, enlarged intervertebral foramina, scalloping of vertebral bodies, etc.).

Myelography demonstrates the presence, location, and extent of most intraspinal abscesses, intramedullary as well as epidural. Complete or incomplete block of the contrast medium is almost always observed.

CT scanning of the spine without myelography but after intravenous administration of meglumine iothalamate (1.5 mg/kg) successfully reveals these abscesses (36). The most common sign is loss of the physiological epidural fat, followed by abnormal focal enhancement of the dural sheath, surrounded by an area of higher density situated between bone and the dural sheath. Discitis can also be detected. The epidural fat reappears a few weeks after treatment (36).

There are few reports of MR in spinal abscess (58). It shows encroachment on the dural sac at the level of the abscess and reveals the full extent of the block; the markedly increased signal intensity of the abscess on the T2-weighted images helps distinguish it from a protruded disc.

Treatment

Antibiotics alone can be very effective in the treatment of spinal epidural abscesses (36,59,60). Treatment consists of parenteral administration of antibiotics for a minimum of 8 weeks, followed by oral antibiotic therapy. The choice of antibiotics is determined by the infectious agent and its sensitivities. Leys et al. (36) used a combination of cefotaxime, fosfomycin, and tobramycin. Kaufman et al. (37) state that patients with *S. aureus* abscess should receive a semisynthetic penicillinase-resistant penicillin such as oxacillin or nafcillin in dosage of 12 to 18 g i.v., daily. Narcotic users can be infected with either *S. aureus* or Gram-negative bacilli and should receive an aminoglycoside such as gentamicin or tobramycin, 60 to 80 mg, i.m., every 8 hr, in addition to a semisynthetic penicillin (37). Appropriate drugs should be used in patients with abscesses due to fungi, brucellosis, nocardiosis, etc. Surgery results in a higher percentage of major and minor sequelae than antibiotic therapy alone (34,61–64). However, patients with a localized spinal epidural abscess with rapid neurologic deterioration probably should be operated on as soon as possible (60,64) with laminectomy to evacuate the pus and for local instillation of antibiotics. Patients who are candidates for purely medical treatment are (36): (a) cases with severe concomitant medical problems, (b) cases with a very extensive abscess or epiduritis, (c) cases without severe loss of spinal cord or cauda equina function, and (d) cases who have had complete paralysis for more than 3 days.

Initial therapy for tuberculous abscess should include isoniazid and two of the following drugs: rifampin, streptomycin, or ethambutol. Good results may be achieved with conservative therapy in these types of abscesses despite the fact that, in the past, some authors have suggested surgery in all cases of tuberculous spondylitis with neurologic signs (65,66).

Intramedullary abscess is a candidate for surgery. All surviving patients with cervical spinal cord abscesses had been treated with laminectomy, myelotomy, and high-dose antibiotics (43). Prompt diagnosis and drainage are the keys to survival and a good neurologic outcome.

Patients should be followed up with serial CT or MR.

SPINAL HYDATID DISEASE (ECHINOCOCCOSIS)

Clinical Findings

Echinococcosis of the spine, spinal cord, or spinal subarachnoid space is uncommon in countries outside the Third World. As is true of cysticercosis, most cases occur in Latin America, North Africa, Asia, or the Arabian countries.

Echinococcal involvement of spinal structures may be observed at any age, including childhood (67–70). It is most frequent in the lumbar spine (68), but it may also affect the dorsal segments (69). Males are more often affected than females (68). The vertebrae are the predominant site of infection. Paravertebral infestation secondary to erosion of the vertebrae, or invasion of extradural space through the intervertebral foramina can also occur. Intradural localization is rare but has been observed in children (67). Three clinicopathologic forms have been reported (70): primitive intraspinal hydatidosis, bone-hydatidosis, and pseudo-Pott's hydatidosis.

The larva of *Taenia echinococcus* is multilocular in form in bone and penetrates into the spongy tissue in all directions. It can spread to adjacent soft tissues. Although the parasite is commonly localized to the spine, neurologic disturbances usually appear sooner or later because of spinal cord lesions caused by infection, fracture, or local swelling. Slow growth of the parasite explains late onset of symptoms. The time elapsed between the onset of symptoms and the diagnosis of vertebral hydatidosis may range from a few months to several years.

Neurologic problems are commonly the presenting signs of the disease. Most patients suffer some type of pain at the onset of their illness, most often back pain and sciatica. Less frequent symptoms are thoracic root pain, dorsal pain, radicular pain, paresis, and paresthesiae. The main clinical manifestations in one of the most extensive series reported (68) were paraparesis, sphincter disturbances, paresthesiae, paraplegia, hypesthesia, paravertebral swelling, monoparesis, lumbosciatica, and axillary swelling. Palpation and percussion almost always cause marked exacerbation symptoms (68).

Eosinophilia is observed in about 30% of the cases of bone echinococcosis (68). Immunological tests, especially immunoelectrophoresis, are of great diagnostic aid.

Radiology

X-ray films are usually not diagnostic. They may show areas of multilocular osteolysis with haziness of the bone, erosion of the vertebral body, and in some cases a typical honeycomb appearance. Paravertebral soft tissue masses may be visualized. The transverse or spinous processes of the vertebrae are sometimes involved or destroyed. Associated mediastinal cysts have been seen (69). The intervertebral discs may occasionally be involved, but very late. Enlargement of the intervertebral foramina is fairly common. The ribs may be involved and destroyed. Tomography may help by showing early signs of bony necrosis. Myelography shows the level of complete or partial block. Intradural hydatidosis may cause the myelographic picture of arachnoiditis (70). CT, and especially metrizamide CT myelography, is superior to conventional radiography and myelography for the assessment of this disease (71). Hydatid cysts appear as hypodense lesions on CT that can be located anywhere.

Treatment

Surgical laminectomy and extirpation of the cyst remains the treatment of choice. Results are generally good in the immediate postoperative period, but long-term results are poor. Repeated interventions are often required in spinal hydatidosis. The average number of surgical interventions per patient was 2.6 in the series of Apt et al. (68).

SPINAL CYSTICERCOSIS

Generalities, Clinical Findings, Radiology

Cysticercosis is a parasitic disease in which humans serve as the intermediate hosts of *T. solium*, the pig tapeworm. This disease is found most frequently in Latin America, Africa, and Asia. It is rare in developed countries. Spinal cysticercosis accounts for only 0.7% to 1.0% of central nervous system (CNS) cysticercosis (72) and is extremely rare in children. Only one case among 18 autopsies in a series of 131 children with cysticercosis of the CNS had spinal cysticercosis (73). Most cases occur in adults or teenagers. This parasitosis may affect either the cord or the leptomeninges. It can occur anywhere along the spinal canal, with about two-thirds in the thoracic region (74). From a pathophysiological point of view, spinal cysticercosis may be classified as (74): (a) primary, which can be either an isolated spinal infestation or multifocal spinal infestation; or (b) secondary, caused by direct spinal extension of massive intracranial cysticercosis or involvement of the spinal cord as a result of severe cervical pachymeningitis accompanying cysticercosis of the posterior fossa.

Cysticercosis can be either intramedullary or extramedullary. Extramedullary cysticercosis can be divided into leptomeningeal and epidural forms. Isolated spinal cysticercosis is very difficult to diagnose neuroradiographically and is usually an autopsy finding (75). Intramedullary cysticercosis is very rare—26 cases had been reported up to 1979 (74), with two-thirds of the cases located in the thoracic spinal cord (74). The course of the disease is usually slow, and with surprising sparing of sensory and motor functions until the disease is quite advanced (76). The clinical diagnosis is usually a spinal cord tumor. Radiologic studies (X-ray and myelography) show widening of the spinal cord. CT and MR may show a cystic lesion, often with calcification in the wall of the cyst. The distribution of intramedullary cysticerci is proportional to blood flow to each region, which suggests a hematogenous route of infection (77).

The leptomeningeal form is the most common form of spinal cysticercosis and is six to eight times more frequent than other spinal locations (77). Epidural and subpial spinal cysticercosis is occasionally described. Myelography shows intradural extramedullary filling defects or arachnoiditis (72,78–80). It is impossible to differentiate spinal cysticercosis from other intradural extramedullary lesions, such as arachnoid cysts, meningiomas, neurofibromas, and metastases, by myelography alone. Occasionally, fluoroscopy during myelography reveals a mobile cyst within the spinal subarachnoid space (78). Awareness of the possibility of migration of the cyst between the time of myelography and of laminectomy is important for the neurosurgeon. Metrizamide-CT studies confirm the existence of the extramedullary and intradural masses. Rupture of a cysticercosis cyst can lead to severe arachnoiditis and distortion of the subarachnoid space. All patients with spinal leptomeningeal cysticercosis in the series of Zee et al. (72) presented with hydrocephalus, which supports the notion that spinal leptomeningeal cysts migrate from the intracranial compartment. When there is doubt about spinal cysticercosis, CT studies of the brain can help in the diagnosis.

Three possible pathophysiological mechanisms may explain the neurologic symptoms and signs in this disorder (74): (a) the mass effect of intraspinal cysts, (b) an inflammatory reaction caused by the metabolites of the parasite or the degenerated larval remains, and (c) cord degeneration secondary to pachymeningitis or vascular insufficiency.

Laboratory

Cysticercosis causes leukocytosis and eosinophilia. The CSF is often moderately xanthochromic, with increased protein, elevated gamma globulin, and eosinophilia without hypercellularity. Serologic tests (blood and CSF), such as indirect immunofluorescence, commonly show an immunoprecipitin reaction to *T. solium*.

Treatment

Primary and isolated spinal lesions, including intramedullary ones, can be removed with few problems and with a favorable outcome (74). Very few cases have been described, however, and, in some of them, necropsy showed severe destruction of the spinal cord by the cyst (77). Currently, cerebral cysticercosis is being treated with the antihelmintic agent pyrazinoisoquinoline, 2-(cyclohexylcarbonyl)-1,2,3,6,7,11b-hexahydro-4H-pyrazino[2,1-a]isoquinolin-4-one, known as praziquantel. The dose is 50 mg/kg body weight in three divided doses daily for 15 days. Improvement by CT occurs in 96% of patients, with a high percentage of total remission demonstrated by CT in 35% of the cases (81). The effectiveness of praziquantel on spinal cysticercosis has yet to be demonstrated. Treatment with corticoids (dexamethasone), associated to praziquantel, is said to be very effective (82).

REFERENCES

1. La Berge JM, Brant-Zawadski M. Evaluation of Pott's disease with computed tomography. *Neuroradiology* 1984;26:429–434.
2. Hsu LCS, Leong JCY. Tuberculosis of the lower cervical spine (C_2 to C_7). A report on 40 cases. *J Bone Joint Surg* 1984;66B:1–5.
3. Fang D, Leong JCY, Fang HSY. Tuberculosis of the upper cervical spine. *J Bone Joint Surg* 1983;65B:47–50.
4. Wang LX. Peroral focal debridement for treatment of tuberculosis of the atlas and axis. *Clin J Orthop* 1981;1:207–209.
5. Medical Research Council Working Party on Tuberculosis of the Spine. A 10-year assessment of a controlled trial comparing debridement and anterior spinal fusion in the management of tuberculosis of the spine in patients on standard chemotherapy in Hong Kong. *J Bone Joint Surg* 1982;64B:393–398.
6. Shaw MDM, Russell JA, Grossart KW. The changing pattern of spinal arachnoiditis. *J Neurol Neurosurg Psychiatry* 1978;41:97–107.
7. Van Dellen JR, Buchanan N. Intrathecal cryptococcal lesion of the cauda equina successfully treated with intrathecal amphotericin B. *S Afr Med J* 1980;58:137–138.
8. Stein SC, Corrado ML, Friedlander M, Farmer P. Chronic mycotic meningitis with spinal involvement (arachnoiditis): a report of five cases. *Ann Neurol* 1982;11:519–524.
9. Takahashi H, Sasaki A, Arai T, et al. Chromoblastomycosis in the cisterna magna and the spinal subarachnoid space. *J Neurosurg* 1973;38:506–509.
10. Jensen TS, Hein O. Intraspinal arachnoiditis and hydrocephalus after lumbar myelography using methylglucamine iocarmate. *J Neurol Neurosurg Psychiatry* 1978;41:108–112.
11. Soulanen J. Adhesive arachnoiditis following myelography with various water soluble contrast media. *Neuroradiology* 1975;9:73–78.
12. Jorgensen J, Hansen PH, Steenskov V, Ovesen N. A clinical and radiological study of chronic lower spinal arachnoiditis. *Neuroradiology* 1975;9:139–144.
13. Feder BH, Smith JL. Roentgen therapy in chronic spinal arachnoiditis. *Radiology* 1962;78:192–197.
14. Rosenfeld JV, Maye AH, Davis S, Gonzales M. Pachymeningitis cervicalis hypertrophica. Case report. *J Neurosurg* 1987;66:137–139.
15. Lopez Ros S, Navarro Gonzalez J. Infección del disco intervertebral en el niño. *An Esp Pediatr* 1982;16:176–180.
16. Alexander CJ. The etiology of juvenile spondyloarthritis (discitis). *Clin Radiol* 1970;21:178–187.
17. Spiegel PG, Kengla KW, Isaacson AS, Wilson JC. Intervertebral disc space inflammation in children. *J Bone Joint Surg* 1972;54A:284–296.
18. Bolivar R, Khol S, Pickering LK. Vertebral osteomyelitis in children: report of four cases. *Pediatrics* 1978;62:549–553.
19. Rocco HD, Eyring EJ. Intervertebral disc infections in children. *Am J Dis Child* 1972;123:448–451.
20. Wenger DR, Bobechko WP, Gilday DL. The spectrum of intervertebral disc-space infection in children. *J Bone Joint Surg* 1978;60A:100–108.
21. Muscher DM, Thorsteinsson SB, Minuth JN, Luchi RJ. Vertebral osteomyelitis. Still a diagnostic pitfall. *Arch Intern Med* 1976;136:105–110.

22. Fischer GW, Popich GA, Sullivan DE, et al. Diskitis: a prospective diagnostic analysis. *Pediatrics* 1978;62:543–548.

23. Gelfant MJ, Silberstein EB. Radionuclide imaging. Use in diagnosis of osteomyelitis in children. *JAMA* 1977;237:245–247.

24. Rubin RC, Jacobs GB, Cooper PR, Wille RL. Disc space infections in children. *Child's Brain* 1977;3:180–190.

25. Gortvai P. Extradural cysts of the spinal canal. *J Neurol Neurosurg Psychiatry* 1963;26:223–230.

26. Jaffe HL, Lichtenstein L, Sutro CJ. Pigmented villonodular synovitis, bursitis and tenosinovitis. A discussion of the synovial and bursal equivalents of the tenosynovial lesion commonly denoted as xanthoma, xanthogranuloma, giant cell tumor, or myeloplaxoma of the tendon sheath, with some explanation of this tendon sheath lesion itself. *Arch Pathol* 1941;31:731–765.

27. Meredith JM. Unusual tumors and tumor-like lesions of the spinal canal and its contents with special reference to pitfalls in diagnosis. *VA Med Month* 1940;67:675–687.

28. Wyllie JC. The stromal cell reaction of pigmented villonodular synovitis: an electron microscopic study. *Arthritis Rheum* 1969;12:205–214.

29. Jergesen HE, Markin HJ, Schiller AL. Diffuse pigmented villonodular synovitis of the knee mimicking primary bone neoplasm. *J Bone Joint Surg* 1978;60A:825–829.

30. Kao CC, Uihlein A, Bickel WH, Soule EH. Lumbar intraspinal extradural ganglion cyst. *J Neurosurg* 1968;29:168–172.

31. Mercader J, Muñoz Gomez J, Cardenal C. Intraspinal synovial cyst: diagnosis by CT. Follow-up and spontaneous remission. *Neuroradiology* 1985;27:346–348.

32. Hemminghytt S, Daniels DL, Williams AL, Haughton VM. Intraspinal synovial cyst: natural history and diagnosis by CT. *Radiology* 1982;145:375–376.

33. Granowitz SP, D'Antonio J, Mankin HL. The pathogenesis and long-term end results of pigmented villonodular synovitis. *Clin Orthop* 1976;114:335–351.

34. Baker AS, Ojemann RG, Swartz MN, Richardson EP Jr. Spinal epidural abscess. *N Engl J Med* 1975;293:463–468.

35. Guerrero IC, Slap GB, MacGregor RR, et al. Anaerobic spinal epidural abscess. *J Neurosurg* 1978;48:465–469.

36. Leys D, Lesoin F, Viaud C, et al. Decreased morbidity from acute bacterial spinal epidural abscesses using computed tomography and nonsurgical treatment in selected patients. *Ann Neurol* 1985;17:350–355.

37. Kaufman DM, Kaplan JG, Litman N. Infectious agents in spinal epidural abscesses. *Neurology* 1980;30:844–850.

38. Aicardi J, Lepinte J. Spinal epidural abscess in a 1-month-old child. *Am J Dis Child* 1967;114:665–667.

39. Baker CJ. Primary spinal epidural abscess. *Am J Dis Child* 1971;121:337–339.

40. Heusner AP. Nontuberculous spinal epidural infections. *N Engl J Med* 1948;239:845–853.

41. Arzt PK. Abscess within the spinal cord. Review of the literature and report of three cases. *Arch Neurol Psychiatry* 1944;51:533–543.

42. Menezes AH, Graf CJ, Perret GE. Spinal cord abscess: a review. *Surg Neurol* 1977;8:461–467.

43. Blacklock JB, Hood TW, Maxwell RE. Intramedullary cervical spinal cord abscess. Case report. *J Neurosurg* 1982;57:270–273.

44. Bean JR, Walsh JW, Blacker HM. Cervical dermal sinus and intramedullary spinal cord abscess: case report. *Neurosurgery* 1979;5:60–62.

45. Morrison RE, Brown J, Goodin RS. Spinal cord abscess caused by listeria monocytogenes. *Arch Neurol* 1980;37:243–244.

46. Rahoria SK, Gulali DR, Mann KS. Epidural intramedullary abscess. A case report. *Neurol India* 1978;26:196–197.

47. Fortuna A, Contratti F, Di Lorenzo N. Cervical intramedullary abscess, extirpation by means of microsurgical techniques. *J Neurol Sci* 1979;23:159–162.

48. Maurice-Williams RS, Pamphilon D, Coakham HB. Intramedullary abscess—a rare complication of spinal disraphism. *J Neurol Neurosurg Psychiatry* 1980;43:1045–1048.

49. Holzman RS, Bishko F. Osteomyelitis in heroin addicts. *Ann Intern Med* 1971;75:693–696.

50. Wiesseman GJ, Wood VE, Kroll LL. Pseudomonas vertebral osteomyelitis in heroin addicts. *J Bone Joint Surg* 1973;55A:1416–1424.

51. Jabbari B, Pierce JF. Spinal cord compression due to pseudomonas in a heroin addict. *Neurology* 1977;27:1034–1037.

52. Ernst J, Ratjen E. Actinomycosis of the spine. *Acta Orthop Scand* 1971;42:35–44.
53. Lane T, Goings S, Fraser DW, et al. Disseminated actinomycosis with spinal cord compression: report of two cases. *Neurology* 1979;29:890–893.
54. Littvinoff J, Nelson M. Extradural lumbar cryptococcosis. *J Neurosurg* 1978;49:921–923.
55. Ganado W, Craig AJ, Malta V. Brucellosis myelopathy. *J Bone Joint Surg* 1958;40A:1380–1388.
56. Causey WA, Lee R. Nocardiosis. In: Vinken PJ, Bruyn GW, eds. *Handbook of neurology*, vol. 35. Amsterdam: North-Holland, 1978;517–531.
57. Kelly PJ, Karlson AG. Musculoskeletal tuberculosis. *Mayo Clin Proc* 1969;44:73–80.
58. Masaryk TJ, Modic MT, Geisinger MA, et al. Cervical myelopathy: a comparison of magnetic resonance and myelography. *J Comput Assist Tomogr* 1986;10:184–194.
59. Gautier J, Luthier F. Epidurite staphilococcique. *Med Interne* 1974;9:509–515.
60. Messer HD, Lenchner GS, Brust JCM, Resor S. Lumbar spinal abscess managed conservatively. *J Neurosurg* 1977;46:825–829.
61. Hancock DO. A study of 49 patients with acute spinal extradural abscess. *Paraplegia* 1973;10:285–288.
62. Russell NA, Vaughan R, Morley TP. Spinal epidural infection. *J Can Sci Med* 1979;6:325–328.
63. Phillips GE, Jefferson A. Acute spinal epidural abscess: observations from fourteen cases. *Postgrad Med J* 1979;55:712–715.
64. Leys D, Lesoin F, Destae A, et al. Les épidurites aiguës à germes banals: 23 observations. *Presse Med* 1984;13:597–599.
65. Kirkaldy-Willis WH, Glyn Thomas T. Anterior approaches in the diagnosis and treatment of infections of the vertebral bodies. *J Bone Joint Surg* 1965;47A:87–110.
66. Ahn BH. Treatment for Pott's paraplegia. *Acta Orthop Scand* 1968;39:145–160.
67. Ciba K. Radiological aspects of spinal echinococcosis. *Neuroradiology* 1975;9:29–31.
68. Apt WA, Fierro JL, Calderon C, et al. Vertebral hydatid disease. Clinical experience with 27 cases. *J Neurosurg* 1976;44:72–76.
69. Bettaieb A, Khaldi M, Ben Rhouma T, Touibi S. L'échinococcose vertébromédullaire à propos de 32 cas. *Neurochirurgie* 1978;24:205–210.
70. Tazi Z, Boujida N, Hamdouch N, Boukhrissi N. Hydatidose vertébromédullaire. Apport de la radiologie et de la tomodensitométrie. A propos de 36 observations. *J Radiol (Paris)* 1935;66:183–188.
71. Braithwaite PA, Lee RF. Vertebral hydatid disease radiological assessment. *Radiology* 1981;140:763–766.
72. Zee C-S, Segall HD, Ahmadi J, et al. CT myelography in spinal cysticercosis. *J Comput Assist Tomogr* 1986;10:195–198.
73. Lopez-Hernandez A. Clinical manifestations and sequential computed tomography scans of cerebral cysticercosis in childhood. *Brain Dev* 1983;5:269–277.
74. Akiguchi I, Fujiwara T, Matsuyama H, et al. Intramedullary spinal cysticercosis. *Neurology* 1979;29:1531–1534.
75. Cabieses F, Vallenas M, Landa R. Cysticercosis of the spinal cord. *J Neurosurg* 1959;16:337–341.
76. Trelles JO, Caceres A, Palomino L. La cysticercose médullaire. *Rev Neurol (Paris)* 1970;123:187–202.
77. De Souza Queiroz L, Filho AP, Callegaro D, Faria LLD. Intramedullary cysticercosis. Case report, literature review and comments on pathogenesis. *J Neurol Sci* 1975;26:61–70.
78. Kim KS, Weinberg PE. Spinal cysticercosis. *Surg Neurol* 1985;24:80–82.
79. Dietemann JL, Gentile A, Dosch JC, et al. Aspects radiologiques de la cysticercose cérébrale et rachidienne. A propos de 2 observations. *J Radiol* 1985;66:143–149.
80. Rodriguez-Carbajal J, Palacios E, Azar-Kia B, Churchill R. Radiology of cysticercosis of the central nervous system including computed tomography. *Radiology* 1977;125:127–131.
81. Sotelo J, Escobedo F, Rodriguez-Carbajal J, et al. Therapy of parenchymal brain cysticercosis with praziquantel. *N Engl J Med* 1984;310:1001–1007.
82. De Ghethaldi LD, Norman RM, Douville AW Jr. Cerebral cysticercosis treated biphasically with dexamethasone and praziquantel. *Ann Intern Med* 1983;99:179–181.

16

Other Spinal Cord Masses in Children

Ignacio Pascual-Castroviejo

INTRASPINAL HEMATOMAS

Idiopathic spinal epidural hematoma refers to a bleed into the spinal epidural space in a person without known predisposition or systemic disease and with negative clinical and radiologic studies. Spontaneous epidural hematoma occurs infrequently in children and adolescents (1–4). Of the cases reported, 18% occurred in patients under 20 years of age (5). Jackson is said to have described the first case in the literature in 1869 (6), in a 14-year-old girl. Determination of the source of the hemorrhage is possible in the great majority of patients with modern radiologic methods. Males and females are equally affected. Any level of the spinal canal can be involved, but in children and adolescents the cervical and cervicothoracic regions (6–9) are the most common sites, followed by the thoracic (5,10,11) and lumbar (5) regions. Signs and symptoms may appear abruptly or be more insidious. Back pain is the main symptom and it precedes neurologic complaints by hours, days, months, or years, although in most cases paraplegia or quadriplegia develops suddenly without warning. The first symptom is local pain or pain and weakness in the legs, and difficulty in walking. The neurologic syndrome is that of acute or subacute cord compression with motor and sensory changes, and sphincter disturbances. A Brown-Séquard syndrome occurs frequently. The Queckenstedt test is usually positive. The cerebrospinal fluid (CSF) protein is elevated. The cause of death commonly is respiratory failure secondary to cervical cord compression. Usually there is no precipitating factor.

Intraspinal hematoma secondary to trauma is uncommon despite the high frequency of traffic accidents and birth injuries (16). Clinical diagnosis of this rare condition is difficult, but computerized tomography (CT) and magnetic resonance (MR) are usually diagnostic.

Spontaneous intraspinal hematomas often occur as a complication of a bleeding diathesis, anticoagulant therapy, or cryptic arteriovenous malformations. Bleeding into the spinal canal as a complication of leukemia (12,13) or hemophilia has been observed in children (14,15), and in most cases is not associated with significant trauma or spinal fracture. The neurologic picture is that of an acute progressive compression of the spinal cord, rarely a chronic one (14,15).

Lumbosacral subarachnoid hematoma may occur as a complication of lumbar puncture in patients with a bleeding diathesis, especially in hemophilia and leukemia (17). Rapid, painful paraparesis following lumbar puncture in a patient with a blood disease should suggest a compressing hematoma. Occasionally, sub-arachnoid hematoma is caused by tearing of radicular vessels by the needle punc-ture. This occurs more frequently in adults than in children (18–20), especially in the presence of thrombocytopenia (21). The hematoma may cause radicular and spinal cord compression, which can be permanent unless early diagnosis leads to immediate surgery. Most intradural hematomas expand and compress adjacent structures. The CSF protein is usually raised and the CSF is bloody when the hematoma is recent.

Radiology

Spinal X-rays are usually negative. Myelography shows a block, which in most cases suggests an extradural mass. CT (13) and, especially, MR may yield better and more complete data about the location, size, extension, and possible cause of the hemorrhage.

Treatment

Decompressive laminectomy is urgently needed. Patients with hemophilia must also receive multiple factor concentrate (22).

HERNIATED DISC

Generalities and Clinical Findings

Intervertebral herniated disc, protruded intervertebral disc, prolapsed disc, her-niated nucleus pulposus, and similar terms are used to describe protrusion of the nucleus pulposus of an intervertebral disc, usually backward and laterally, but sometimes anteriorly. The disease occurs most often in the lumbar region. Disc extrusion is frequent in adults but is rare in children. Among 6,500 patients oper-ated on for herniated lumbar intervertebral discs by Webb et al. (23), only five were below 16 years of age. Cases between 9 and 15 years of age have occa-sionally been reported (23–26).

Clinical features in children do not differ from those of adults with lumbosacral disc disease, although low back pain, with or without sciatica—which is a fre-quent complaint and cause of disability in adults—is rarely encountered in chil-dren or adolescents (25). The most common symptom is pain, unilateral or in the midline, which, in severe cases, may extend into the buttock, thigh, or leg. It is seldom aggravated by coughing, sneezing, or straining at stool but is usually worse in the evening or after activities such as stooping, lifting, or even prolonged standing. It can be relieved by bed rest. There may also be numbness, paresthesia, or muscle weakness. The most common physical findings are local pain on deep pressure, limitation of straight leg raising on one or both sides, and pain and limitation of movement in the lower back. All symptoms and signs vary with the severity of the disease. Herniated discs are more frequent in boys than in girls, especially in those competing athletically.

Thoracic disc herniation is uncommon, especially in children. Back pain is the most usual presenting symptom, followed by sensory disturbances. A significant number of patients have signs of spinal cord compression at the time of diagnosis. CT has improved the diagnosis and prognosis of a protruding disc of this region, a diagnosis that was very difficult prior to CT (27).

Eight patients between 10 and 20 years of age with cervical herniated disc were studied by Jomin et al. (28). Their main symptoms and signs were cervicobrachial neuralgia, motor deficit, sensory deficit, abnormal reflexes, and muscular atrophy when the roots were involved.

Radiology

Plain X-ray films are seldom diagnostic. Myelography will show the protruded disc. The advent of CT and MR, which provide well-defined images uninvasively, has considerably lessened the need for myelography.

CT regularly shows the extruded disc. Herniation is most frequently intraforaminal (Fig. 1). The disc appears hyperdense in comparison with the dural sac and has broad contact with the intervertebral disc space (29). The size and shape

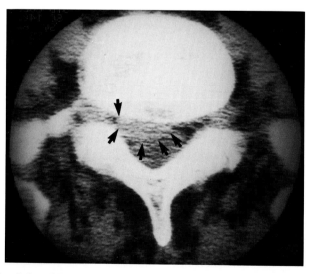

FIG. 1. Herniated disc. CT shows the protruded disc (*arrows*) in the spinal canal and in the foramen on the left side.

of the foramen are usually normal. Differential diagnosis with benign tumors, which often cause bone erosion with enlargement of the foramen, is rarely difficult. Differential diagnosis includes conjoined nerve roots. In this condition, asymmetry of the bony spinal canal, seen as slight dilatation of the ipsilateral lateral recess, is always present (30), a finding not associated with extruded free intervertebral disc fragments. CT is more specific than MR for distinguishing herniated disc from disc bulge and for localizing disc herniation. CT is the preferred method for evaluating degenerative disc disease of the lumbar spine (31). MR is more sensitive than CT for detecting early disc disease, which appears as decreased signal intensity within the disc.

Treatment

Conservative therapy with physiotherapy may be tried initially. Surgical removal of the extruded disc is necessary only when conservative methods have failed.

Full recovery with minimal or no neurologic deficit has been recorded in 85% of patients, including those having ruptured median and paramedian lumbar discs and complete or partial myelographic block (seen in 72% of the patients). A recurrence rate of 6% has been achieved with an adequate laminectomy (32). Cloward (33) reported long-term cure in over 85% of lumbar discs using vertebral body fusion. There are several surgically different exposures. A mixed exposure may be necessary in some cases, especially when there are more than one protruded discs (34). A new technique for percutaneous lumbar disc removal has recently been described (35).

Severe muscle spasm of the back and the hamstrings, limited flexion, and severely restricted straight leg raising are typical postsurgical signs in patients below 30 years of age. These findings are less severe in older people (36).

Chymopapain (chemonucleolysis) has been extensively used as a treatment since 1964 in Canada and Europe. This method is only applicable to lumbar disc disease and is not indicated in patients less than 15 years of age, in those with extruded nucleus pulposus and broken fibrous annulus, or in cases where there is hypersensitivity to the substance. Post-chymopapain study by CT has shown that (37): (a) disc space narrowing occurs almost invariably, (b) retraction of the prolapsed or extruded disc is common, (c) clinical improvement is closely related to retraction of the extruded disc, and (d) the best clinical results are obtained in patients who are injected at a single level.

The preoperative chymopapain sensitivity test, a fluorescence enzyme immunoassay for the quantitation of chymopapain-specific IgE antibody concentration in human serum (38), avoids or minimizes the risks associated with chemonucleolysis. Chymopapain treatment of lumbar disc disease is controversial. Very favorable results have been obtained with it (39,40), but complications have also been reported (41).

Other Types of Disc Herniations

Anterior intervertebral disc herniations, unlike posterior and lateral disc extrusions, are not common in adults, but they occur quite often in children and adolescents. They occur most often in children who are active in sports (42–44) and are probably secondary to chronic trauma caused by active physical exercise. Their main clinical symptom is back pain. They also occur in children with osteoporosis (42). The diagnosis may be made on plain X-ray. The radiologic changes include erosion or fracture with sclerotic margins of adjacent end plates, narrowing of the intervertebral space, increase in the sagittal diameter of the vertebral body, and loss of the lumbar lordosis (43–45). CT and MR may also help in the diagnosis. The differential diagnosis is with fracture (old or acute), discitis, tuberculosis, eosinophilic granuloma, and Scheuermann's disease. Scheuermann's disease and anterior disc herniations are similar and may coexist. Complete blood count and erythrocyte sedimentation rate may help to differentiate anterior disc herniation from discitis and tuberculosis. Follow-up on most of these patients shows minimal morbidity. Surgery, when necessary, also gives good results (45).

Intraosseous disc herniation often occurs after acute trauma. The syndrome is a consideration in adolescent patients having severe back pain with limited radiation to the upper thigh, following significant compression/flexion stress to the spine (46). Discography can confirm this condition. CT and MR can show the lesion as well. Conservative management and use of analgesics are indicated.

SPINAL EPIDURAL LIPOMATOSIS

Spinal epidural lipomatosis appears after prolonged exposure to large amounts of glucocorticoids. Excessive deposition of fat about the head, neck, trunk, mediastinum, episternum, and presacral region is also observed in patients of Cushing's syndrome (47). The first case of spinal epidural lipomatosis was reported by Lee et al. (48) in a patient treated with glucocorticoids for renal transplantation. Recent reviews of additional cases of steroid-induced epidural lipomatosis at various ages have appeared (49,50). All patients presented severe back and leg pain and developed spinal cord or cauda equina compression. Administration of steroids averaged about 1.5 years before the appearance of neurologic disease. High dose steroid, usually exceeding 40 mg/day, or low dose used for prolonged periods, can induce spinal epidural lipomatosis. Improvement of the pain and other neurologic problems, as well as a decrease in the amount of epidural fat on CT scan, may be observed when the dose of corticoid is reduced (49,51).

X-ray films are usually normal. Myelography may show concentric extradural compression in some cases (50). CT scan demonstrates the compression of the spinal cord by a mass with the pathognomonic low specific density of fat (Fig. 2) (52). We have observed an important increase in the amount of extradural fat in children treated for prolonged periods with high corticoid dose, for example, for

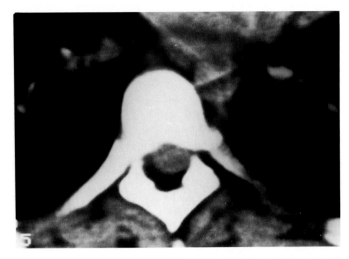

FIG. 2. Spinal epidural lipomatosis in a 14-year-old girl 6 months after suffering from transverse myelitis treated with high dose steroid. CT shows excessive epidural fat with an atrophic spinal cord in the dorsal region.

dermatomyositis or relapsing chronic polyneuropathy. Failure to improve after adequate surgical decompression indicates that epidural lipomatosis may cause irreversible, or at least partially irreversible (53), neurologic damage if the compression is severe or long-standing (50,51,54).

In our experience, surgical decompression rarely improves the patient's condition. Consequently, surgery should be performed only when spinal cord compression is progressive with worsening neurologic symptomatology. Conservative treatment with steroid reduction and restriction of carbohydrates and total calories may help promote fat mobilization in the epidural space. Reduction of the epidural fat can be followed by serial CT scans.

TUMORS OF THE FORAMEN MAGNUM

Generalities

The region of the foramen magnum may be the site of several tumors at any age, although usually in adults. The foramen magnum, also known as the craniovertebral junction or the transitional zone, is the site of communication between the posterior fossa and the spinal canal. Tumors may be craniospinal or spinocranial (originating at C1 or C2). Benign and, less often, malignant tumors are observed in this region (55–59). Most of these masses are slow growing ones, such as meningiomas and neurofibromas. Von Recklinghausen disease is frequently associated with neurofibromas. Chordomas, teratomas, metastases, and other more rare tumors have also been described.

The female to male ratio in tumors of the foramen magnum is 2:1. The tumor is located ventrally to the spinal cord in more than half the cases and, less frequently, laterally or posteriorly. Intrinsic tumors of the brainstem, cerebellum, or spinal cord extending downward or upward beyond the level of the occipitocervical joint are not considered to be tumors of the foramen magnum.

Clinical Findings

The most frequent presenting complaints (56) are suboccipital neck pain, dysesthesias, gait disturbances, weakness, and clumsiness. The neck pain often has a radicular distribution, commonly presents on waking, and is exacerbated by movement of the head or neck. Neck pain may be present for a long time—months or even years—prior to the development of other symptoms or signs since it can usually be relieved with mild analgesics. Dysesthesia occurs predominantly in the hand, followed by the arm, leg, and face. Gait disturbance, generalized weakness, hand clumsiness or astereognosis, bladder dysfunction, dysphagia, respiratory dysfunction, and dizziness may occur. Hyperreflexia is the most frequent neurologic sign, followed by weakness in both arms, or less often in one arm, or by quadriparesis, hemiparesis, triparesis, or paresis in one leg. Atrophy of the hand, arm, or leg may occasionally be seen. A Babinski sign, spastic gait, various sensory disorders (most frequently affecting pain and temperature, less often position sense and touch), dissociated sensory loss, C2 hypalgesia, incoordination of the hands, and Brown-Séquard syndrome are more common. Signs of intracranial disease are frequent, most often nystagmus, stiff neck, and cranial nerve palsies, especially of the eleventh nerve, followed by the twelfth, ninth, tenth, and fifth. Porras (60) described an 8-year-old child who presented hemitongue atrophy, hemiparesis on the same side, dysarthria, apathy, vomiting, and, finally, tetraparesis. Eleventh cranial nerve involvement is highly suggestive of a foramen magnum tumor (56). Papilledema, Horner's syndrome, dysarthria, and hiccups are also seen occasionally. Neurologic signs appear late and only 40% of the patients have an abnormal neurologic examination on first evaluation. The average time from initial symptoms to diagnosis is usually more than 2 years. The CSF protein is elevated in half of the patients.

Radiology

Plain X-rays show enlargement of the intervertebral foramina in many cases of neurofibroma. Chordomas of the clivus may show the typical image of bony destruction and proliferation.

The usefulness of myelography is controversial, often because of an incomplete or inadequate study, or because the films were incorrectly interpreted as negative because they did not include complete examination of the foramen magnum in both the prone and supine positions.

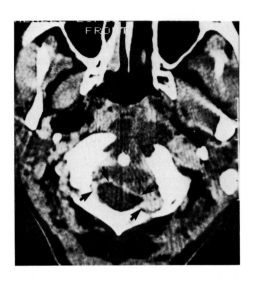

FIG. 3. Chordoma affecting the foramen magnum. The MR in axial projection shows anterior destruction of the atlas with sparing of the odontoid. The lumen of the foramen magnum is severely narrowed by the tumor (*arrows*).

CT scanning enhanced with intravenous contrast or combined with metrizamide myelography may be highly informative. MR is the procedure of choice because it provides complete visualization of the upper cervical spinal canal and posterior fossa in three views—frontal, lateral, and axial—and delineates the tumor from nervous tissue (Fig. 3).

Differential Diagnosis

Many patients with tumors of the foramen magnum are misdiagnosed as having multiple sclerosis, syringomyelia, a ruptured disc, cervical spondylosis, an intramedullary tumor, Arnold-Chiari malformation, carpal tunnel syndrome, normal-pressure hydrocephalus, or some other disease before the correct diagnosis is made (56,59). This error is due to an inadequate imaging study.

Treatment and Prognosis

Surgical removal of foramen magnum tumors can be curative. Large tumors situated anterior to the spinal cord are difficult to remove, although removal by an anterior transoral approach has improved their outlook (61). An operative mortality rate of 5% was reported in the largest series published to date (56). Functional recovery depends on the preoperative neurologic status, size, location, and nature of the tumor. Prognosis is best in patients in whom the tumor is diagnosed early and can be totally removed. In the series of Meyer et al. (56), approximately 75% of the patients were able to maintain full productive lives, 12% were mildly impaired, and 13% had marked impairment.

TUMORS OF THE LUMBOSACRAL REGION

Tumors located in the lumbosacral area can be divided into two groups: tumors of the cauda equina and tumors of the sacral and presacral zones.

Tumors of the Cauda Equina

Neurofibromas and ependymomas are the most frequent tumors in adults (62,63). Lipomas and epidermoid cysts are the most numerous in children, as was the case in our series. These tumors are often associated with the tethered cord syndrome (64–66). Other tumors, such as astrocytomas, hemangioblastomas, meningiomas, neuroblastomas, metastases, aneurysmal cysts, and histiocytosis X, occasionally involve the cauda equina. Paraganglioma of the cauda equina usually occurs in adults (67), but it can occasionally be found in children (68). Neurofibrosarcoma of the cauda equina is also rare (69).

Symptoms of these tumors consist mainly of back pain, most often with unilateral sciatica and, occasionally, with bilateral sciatica, painless weakness in the legs, sphincter disturbance, sensory disturbance, anterior thigh pain, back and buttock pain, subarachnoid hemorrhage, and raised intracranial pressure with papilledema. Nocturnal pain is a classical characteristic of cauda equina tumors. Nocturnal pain occurs in 25% (63) to 50% (62) of cases. Early on, the symptoms and signs caused by these tumors are similar to those of prolapsed intervertebral disc. The CSF protein content is usually raised.

Plain radiographs of the lumbar spine are normal in most cases. Vertebral body erosion and widened interpedicular distances are found in some patients. Myelography, CT scan, or MR correctly locates the tumor and may provide clues as to its nature.

The treatment of choice is surgery, and when complete removal is carried out and the tumor is benign, cure is often achieved and recurrence unusual. Some masses require radiotherapy as well as excision, for example, histiocytosis X. Prognosis is usually favorable.

Tumors of the Sacral and Presacral Area

A considerable number of masses may be located in the sacral and presacral region. These masses may or may not be tumorous, but their symptoms and signs are similar. Several expansive processes located in the sacrum may affect the cauda equina, as discussed earlier. Others, located in the presacral region, affect the roots and nerves in addition to other local tissues and organs.

The complex of anorectal malformation, abnormality of the sacrum, and presacral mass is known as the Currarino triad (70,71). Occult intrasacral meningocele, a rare disease of this region, has the same symptomatology as presacral masses (72).

There are a number of presacral masses (73):

1. *Masses of congenital origin:* anterior meningocele, chordoma, dermoid and developmental cysts, ectopic kidney, hamartoma, neurenteric cyst, teratoma
2. *Neurogenic masses:* ependymoma, ganglioneuroma, neuroblastoma, neurofibroma, neurilemmoma, neurinoma, paraganglioma
3. *Inflammatory masses:* abscess, granuloma, osteomyelitis of sacrum, ulcerative colitis
4. *Osteocartilaginous tumors:* aneurysmal bone cyst, chondroma, chondrosarcoma, giant cell tumor, osteogenic sarcoma, osteoma
5. *Miscellaneous masses:* fibroma, fibrosarcoma, hemangioendothelioma, hematoma, leiomyoma, leiomyosarcoma, lipoma, lymphoma, metastatic tumors, ovarian tumor

Other tumors have been also described (74) and we have encountered several of them in our series. Most of them are discussed elsewhere in this book.

We observed a patient with a tumor not mentioned previously. A 5-year-old boy complained of weakness and gait disturbance in the left leg for 3 months. Plain films of the lumbosacral region were normal, but abdominal X-ray showed displacement of the rectum to the right (Fig. 4). CT scan revealed a tumor affecting the gluteus and psoas muscles and bones of the left hip (Fig. 5); it turned out to be a hemangioma on histologic study. A postoperative angiogram showed the characteristic abundant vascularization of a hemangioma.

Symptoms and signs most frequently caused by sacral and presacral tumors are lumbosacral pain, a malformation of the anorectal region, weakness, gait distur-

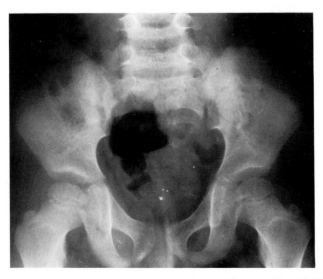

FIG. 4. A 5-year-old boy with hemangioma in muscles and bones of the left hip. The X-ray film shows marked displacement of the rectum to the right.

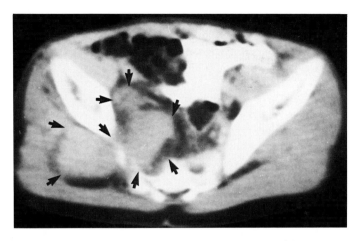

FIG. 5. Same case as Fig. 4. CT shows destruction of the left side of the sacrum, and bones and muscles of the left hip (*arrows*).

bance, occasionally muscular atrophy in one or both lower limbs (Fig. 6), as well as constipation and other bowel and bladder problems due to local pressure effects. Many of these masses remain clinically asymptomatic for a long time.

X-ray films are usually abnormal in most cases with congenital neurogenic tumors and osteocartilaginous ones, although it is crucial to obtain the radiographs after an excellent lower bowel preparation. Myelography has lost most of its importance because CT scan and MR studies permit one to visualize masses located not only in the spinal canal and in bones but also in the soft tissues of the presacral area and to see the relationship of the tumor with the adjacent structures.

Treatment is surgical in most cases, with or without radiotherapy and chemotherapy.

LUMBOSACRAL SPINAL STENOSIS

The syndrome of cauda equina compression resulting from a narrow spinal canal or lumbosacral spinal stenosis is well known. This disorder may be the result of bone disease or result from a developmental anomaly. It has distinctive features that distinguish it from other causes of lower back and leg pain. Although quite frequent in adults (75), it has seldom been described in childhood or adolescence (76). The syndrome consists of a stereotyped, intermittent, and reversible disorder of the cauda equina, commonly bilateral and multisegmental. Symptoms usually appear or increase with exercise and posture. No neurologic abnormalities are usually found when examining the patient at rest. Spinal levels L_3-L_4-L_5 are the most frequently affected.

The differential diagnosis of cauda equina compression includes herniated disc, neoplasm, spina bifida, tethered conus, spondylolisthesis, and ventral congenital

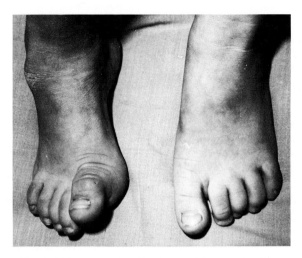

FIG. 6. A 7-year-old girl with intra-extradural lumbosacral lipoma who shows muscular atrophy and right foot deformity.

bony ridge. Claudication of the lower limbs is thought to result from ectopic nerve discharges elicited by rapid changes in the blood supply following exertion (77). Epidural venous engorgement has been visualized in association with spinal stenosis (78). According to one theory, compression of the nutrient arteries may preclude increased blood flow to the nerve roots required during increased activity. Another theory suggests that disturbances are caused by heightened postural pressure on nerve roots through one or more of the following mechanisms: (a) increased lordosis, (b) disc protrusion or thickening of the ligamentum flavum, (c) increased cross-sectional diameter of the caudal nerve roots during extension of the spine, (d) unequal distribution of CSF pressure above and below the area of stenosis, or (e) increased internal pressure in the epidural venous plexus.

X-ray films, and especially CT, reveal the existence and degree of narrowing of the lumbar canal, as well as its cause (79). Segmental epidural venous stasis is a CT sign of clinically significant narrowing of the spinal canal. Myelography may show partial or total block in the lumbar region but may require flexion extension studies to do so (80).

Treatment of spinal stenosis is directed at widening the canal by decompressive laminectomy limited to the extent of the compression demonstrated by radiologic study.

REFERENCES

1. Dauch WA. Spinale epidural-Hämatome bei Kindern und Jugendlichen. *Neurochirurgia (Stuttg)* 1986;29:83–89.
2. Ghanem Q, Ivan LP. Spontaneous spinal epidural hematoma in an 8-year-old boy. *Neurology* 1978;28:829–832.

3. Vallés B, Besson G, Gaudin J, et al. Spontaneous spinal epidural hematoma in a 22-month-old girl. *J Neurosurg* 1982;56:135–138.
4. Robertson WC Jr, Lee YE, Edmonson MB. Spontaneous spinal epidural hematoma in the young. *Neurology* 1979;29:120–122.
5. Tsai FY, Popp AJ, Waldman J. Spontaneous spinal epidural hematoma. *Neuroradiology* 1975;10: 15–30.
6. Jackson R. Case of spinal apoplexy. *Lancet* 1869;ii:56.
7. Cooper DW. Spontaneous spinal epidural hematoma. Case report. *J Neurosurg* 1967;26:343–345.
8. Nichols P Jr, Manganiello LOJ. Extradural hematoma of the spinal canal. Report of a case. *J Neurosurg* 1956;13:638–640.
9. Posnikoff J. Spontaneous spinal epidural hematoma of childhood. *J Pediatr* 1968;73:178–183.
10. Maxwell GM, Puletti F. Chronic spinal hematoma in a child. *Neurology* 1957;7:596–600.
11. Pear BL. Spinal epidural hematoma. *Am J Roentgenol* 1972;115:155–164.
12. Wolcott CJ, Grunnet ML, Lahey ME. Spinal subdural hematoma in a leukemic child. *J Pediatr* 1970;77:1060–1062.
13. Tantana S, Pilla TJ, Luisiri A. Computed tomography of acute spinal subdural hematoma. *J Comput Assist Tomogr* 1986;10:891–892.
14. Keely ML, Taylor N, Chard RL Jr. Spinal cord compression as a complication of haemophilia. *Arch Dis Child* 1972;47:826–828.
15. Stanley P, McComb JG. Chronic spinal epidural hematoma in hemophilia A in a child. *Pediatr Radiol* 1983;13:241–243.
16. Aufdermaur M. Spinal injuries in juveniles. Necropsy findings in twelve cases. *J Bone Joint Surg* 1974;56B:513–519.
17. Walsh R, Crawford P, Kendall B. Lumbosacral subarachnoid haematoma following lumbar puncture: characteristic myelographic appearances. *Br J Radiol* 1983;56:423–425.
18. Rengarachy SS, Murphy D. Subarachnoid hematoma following lumbar puncture causing compression of the cauda equina. A case report. *J Neurosurg* 1974;41:252–254.
19. Masdeu JC, Breuer AC, Schoene WC. Spinal subarachnoid hematomas: due to a source of bleeding in traumatic lumbar puncture. *Neurology* 1979;29:872–876.
20. Brem SS, Hafler DA, Van Witert RL, et al. Spinal subarachnoid hematoma. A hazard of lumbar puncture resulting in reversible paraplegia. *N Engl J Med* 1981;30:1020–1021.
21. Edelson RN, Chermick NL, Posner JB. Spinal subdural hematomas complicating lumbar puncture. Occurrence in thrombocytopenic patients. *Arch Neurol* 1974;31:134–137.
22. Goodnight SH Jr, Common HH, Lovrien EW. Factor VIII inhibitor following surgery for epidural hemorrhage in hemophilia: successful therapy with a concentrate containing factors II, VII, IX, and X. *J Pediatr* 1976;88:356–357.
23. Webb JH, Svien HJ, Kennedy RLJ. Protruded lumbar intervertebral disc in children. *JAMA* 1954; 154:1153–1154.
24. Lins E, Basedow H. Bandscheibenvorfall im Jugendalter. Beshreibung eines Falles. *Neuropädiatrie* 1976;7:122–125.
25. Key JA. Intervertebral-disc lesions in children and adolescents. *J Bone Joint Surg* 1950;32A:97–102.
26. Wahren H. Herniated nucleus pulposus in a child of 12 years. *Acta Orthop Scand* 1946;16:40–42.
27. Arce CA, Dohrmann GJ. Thoracic disc herniation. Improved diagnosis with computed tomography scanning and a review of the literature. *Surg Neurol* 1985;23:356–361.
28. Jomin M, Lesoin F, Lozes G, et al. Herniated cervical discs. Analysis of a series of 230 cases. *Acta Neurochir (Wien)* 1986;79:107–113.
29. Schubiger O, Valavanis A, Hollmann J. Computed tomography of the intervertebral foramen. *Neuroradiology* 1984;26:439–444.
30. Hoddick WK, Helms CA. Bony spinal canal changes that differentiate conjoined nerve roots from a herniated nucleus pulposus. *Radiology* 1985;154:119–120.
31. Maravilla KR, Lesh P, Weinreb JC, et al. Magnetic resonance imaging of the lumbar spine with CT correlation. *AJNR* 1985;6:237–245.
32. Fager CA. Ruptured median and paramedian lumbar disk. *Surg Neurol* 1985;23:309–323.
33. Cloward RB. The treatment of ruptured lumbar intervertebral discs by vertebral body fusion. I. Indications, operative technique, after cure. *Clin Orthop* 1985;193:5–15.
34. Recoules-Arche D. La chirurgie de la hernie discale du canal de conjugaison lombaire. *Neurochirurgie (Paris)* 1985;31:61–64.

35. Maroon JC, Onik G. Percutaneous automated discectomy: a new method for lumbar disc removal. Technical note. *J Neurosurg* 1987;66:143–146.
36. Halperin N, Arbel R, Aner A, Axer A. Herniated lumbar disk syndrome. Report of 108 patients treated surgically. *Orthop Rev* 1985;14:240–275.
37. Mall JC, Kaiser JC. Post-chymopapain (chemonucleolysis)—clinical and computed tomography correlation: preliminary results. *Skeletal Radiol* 1984;12:270–275.
38. Tsay Y-G, Jones R, Calenoff E, et al. A preoperative chymopapain sensitivity test for chemonucleolysis candidates. *Spine* 1984;9:764–768.
39. Maciunas RJ, Onofrio BM. The long-term results of chymopapain chemonucleolysis for lumbar disc disease. Ten-year follow up results in 268 patients injected at the Mayo Clinic. *J Neurosurg* 1986;65:1–8.
40. David MJ. Efficacy of chymopapain chemonucleolysis. A long-term review of 105 patients. *J Neurosurg* 1985;62:662–666.
41. Artigas J, Brock M, Mayer H-M. Complications following chemonucleolysis with collagenase. *J Neurosurg* 1984;61:679–685.
42. Kozlowski K. Anterior intervertebral disc herniations in children: unrecognised chronic trauma to spine. *Austral Radiol* 1979;23:67–71.
43. Kozlowski K. Anterior intervertebral disc herniations in children. Report of four cases. *Pediatr Radiol* 1977;6:32–35.
44. Haapanen A, Latvala A, Ala-Ketola L. Anterior intervertebral disc herniation in young athletes. *Scan J Sport Sci* 1985;7:41–44.
45. Fitzer PM. Anterior herniation of the nucleus pulposus: radiologic and clinical features. *South Med J* 1985;78:1296–1300.
46. McCall IW, Park WM, O'Brien JP, Seal V. Acute traumatic intraosseous disc herniation. *Spine* 1985;10:134–137.
47. Gold EM. The Cushing syndromes: changing views of diagnosis and treatment. *Ann Intern Med* 1979;90:829–844.
48. Lee M, Lekias J, Gubbay SS, Hurst PE. Spinal cord compression by extradural fat after renal transplantation. *Med J Aust* 1975;1:201–203.
49. George WE Jr, Wilmot M, Greenhouse A, Hammeke M. Medical management of steroid-induced epidural lipomatosis. *N Engl J Med* 1983;308:316–319.
50. Russell NA, Belanger G, Benoit BG, et al. Spinal epidural lipomatosis: a complication of glucocorticoid therapy. *Can J Neurol Sci* 1984;11:383–386.
51. Butcher DL, Sahn SA. Epidural lipomatosis: a complication of corticosteroid therapy. *Ann Intern Med* 1979;90:60.
52. Pennisi AK, Meisler WJ, Dina TS. Lymphomatous meningitis and steroid induced epidural lipomatosis: CT evaluation. *J Comput Assist Tomogr* 1985;9:595–598.
53. Archer CR, Smith KR Jr. Extradural lipomatosis simulating an acute herniated nucleus pulposus. *J Neurosurg* 1982;57:559–562.
54. Chapman PH, Martuza RL, Poletti CE, Karchmer AW. Symptomatic spinal epidural lipomatosis associated with Cushing's syndrome. *Neurosurgery* 1981;8:724–727.
55. Love JG, Thelen EP, Dodge HW Jr. Tumors of the foramen magnum. *J Int Coll Surg* 1954;22:1–17.
56. Meyer FB, Ebersold MJ, Reese DF. Benign tumors of the foramen magnum. *J Neurosurg* 1984;61:136–142.
57. Yasnoka S, Okazaki H, Daube JR, McCarty CS. Foramen magnum tumors. Analysis of 57 cases of benign extramedullary tumors. *J Neurosurg* 1978;49:828–838.
58. Marc JA, Schecter MM. Radiological diagnosis of mass lesions within and adjacent to the foramen magnum. *Radiology* 1975;114:351–365.
59. Howe JR, Taren JA. Foramen magnum tumors. Pitfalls in diagnosis. *JAMA* 1973;225:1061–1066.
60. Porras CL. Meningioma in the foramen magnum in a boy aged 8 years. *J Neurosurg* 1963;20:167–168.
61. Mullan S, Naunton R, Hekmat-panah J, et al. The use of an anterior approach to ventrally placed tumors in the foramen magnum and vertebral column. *J Neurosurg* 1966;24:536–543.
62. Fearnside MR, Adams CBT. Tumours of the cauda equina. *J Neurol Neurosurg Psychiatry* 1978;41:24–31.
63. Ker NB, Jones CB. Tumours of the cauda equina. The problem of differential diagnosis. *J Bone Joint Surg* 1985;67B:358–362.

64. Lapras C, Patet JD, Huppert J, Bret P. Syndrome de traction du cône terminal ou syndrome de la moelle attachée. Lipomes lombo-sacrés. *Rev Neurol (Paris)* 1985;141:207–215.
65. Yamada S, Zinke DE, Sanders D. Pathophysiology of "tethered cord syndrome." *J Neurosurg* 1981;54:494–503.
66. Pierre-Kahn A, Reiner D, Sainte-Rose C, Hirsch JF. Les lipomes lombo-sacrés avec spina bifida. Corrélations anatomo-cliniques. Résultats thérapeutiques. *Neurochirurgie* 1983;29:359–363.
67. Sonneland PRL, Scheithauer BW, Lechago J, et al. Paraganglioma of the cauda equina region. Clinico-pathologic study of 31 cases with special reference to immunocytology and ultrastructure. *Cancer* 1986;58:1720–1735.
68. Soffer D, Pittaluga S, Caine Y, Feinsod M. Paraganglioma of cauda equina: a report of a case and review of the literature. *Cancer* 1983;51:1907–1910.
69. Thomeer RTWM, Bots GTAM, Van Dulken H, et al. Neurofibrosarcoma of the cauda equina. Case report. *J Neurosurg* 1981;54:409–411.
70. Currarino G, Coln D, Votteler T. Triad of anorectal, sacral, and presacral anomalies. *Am J Roentgenol* 1981;137:395–398.
71. Kirks DR, Merten DF, Filston HC, Oakes WJ. The Currarino triad: complex of anorectal malformation, sacral bony abnormality, and presacral mass. *Pediatr Radiol* 1984;14:220–225.
72. Genest AS. Occult intrasacral meningocele. *Spine* 1984;9:101–103.
73. Werner JI, Taybi H. Presacral masses in childhood. *Am J Roentgenol* 1970;109:403–410.
74. Shulman L, Bale P, de Silva M. Sacral chondromyxoid fibroma. *Pediatr Radiol* 1985;15:138–140.
75. Verbiest H. A radicular syndrome from developmental narrowing of the lumbar vertebral canal. *J Bone Joint Surg* 1954;36B:230–237.
76. Birkenfeld R, Kasdon DL. Congenital lumbar ridge causing spinal claudication in adolescents. Report of two cases. *J Neurosurg* 1978;49:441–444.
77. Watanabe R, Parke WW. Vascular and neural pathology of lumbosacral spinal stenosis. *J Neurosurg* 1986;64:64–70.
78. Kaiser MC, Capesius P, Roilgen A, et al. Epidural venous stasis in spinal stenosis. CT appearance. *Neuroradiology* 1984;26:435–438.
79. Crouzet G, Vasdev A, Chirossell JP, et al. Réflexions sur les aspects tomodensitométriques du canal lombaire étroit. *J Radiol* 1983;64:405–414.
80. Wilmink JT, Penning L, van den Burg W. Role of stenosis of spinal canal in L_4–L_5 nerve root compression assessed by flexion-extension myelography. *Neuroradiology* 1984;26:173–181.

SUBJECT INDEX

Subject Index